New Perspectives in Basic and Applied Immunology

New Perspectives in Basic and Applied Immunology

Lakshmi Prasanna Jakka

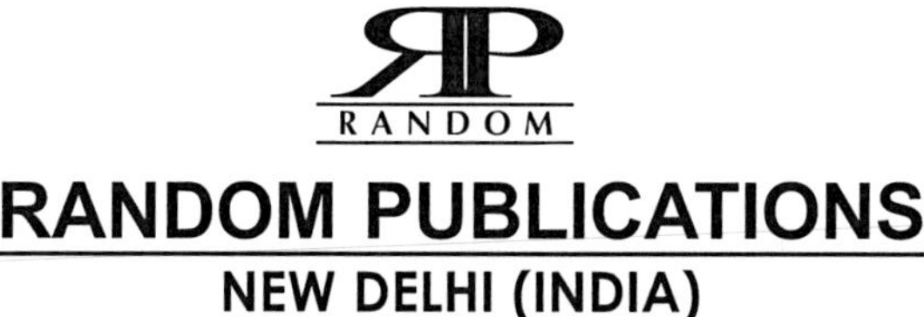

RANDOM PUBLICATIONS
NEW DELHI (INDIA)

New Perspectives in Basic and Applied Immunology

ISBN 978-93-5111-796-4

Published in 2016 in India by

Reprint 2019

RANDOM PUBLICATIONS

4376-A/4B, Gali Murari Lal, Ansari Road
New Delhi-110 002
Phone : +9111-43580356, 011-23289044, 011-43142548
e-mail: sales@randompublications.com,
info@randompublications.com, randomexports@gmail.com

Type Setting by : Friends Media, Delhi-110089
Printed at : Mehra Printers, Delhi-110 092

Preface

Immunology is a branch of biomedical science that covers the study of all aspects of the immune system in all organisms. It deals with the physiological functioning of the immune system in states of both health and diseases; malfunctions of the immune system in immunological disorders; the physical, chemical and physiological characteristics of the components of the immune system in vitro, in situ and in vivo. Immunology has applications in several disciplines of science, and as such is further divided. Even before the concept of immunity was developed, numerous early physicians characterized organs that would later prove to be part of the immune system.

The key primary lymphoid organs of the immune system are the thymus and bone marrow, and secondary lymphatic tissues such as spleen, tonsils, lymph vessels, lymph nodes, adenoids, and skin and liver. When health conditions warrant, immune system organs including the thymus, spleen, portions of bone marrow, lymph nodes and secondary lymphatic tissues can be surgically excised for examination while patients are still alive. Many components of the immune system are actually cellular in nature and not associated with any specific organ but rather are embedded or circulating in various tissues located throughout the body.

– Author

Contents

Preface .... *v-vi*

1. Introduction **1**

Historical Background of Immunology 8
Innate immune system 10
Alternative adaptive immune system 15
Vaccination Application of Immunology 22
Characteristics of the Immune System 31
Antigens 33
Specific Immune Response 35
Monoclonal Antibodies 37

2. Applied Immune System in Health and Disease **40**

Basic Concepts in Immunology 40
Effects of Exercise on The Immune System 45
Infectious Disease 64
Human Body and Immune System 65
Immunology in Allergic Disease 86
Cells Important for Allergic Response 87
Immune Response to Vaccines 109
Multiplicity of Immune Defences and Stress 115
Cell-Mediated Immunity 118
Stress and the Immune System 124
Other Factors Affecting Stress Nd Immunity 137

3. Genetics, Immunology and Diseases Resistance of Animals **141**

Genetics of Scrapie Resistance In Sheep 141
Genomics, Immunology and Diseases in non- salmonid fish 146
Cloned and Genetically Modified Animals 157
Cloning and Genetically Altered Animals 162
Animal Models of Disease 166
Current Context of Genetically Engineered Animals 173

4. **Cell Physiology** **177**

Human Body Structure 177
Anatomical Terminology 178
Planes of the Body 178
Body Functions and Life Process 179
Levels of Structural Organization 181
Planes in the Human Body 185
Cell Structure and Function 188
Body Tissues 201
Membranes 203
Organ Systems, Body Cavities, and Body Memranes 208
Physiology of the Heart 211
An Electrocardiogram (ECG) 213
Anatomy of the Heart 220
The Physiology of the Human Heart 225
Electro Physiology of Human Heart 227
Survey of Literature on Electro Physiology of Heart 247
The Cardiovascular System 256
The Heart's Electrical Conduction System 262
Anatomy and Physiology of The Heart 266
Electric Activation of The Heart 268
The Genesis of The Electrocardiogram 273

Bibliography **277**

Index ***279***

1

Introduction

Immunology is the study of the organs, cells, and chemical components of the immune system. The immune system creates both *innate* and *adaptive* immune responses. The innate response exists in many lower species, all the way up the evolutionary ladder to humans, and it acts through relatively crude means against large classes of pathogens.

The adaptive response is unique to vertebrates, reacting to foreign invaders with specificity and selectivity.

The immune system must maintain a delicate balance, with potent defensive responses capable of destroying large numbers of foreign cells and viruses while refraining from undue destruction of the host's body. When the immune system cannot mount a sufficient defence of the host, there is an immune deficiency; this is seen in HIV infection and SCID. If, on the other hand, the immune system acts too vigourously and begins to attack the host, we have autoimmunity.

This is a defiance of the integral immune system property of self/non-self recognition. That is, the immune system begins attacking or forming antibodies against the host's own body tissues. Examples of autoimmune diseases include Graves' disease, Hashimoto's thyroiditis, *myaesthenia gravis* and type I diabetes mellitus.

The human immune system recognizes non-self entities and mounts an effector response to neutralize the organism. A faster and stronger memory response may occur upon later exposure.

The memory response has been used throughout history to confer immunity upon several populations, even previous to our understanding of the physiological basis for such a response. Thucydides wrote in his History of the Peloponnesian War that persons who had been exposed to plague previously could care for the sick without danger. In the 19th century, variolation was commonplace; this was the removal of smallpox (variola virus) skin pustules which were subsequently put into small cuts in the skin of healthy people. This was itself a crude form of vaccination, with the crusty dry pustules acting as an incubator of attenuated virus.

Edward Jenner would later use the cowpox virus to vaccinate (from *vacca*, Latin for "cow") patients against smallpox, and Louis Pasteur attenuated rabies and injected it into a small boy, naming this substance a vaccine in honour of Jenner's earlier studies in the science of immunology.

As immunology progressed, many people began to question how these vaccines worked. Why should exposure to plague in Thucycides' time confer protection only against plague and not all disease? Why should cowpox, a similar disease to smallpox but clearly a less severe virus, give milk maids sufficient immunity to resist full smallpox infection? In short, what has caused this memory response to be relatively (yet not absolutely) specific as well as selective?

THE BASICS

First, some vocabulary:

- Serum—liquid, noncellular component of blood after coagulation has occurred (and thus devoid of clotting factors).
- Immunoglobulin—a serum fraction (aka gamma globulin) that has antitoxin, precipitin, and agglutin factors (abbreviation: Ig)
- Antigen—"Antibody Generator"; a foreign organism or molecule that generates a humoral immune response, causing the release of antibodies (abbreviation: Ag)
- Epitope—the molecular sidechain of an antigen that each antibody attaches to; there can be many epitopes on a single antigen
- Antibody—refined, Y-shaped proteins that make up the immunoglobulin fraction of serum; antibodies are specific to certain foreign bodies; antibodies can be membrane-bound or free in the serum (abbreviation: Ab)

Note: Often, antibody and immunoglobulin are used interchangably.

There have been several competing theories of the immune response mechanism. The instructional theory of antigen interaction postulated that the antigen itself caused antibodies to fold around the antigen in a certain way; this theory was later disproven.

The selection theory states that the body creates many different sidechains on antibodies, and the antigen "selects" the correct antibody; in other words, the body creates every possible permutation of chemical sidechain-specific antibodies, and when an antigen enters the body, it is matched up with antibodies that correspond to its epitopes. The current theory of immune response is known as the clonal selection theory, which states that an individual lymphocyte (specifically, a B cell) expresses receptors specific to the distinct antigen, determined before the antibody ever encounters the antigen. Binding of Ag to a cell activates the cell, causing a proliferation of clone daughter cells.

INNATE IMMUNITY

Innate immunity is basic and non-specific. It includes:

- Phagocytic cells (macrophages, neutrophils; more generally, antigen-presenting cells (APCs))
- Barriers (*e.g.* skin)
- Antimicrobial compounds
- Inflammation

PHAGOCYTIC CELLS

Certain cells "eat up" foreign invaders; this is termed phagocytosis. Many of these cells are known as Antigen-Presenting Cells (APCs) because they break apart the ingested pathogen and display certain epitopes of the antigen on their surface. In this way, they localize the presentation of antigen, forming a vital link between the innate response and the adaptive response. Lymphocytes (such as B cells and T-helper cells) will have antigen presented to them, initiating the adaptive response. Monocyte-derived cells are common APCs, and they include tissue macrophages and monocytes within the blood; neutrophils are also APCs.

BARRIERS

The skin contains epidermis and dermis. The epidermis contains tightly packed epithelial (cytokeratin positive) cells with keratin waterproofing. The dermis contains connective tissue blood vessels hair follicles, sweat glands, and sebaceous glands. Sebaceous glands secrete sebum; this contains fatty acids and lactic acid, lowering skin pH to 3-5.

Mucous membranes contain normal flora, mucus, and cilia. Mucous membranes are found in the nose, eyes, mouth, urogenital, and anal regions of the body. Flora refers to bacteria that inhabit the human body in a relative steady-state; the gastro-intestinal tract contains a large number of these bacteria, and different areas of the world contain different flora. It is for this reason that people contract Traveller's Diarrhea; in short, flora from one region of the world are more dangerous because the body has not acclimated to their presence. Mucus contains certain mucin proteins, inorganic salts, and water; it is secreted from goblet cells.

Cilia acts to sway back and forth during two phases, known as the power stroke and the recovery stroke; this allows mucus to be swept out of the body, either proximodistally from the lungs up the respiratory tract, or down the GI tract through the intestines, culminating in defecation. The enteric nervous system causes contractions of the gut, moving foodstuffs, waste, and bacteria/toxins down the digestive tract. This is just one example of disparate systems of the body working together with the immune system proper. Other examples are skeletal muscles, which squeeze blood along the veins and lymph along the lymph vessels, or the nervous system, which supports a rise in body temperature in response to infection. Some bacteria can attach to mucous membranes via fimbriae or pili, which attach to special glyoproteins/glycolipids on the epithelial cells of mucous membranes.

ANTIMICROBIAL COMPOUNDS

Several antimicrobial compounds mediate the innate response.

- Lysozyme—hydrolytic enzyme in tears and mucous; cleaves peptidoglycan in bacterial cell walls
- Interferon—produced by virus-infected cells; binds to nearby cells (it is a paracrine factor), inducing a generalized antiviral state
- Complement—inactive circulating serum proteins that act on pathogen cell membranes
- Collectins—surfactant materials; kills bacteria by disrupting their lipid membranes or agglutinating them
- Toll-Like Receptors—(TLRs) membrane-bound receptors that react via pattern recognition to certain classes of molecules; TLR4, for example, recognizes lipopolysaccharide (LPS) on gram-negative bacteria

INFLAMMATION

Classical biology put several characteristics together as an inflammatory response. These included redness (erythema, *rubor*), heat (*calor*), swelling (edema, *tumor*), pain (*dolor*), and loss of function (*functio laesa*). The physiological processes that bring about these symptoms are central to the innate immune response.

Erythema results from constriction of post-capillary venules in tissue beds and vasodilation in pre-capillary arterioles/metarterioles. This results in an increase of hydrostatic pressure in the capillary bed, overcoming the osmotic pressure of the interstitial fluid and causing exudate (high-protein fluid with acute-phase proteins like C-reactive protein and macrophages) to flow into the interstitial tissue. This flowing of exudate also allows the factors of the clotting cascade to enter areas of tissue damage, forming clots and, eventually, scars. Certain inflammatory factors also cause phagocytic cells to enter the damaged tissue.

The now-permeable capillaries are traversed by these phagocytes in response to chemotaxis, the release of factors that lure the cells to the site of injury. The cells first approach the side of a capillary (margination), move through the spaces between capillary endothelial cells (diapedesis), and then enter the tissue itself. Histamine helps to mediate this response, and certain factors (such as bradykinin and possibly prostaglandins) stimulate skin pain receptors. Thus, blood flows into the tissue, causing redness, warmer steady-state temperature, swelling, and pain; loss of function is a secondary effect of these four states.

ADAPTIVE IMMUNITY

Adaptive immunity occurs in response to antigen exposure. It is specific, and it shows memory. As long as an antigen is made of the normal chemical elements we experience in biological systems (*e.g.* Carbon, Nitrogen, Sulfur, Hydrogen, Oxygen), we can form an adaptive response to it. This is how we fight off new diseases, and it has even been shown that we can create antigens in the laboratory that have never before existed on Earth, only to have animals mount competent immune reactions to them. As stated earlier, the adaptive immune system's specificity is tempered with an ability to differentiate between self and non-self antigen; simply put, the body doesn't attack its own cells, unless they have been invaded by virus and ask to be sacrificed for the sake of the host. When the immune system does attack the body, this is a disease state: autoimmunity.

The primary response takes 5-6 days, but the memory (secondary) response will be swifter and deadlier. It includes:

LYMPHOCYTES

Blood cells are made in the bone marrow of adults. Leukocytes are white blood cells (WBCs). This includes monocytes (which become myriad cell types in the body, most importantly macrophages), granulocytes (neutrophils, basophils, eosinophils), and lymphocytes. Of all the leukocytes, the lymphocyte class are the most preeminent in the adaptive immune response. On a peripheral blood smear, lymphocytes are approximately the size of erythrocytes (red blood cells, RBCs), although they can be larger if activated and have a characteristic "clock-face" nucleus if they are B cells. Lymphocytes are so named because fewer than 1 per cent are present in the circulating blood; the rest lie in the lymph nodes, spleen and other lymphoid organs.

T lymphocytes leave the bone marrow, travelling to the thymus gland, where they mature and gain their specificity for the diverse antigens the body might come into contact with; additionally, any T cells that react against the body's own epitopes are selected against (killed) in the thymus, in an effort to stop any possible autoimmunity. A similar process occurs in the bone marrow in the case of B lymphocytes. B cells are conveniently named ("B for bone marrow"), but this is just a coincidence; it turns out that they are named B cells after the Bursa of Fabricius, a small pouch in the cloaca (lower large intestine, *cloaca* Latin for "sewer") of birds.

B cells leave the bone marrow with their specific membrane bound Ig (antibody) already specified. The Ig itself is made up of two medial heavy chains (both identical) with two lateral light chains (also identical) attached to the "top" of the heavy chains, which form a Y shape. Before they encounter antigen, B cells are known as "naive." Once they encounter antigen, the naive B cells will undergo clonal expansion; an activated B cell will form some daughter memory B cells and some plasma cells. The memory cells will lie in wait for a second encounter with the antigen, while the plasma cells will begin a *massive* secretion of antibody (Ig). B cells can bind to antigen when it is free and unprocessed in the body, much like APCs can.

Before moving on to T lymphocytes, it should be noted that certain cell surface molecules distinguish each person's unique immune system profile.

The Major Histocompatibility Complex(MHC, or HLA) is a type of protein expressed on the surface of host cells that interacts with T-cell receptors (TCRs) of T cells. Virtually all the body's cells, including APCs, express class I MHC (MHC-I) on their surface.

Only APCs express class II MHC (MHC-II). Thus, most body cells express MHC-I, while APCs express both MHC-I *and* MHC-II. When antigen enters a body cell and is broken down, the products of this breakdown are sent to the surface of the cell coupled with MHC-I. This forms the MHC-I/Ag complex, and usually occurs when a virus or bacterium enter a cell and are broken down by intracellular defences. This can also occur in APCs, but APCs additionally process the antigen that they phagocytose, presenting it as an MHC-II/Ag complex on the surface of their cells.

T cells can be subdivided into two broad types: T helper cells and T cytotoxic cells. T helper cells express a T-Cell Receptor (TCR) that will interact with APC surfaces. Specifically, they interact with the MHC-II/Ag complex on the surface of APCs, and the TCR is stabilized in its binding by a CD4 receptor. CD stands for "cluster of differentiation," and is simply a class of cell receptor which occurs predominantly on T cells. T helper cells contain CD4 receptors and T cytoxic cells contain CD8 receptors. Upon binding, T helper cells release cytokines, which act as chemotactic agents to call for more T helper cells, T cytotoxic cells, APCs, and B cells.

T cytotoxic cells encounter body cells that have been invaded and are presenting MHC-I/Ag on their surface. Tc cells extend their TCR to the MHC-I/Ag complex and stabilize this interaction with their CD8 receptor arms.

Upon binding, the CD8+ cells differentiate, much like naive B cells, into memory T cells and cytotoxic T lymphocytes (CTLs), effector cells that cause the MHC-I/Ag-presenting cell (the "altered self cell") to die (apoptose). CTLs trigger apoptosis by secreting a perforin that allows the entry of a serine protease (Granzyme B) which activates intracellular executioner caspases. It should be noted that cancer cells can also become altered self cells, and CTLs are very important in the destruction of cancerous cells. T cells can interact with antigen *only* after it has been processed, either by a normal body cell (MHC-I) or by an APC (MHC-II).

Difference between the two types of T cells:

- T helper cells react to exogenous antigen, phagocytosed by APCs, presented on MHC-II, via binding with TCR and CD4.
- T cytotoxic cells react to endogenous antigen (such as viral or cancer proteins), broken down by lysosomes in many types of body cells, presented on MHC-I, via binding with TCR and CD8.

Note that it is both the antigen and the MHC that is presented to T cells; each person has a unique MHC. This is why we must type for bone marrow transplants—we don't want people producing tons of new immune cells in bone marrow that think every MHC in the body is actually just antigen; when this does occur, it is called graft-vs.-host disease. Not only would the new bone marrow make cells that attacked every body cell's MHC, but when the body did present Ag on MHC, the lymphocytes from the transplant would not be able to recognize this MHC-I/Ag complex (although the MHC-II complex cells would be made in the new bone marrow, and thus APCs could, in some cases, still present).

Unfortunately, these APCs would be very busy presenting the host's own body cells; clearly MHC typing (also known as HLA typing) for bone marrow transplants is a necessary result of the elegant self-non-self recognition of the human immune system. It is also worth noting that we are only as good as our presenting molecules. Some people have MHC genes that are not as good at presenting antigen, and thus some people have more vigourous immune respones than others.

ANTIBODIES

The cellular and humoral responses of the adaptive immune system are linked via the T helper cell-B cell interaction. The T helper cell secretes cytokine factors to encourage chemotaxis of B cells to the site of infection as well as B cell differentiation and growth.

B cells themselves, in their effector plasma B cell form, release antibodies into the blood. Antigens, or foreign substances that enter the body,are very harmful to the Immune System. But when specific antibodies are produced to bind with an antigen, the foreign substance becomes harmless and is delivered to the lymph.

Antibodies are also very important in the complement system; this is an example of the vertebral adaptive immune response making good use of the relatively primitive innate immune response. Antibodies to the body's own cells are a very real danger. Type I diabetes may be caused by an autoimmune response, where the body makes antibodies to its own Beta cells in the pancreatic Islets of Langerhans.

Graves' disease is a condition where the body produces antibodies to receptors in the follicular cells of the thyroid; these Ab keep the cells constantly activated, giving the patient hyperthyroidism and increasing their metabolism, to adverse effect. The interesting counterpoint to this is Hashimoto's thyroiditis; here the body makes antibodies to thyroid follicular cells' receptors, but in this case the cells are shut down by the Ab, and the patient endures*hypo*thyroidism.

Autoimmunity due to antibody overreaction (hypersensitivity) is a huge problem, and it is a much greater problem in women than in men. Women tend to have a higher titer of immunoglobulin (antibody), and thus they exert a stronger (and sometimes overwhelming) immune response. For example, for every one man who gets Graves' disease, 8 women will contract it. Antibodies are often given to produce a short-lived humoral immunity in emergency situations. Many antivenoms are actually horse immunoglobulin, produced in order to bind the venom until it can be cleared from the body.

THEORY MEETS FUNCTION

It should be noted that all of the above-mentioned immune responses result in the destruction or agglutination of foreign pathogen. The goal of the immune response is three-fold:

1. Destroy foreign antigen via innate or humoral responses such as complement fixation or endocytosis by macrophages.
2. Attract immune cells to the site of infection so they can engulf, process and present the antigen to T cells
3. Move the antigen to the site of differentiation (*e.g.* lymph nodes, thymus) via the lymphatic system, so that it can interact with naive B cell. This process creates new effector and memory cells which can return to the site of infection and destroy the foreign cells in a highly effective fashion via the adaptive response.

The immune responses listed above show the intimate interaction between the innate and adaptive immune systems, as well as the subclasses of adaptive responses. The clonal selectiontheory of immune response, introduced above, is clear in the action of lymphocytes. Clonal selection simply means that antigen is presented to many circulating naive B and (via MHC) T cells, and the lymphocytes that match the antigen are "selected" to form clones of themselves, both memory and effector. This mass production of daughter cells is termed clonal expansion, and it is essential in the understanding of the theoretical basis of immunology. Not only this; clonal selection is used negatively in the lymphoid organs. Here, the body's own epitopes are presented to the infant lymphocytes; those that react are recognized as traitors and destroyed before they (and their future cloned daughters) can leave and wreak havoc in the body.

HISTORICAL BACKGROUND OF IMMUNOLOGY

Immunology is a science that examines the structure and function of the immune system. It originates from medicine and early studies on the causes of immunity to disease. The earliest known reference to immunity was during the plague of Athens in 430 BC. Thucydides noted that people who had recovered from a previous bout of the disease could nurse the sick without contracting the illness a second time. In the 18th century, Pierre-Louis Moreau de Maupertuis made experiments with scorpion venom and observed that certain dogs and mice were immune to this venom. This and other observations of acquired immunity were later exploited by Louis Pasteur in his development of vaccination and his proposed germ theory of disease. Pasteur's theory was in direct opposition to contemporary theories of disease, such as the miasma theory. It was not until Robert Koch's 1891 proofs, for which he was awarded aNobel Prize in 1905, that microorganisms were confirmed as the cause of infectious disease. Viruses were confirmed as human pathogens in 1901, with the discovery of the yellow fever virus by Walter Reed.

Immunology made a great advance towards the end of the 19th century, through rapid developments, in the study of humoral immunity and cellular immunity. Particularly important was the work of Paul Ehrlich, who proposed the side-chain theory to explain the specificity of the antigen-antibody reaction; his contributions to the understanding of humoral immunity were recognized by the award of a Nobel Prize in 1908, which was jointly awarded to the founder of cellular immunology, Elie Metchnikoff.

LAYERED DEFENCE

The immune system protects organisms from infection with layered defences of increasing specificity. In simple terms, physical barriers prevent pathogens such as bacteria and viruses from entering the organism. If a pathogen breaches these barriers, the innate immune system provides an immediate, but non-specific response. Innate immune systems are found in all plants and animals. If pathogens successfully evade the innate response, vertebrates possess a second layer of protection, the adaptive immune system, which is activated by the innate response.

Here, the immune system adapts its response during an infection to improve its recognition of the pathogen. This improved response is then retained after the pathogen has been eliminated, in the form of an immunological memory, and allows the adaptive immune system to mount faster and stronger attacks each time this pathogen is encountered. Both innate and adaptive immunity depend on the ability of the immune system to distinguish between self and non-self molecules. In immunology, *self* molecules are those components of an organism's body that can be distinguished from foreign substances by the immune system. Conversely, *non-self* molecules are those recognized as foreign molecules. One class of non-self molecules are called antigens (short for *anti*body *gen*erators) and are defined as substances that bind to specific immune receptors and elicit an immune response.

Surface Barriers

Several barriers protect organisms from infection, including mechanical, chemical, and biological barriers. The waxy cuticle of many leaves, the exoskeleton of insects, the shells and membranes of externally deposited eggs, and skin are examples of mechanical barriers that are the first line of defence against infection. However, as organisms cannot be completely sealed against their environments, other systems act to protect body openings such as the lungs, intestines, and the genitourinary tract. In the lungs, coughing and sneezing mechanically eject pathogens and otherirritants from the respiratory tract. The flushing action of tears and urine also mechanically expels pathogens, while mucus secreted by the respiratory and gastrointestinal tract serves to trap and entangle microorganisms.

Chemical barriers also protect against infection. The skin and respiratory tract secrete antimicrobial peptides such as the β-defensins. Enzymes such as lysozyme and phospholipase A2 insaliva, tears, and breast milk are also antibacterials. Vaginal secretions serve as a chemical barrier following menarche, when they become slightly acidic, while semen contains defensins and zinc to kill pathogens. In the stomach, gastric acid and proteases serve as powerful chemical defences against ingested pathogens.

Within the genitourinary and gastrointestinal tracts, commensal flora serve as biological barriers by competing with pathogenic bacteria for food and space and, in some cases, by changing the conditions in their environment, such as pH or available iron. This reduces the probability that pathogens will reach sufficient numbers to cause illness. However, since most antibiotics non-specifically target bacteria and do not affect fungi, oral antibiotics can lead to an "overgrowth" of fungi and cause conditions such as a vaginal candidiasis (a yeast infection). There is good evidence that re-introduction of probiotic flora, such as pure cultures of the lactobacilli normally found in unpasteurized yogurt, helps restore a healthy balance of microbial populations in intestinal infections in children and encouraging preliminary data in studies on bacterial gastroenteritis, inflammatory bowel diseases, urinary tract infection and post-surgical infections.

INNATE IMMUNE SYSTEM

Microorganisms or toxins that successfully enter an organism encounter the cells and mechanisms of the innate immune system. The innate response is usually triggered when microbes are identified by pattern recognition receptors, which recognize components that are conserved among broad groups of microorganisms, or when damaged, injured or stressed cells send out alarm signals, many of which (but not all) are recognized by the same receptors as those that recognize pathogens. Innate immune defences are non-specific, meaning these systems respond to pathogens in a generic way. This system does not confer long-lasting immunity against a pathogen. The innate immune system is the dominant system of host defence in most organisms.

ADAPTIVE IMMUNE SYSTEM

The adaptive immune system evolved in early vertebrates and allows for a stronger immune response as well as immunological memory, where each pathogen is "remembered" by a signature antigen. The adaptive immune response is antigen-specific and requires the recognition of specific "non-self" antigens during a process called antigen presentation. Antigen specificity allows for the generation of responses that are tailored to specific pathogens or pathogen-infected cells. The ability to mount these tailored responses is maintained in the body by "memory cells". Should a pathogen infect the body more than once, these specific memory cells are used to quickly eliminate it.

Lymphocytes

The cells of the adaptive immune system are special types of leukocytes, called lymphocytes. B cells and T cells are the major types of lymphocytes and are derived from hematopoietic stem cells in the bone marrow. B cells are involved in the humoral immune response, whereas T cells are involved in cell-mediated immune response. Both B cells and T cells carry receptor molecules that recognize specific targets. T cells recognize a "non-self" target, such as a pathogen, only after antigens (small fragments of the pathogen) have been processed and presented in combination with a "self" receptor called a major histocompatibility complex (MHC) molecule. There are two major subtypes of T cells: the killer T cell and the helper T cell. Killer T cells only recognize antigens coupled to Class I MHC molecules, while helper T cells only recognize antigens coupled to Class II MHC molecules. These two mechanisms of antigen presentation reflect the different roles of the two types of T cell. A third, minor subtype are the γδ T cells that recognize intact antigens that are not bound to MHC receptors.

In contrast, the B cell antigen-specific receptor is an antibody molecule on the B cell surface, and recognizes whole pathogens without any need for antigen processing. Each lineage of B cell expresses a different antibody, so the complete set of B cell antigen receptors represent all the antibodies that the body can manufacture.

Killer T cells

Killer T cells are a sub-group of T cells that kill cells that are infected with viruses (and other pathogens), or are otherwise damaged or dysfunctional. As with B cells, each type of T cell recognizes a different antigen. Killer T cells are activated when their T cell receptor (TCR) binds to this specific antigen in a complex with the MHC Class I receptor of another cell. Recognition of this MHC:antigen complex is aided by a co-receptor on the T cell, called CD8. The

T cell then travels throughout the body in search of cells where the MHC I receptors bear this antigen. When an activated T cell contacts such cells, it releases cytotoxins, such as perforin, which form pores in the target cell's plasma membrane, allowing ions, water and toxins to enter. The entry of another toxin called granulysin (a protease) induces the target cell to undergo apoptosis. T cell killing of host cells is particularly important in preventing the replication of viruses. T cell activation is tightly controlled and generally requires a very strong MHC/antigen activation signal, or additional activation signals provided by "helper" T cells.

Helper T cells

Helper T cells regulate both the innate and adaptive immune responses and help determine which immune responses the body makes to a particular pathogen. These cells have no cytotoxic activity and do not kill infected cells or clear pathogens directly. They instead control the immune response by directing other cells to perform these tasks.

Helper T cells express T cell receptors (TCR) that recognize antigen bound to Class II MHC molecules. The MHC:antigen complex is also recognized by the helper cell's CD4 co-receptor, which recruits molecules inside the T cell (*e.g.*, Lck) that are responsible for the T cell's activation. Helper T cells have a weaker association with the MHC:antigen complex than observed for killer T cells, meaning many receptors (around 200–300) on the helper T cell must be bound by an MHC:antigen in order to activate the helper cell, while killer T cells can be activated by engagement of a single MHC:antigen molecule. Helper T cell activation also requires longer duration of engagement with an antigen-presenting cell. The activation of a resting helper T cell causes it to release cytokines that influence the activity of many cell types. Cytokine signals produced by helper T cells enhance the microbicidal function of macrophages and the activity of killer T cells. In addition, helper T cell activation causes an upregulation of molecules expressed on the T cell's surface, such as CD40 ligand (also called CD154), which provide extra stimulatory signals typically required to activate antibody-producing B cells.

B lymphocytes and antibodies

A B cell identifies pathogens when antibodies on its surface bind to a specific foreign antigen. This antigen/antibody complex is taken up by the B cell and processed by proteolysis into peptides. The B cell then displays these antigenic peptides on its surface MHC class II molecules. This combination of MHC and antigen attracts a matching helper T cell, which releases lymphokines and activates the B cell. As the activated B cell then begins to divide, its offspring (plasma cells) secrete millions of copies of the antibody that recognizes this antigen. These antibodies circulate in blood plasma and lymph, bind to pathogens expressing the antigen and mark them for destruction by complement activation or for uptake and destruction by phagocytes. Antibodies can also neutralize challenges directly, by binding to bacterial toxins or by interfering with the receptors that viruses and bacteria use to infect cells.

HUMORAL AND CHEMICAL BARRIERS

Complement System

The complement system is a biochemical cascade that attacks the surfaces of foreign cells. It contains over 20 different proteins and is named for its ability to "complement" the killing of pathogens by antibodies. Complement is the major humoral component of the innate immune response. Many species have complement systems, including non-mammals like plants, fish, and some invertebrates.

In humans, this response is activated by complement binding to antibodies that have attached to these microbes or the binding of complement proteins to carbohydrates on the surfaces of microbes. This recognition signal triggers a rapid killing response. The speed of the response is a result of signal amplification that occurs following sequential proteolytic activation of complement molecules, which are also proteases. After complement proteins initially bind to the microbe, they activate their protease activity, which in turn activates other complement proteases, and so on. This produces a catalytic cascade that amplifies the initial signal by controlled positive feedback. The cascade results in the production of peptides that attract immune cells, increase vascular permeability, and opsonize (coat) the surface of a pathogen, marking it for destruction. This deposition of complement can also kill cells directly by disrupting their plasma membrane.

Inflammation

Inflammation is one of the first responses of the immune system to infection. The symptoms of inflammation are redness, swelling, heat, and pain, which are caused by increased blood flow into tissue. Inflammation is produced by eicosanoids and cytokines, which are released by injured or infected cells. Eicosanoids include prostaglandins that produce fever and the dilation of blood vessels associated with inflammation, and leukotrienes that attract certain white blood cells (leukocytes). Common cytokines include interleukins that are responsible for communication between white blood cells; chemokines that promote chemotaxis; and interferons that have anti-viral effects, such as shutting down protein synthesis in the host cell. Growth factors and cytotoxic factors may also be released. These cytokines and other chemicals recruit immune cells to the site of infection and promote healing of any damaged tissue following the removal of pathogens.

Cellular barriers

Leukocytes (white blood cells) act like independent, single-celled organisms and are the second arm of the innate immune system. The innate leukocytes include the phagocytes (macrophages, neutrophils, and dendritic cells), mast cells, eosinophils, basophils, and natural killer cells. These cells identify and eliminate pathogens, either by attacking larger pathogens through contact or by engulfing and then killing microorganisms. Innate cells are also important mediators in the activation of the adaptive immune system.

Phagocytosis is an important feature of cellular innate immunity performed by cells called 'phagocytes' that engulf, or eat, pathogens or particles. Phagocytes generally patrol the body searching for pathogens, but can be called to specific locations by cytokines. Once a pathogen has been engulfed by a phagocyte, it becomes trapped in an intracellular vesicle called a phagosome, which subsequently fuses with another vesicle called alysosome to form a phagolysosome.

The pathogen is killed by the activity of digestive enzymes or following a respiratory burst that releases free radicals into the phagolysosome. Phagocytosis evolved as a means of acquiring nutrients, but this role was extended in phagocytes to include engulfment of pathogens as a defence mechanism. Phagocytosis probably represents the oldest form of host defence, as phagocytes have been identified in both vertebrate and invertebrate animals.

Neutrophils and macrophages are phagocytes that travel throughout the body in pursuit of invading pathogens. Neutrophils are normally found in the blood stream and are the most abundant type of phagocyte, normally representing 50 per cent to 60 per cent of the total circulating leukocytes. During the acute phase of inflammation, particularly as a result of bacterial infection, neutrophils migrate towards the site of inflammation in a process called chemotaxis, and are usually the first cells to arrive at the scene of infection. Macrophages are versatile cells that reside within tissues and produce a wide array of chemicals including enzymes, complement proteins, and regulatory factors such as interleukin 1.

Macrophages also act as scavengers, ridding the body of worn-out cells and other debris, and as antigen-presenting cells that activate the adaptive immune system.

Dendritic cells (DC) are phagocytes in tissues that are in contact with the external environment; therefore, they are located mainly in the skin, nose, lungs, stomach, and intestines. They are named for their resemblance to neuronal dendrites, as both have many spine-like projections, but dendritic cells are in no way connected to the nervous system. Dendritic cells serve as a link between the bodily tissues and the innate and adaptive immune systems, as they present antigen to T cells, one of the key cell types of the adaptive immune system. Mast cells reside in connective tissues and mucous membranes, and regulate the inflammatory response. They are most often associated with allergy and anaphylaxis. Basophils and eosinophils are related to neutrophils. They secrete chemical mediators that are involved in defending against parasites and play a role in allergic reactions, such as asthma. Natural killer (NK cells) cells are leukocytes that attack and destroy tumor cells, or cells that have been infected by viruses.

ALTERNATIVE ADAPTIVE IMMUNE SYSTEM

Although the classical molecules of the adaptive immune system (*e.g.*, antibodies and T cell receptors) exist only in jawed vertebrates, a distinctlymphocyte-derived molecule has been discovered in primitive jawless vertebrates, such as the lamprey and hagfish. These animals possess a large array of molecules called variable lymphocyte receptors (VLRs) that, like the antigen receptors of jawed vertebrates, are produced from only a small number (one or two) of genes. These molecules are believed to bind pathogenic antigens in a similar way to antibodies, and with the same degree of specificity.

IMMUNOLOGICAL MEMORY

When B cells and T cells are activated and begin to replicate, some of their offspring become long-lived memory cells. Throughout the lifetime of an animal, these memory cells remember each specific pathogen encountered and can mount a strong response if the pathogen is detected again. This is "adaptive" because it occurs during the lifetime of an individual as an adaptation to infection with that pathogen and prepares the immune system for future challenges. Immunological memory can be in the form of either passive short-term memory or active long-term memory.

Passive Memory

Newborn infants have no prior exposure to microbes and are particularly vulnerable to infection. Several layers of passive protection are provided by the mother. During pregnancy, a particular type of antibody, called IgG, is transported from mother to baby directly across the placenta, so human babies have high levels of antibodies even at birth, with the same range of antigen specificities as their mother.

Breast milk or colostrum also contains antibodies that are transferred to the gut of the infant and protect against bacterial infections until the newborn can synthesize its own antibodies.

This is passive immunity because the fetus does not actually make any memory cells or antibodies—it only borrows them. This passive immunity is usually short-term, lasting from a few days up to several months. In medicine, protective passive immunity can also be transferred artificially from one individual to another via antibody-rich serum.

Active Memory and Immunization

Long-term *active* memory is acquired following infection by activation of B and T cells. Active immunity can also be generated artificially, through vaccination. The principle behind vaccination (also called immunization) is to introduce an antigen from a pathogen in order to stimulate the immune system and develop specific immunity against that particular pathogen without causing disease associated with that organism.

This deliberate induction of an immune response is successful because it exploits the natural specificity of the immune system, as well as its inducibility. With infectious disease remaining one of the leading causes of death in the human population, vaccination represents the most effective manipulation of the immune system mankind has developed.

Most viral vaccines are based on live attenuated viruses, while many bacterial vaccines are based on acellular components of micro-organisms, including harmless toxin components. Since many antigens derived from acellular vaccines do not strongly induce the adaptive response, most bacterial vaccines are provided with additional adjuvants that activate the antigen-presenting cells of the innate immune system and maximize immunogenicity.

Disorders of Human Immunity

The immune system is a remarkably effective structure that incorporates specificity, inducibility and adaptation. Failures of host defence do occur, however, and fall into three broad categories: immunodeficiencies, autoimmunity, and hypersensitivities.

Immunodeficiencies

Immunodeficiencies occur when one or more of the components of the immune system are inactive. The ability of the immune system to respond to pathogens is diminished in both the young and the elderly, with immune responses beginning to decline at around 50 years of age due to immunosenescence. In developed countries, obesity, alcoholism, and drug use are common causes of poor immune function. However, malnutrition is the most common cause of immunodeficiency in developing countries. Diets lacking sufficient protein are associated with impaired cell-mediated immunity, complement activity, phagocyte function, IgA antibody concentrations, and cytokine production. Additionally, the loss of the thymus at an early age through genetic mutation or surgical removal results in severe immunodeficiency and a high susceptibility to infection. Immunodeficiencies can also be inherited or 'acquired'. Chronic granulomatous disease, where phagocytes have a reduced ability to destroy pathogens, is an example of an inherited, orcongenital, immunodeficiency. AIDS and some types of cancer cause acquired immunodeficiency.

Autoimmunity

Overactive immune responses comprise the other end of immune dysfunction, particularly the autoimmune disorders. Here, the immune system fails to properly distinguish between self and non-self, and attacks part of the body. Under normal circumstances, many T cells and antibodies react with "self" peptides. One of the functions of specialized cells (located in the thymus andbone marrow) is to present young lymphocytes with self antigens produced throughout the body and to eliminate those cells that recognize self-antigens, preventing autoimmunity.

Hypersensitivity

Hypersensitivity is an immune response that damages the body's own tissues. They are divided into four classes (Type I – IV) based on the mechanisms involved and the time course of the hypersensitive reaction. Type I hypersensitivity is an immediate or anaphylactic reaction, often associated with allergy. Symptoms can range from mild discomfort to death. Type I hypersensitivity is mediated by IgE, which triggers degranulation of mast cells and basophils when cross-linked by antigen. Type II hypersensitivity occurs when antibodies bind to antigens on the patient's own cells, marking them for destruction.

This is also called antibody-dependent (or cytotoxic) hypersensitivity, and is mediated by IgG and IgM antibodies. Immune complexes (aggregations of antigens, complement proteins, and IgG and IgM antibodies) deposited in various tissues trigger Type III hypersensitivity reactions. Type IV hypersensitivity (also known as cell-mediated or*delayed type hypersensitivity*) usually takes between two and three days to develop. Type IV reactions are involved in many autoimmune and infectious diseases, but may also involve *contact dermatitis* (poison ivy). These reactions are mediated by T cells, monocytes, and macrophages.

Other Mechanisms

It is likely that a multicomponent, adaptive immune system arose with the first vertebrates, as invertebrates do not generate lymphocytes or an antibody-based humoral response. Many species, however, utilize mechanisms that appear to be precursors of these aspects of vertebrate immunity. Immune systems appear even in the structurally most simple forms of life, with bacteria using a unique defence mechanism, called the restriction modification system to protect themselves from viral pathogens, called bacteriophages. Prokaryotes also possess acquired immunity, through a system that uses CRISPR sequences to retain fragments of the genomes of phage that they have come into contact with in the past, which allows them to block virus replication through a form of RNA interference.

Pattern recognition receptors are proteins used by nearly all organisms to identify molecules associated with pathogens. Antimicrobial peptides called defensins are an evolutionarily conserved component of the innate immune response found in all animals and plants, and represent the main form of invertebrate systemic immunity.

The complement system and phagocytic cells are also used by most forms of invertebrate life. Ribonucleases and the RNA interference pathway are conserved across all eukaryotes, and are thought to play a role in the immune response to viruses.

Unlike animals, plants lack phagocytic cells, but many plant immune responses involve systemic chemical signals that are sent through a plant. Individual plant cells respond to molecules associated with pathogens known as Pathogen-associated molecular patterns or PAMPs. When a part of a plant becomes infected, the plant produces a localized hypersensitive response, whereby cells at the site of infection undergo rapid apoptosis to prevent the spread of the disease to other parts of the plant. Systemic acquired resistance (SAR) is a type of defensive response used by plants that renders the entire plant resistant to a particular infectious agent. RNA silencing mechanisms are particularly important in this systemic response as they can block virus replication.

TUMOR IMMUNOLOGY

Another important role of the immune system is to identify and eliminate tumors. The *transformed cells* of tumors express antigens that are not found on normal cells. To the immune system, these antigens appear foreign, and their presence causes immune cells to attack the transformed tumor cells. The antigens expressed by tumors have several sources; some are derived from oncogenic viruses like human papillomavirus, which causes cervical cancer, while others are the organism's own proteins that occur at low levels in normal cells but reach high levels in tumor cells. One example is an enzyme called tyrosinase that, when expressed at high levels, transforms certain skin cells (*e.g.* melanocytes) into tumors called melanomas. A third possible source of tumor antigens are proteins normally important for regulating cell growth and survival, that commonly mutate into cancer inducing molecules called oncogenes.

The main response of the immune system to tumors is to destroy the abnormal cells using killer T cells, sometimes with the assistance of helper T cells. Tumor antigens are presented on MHC class I molecules in a similar way to viral antigens. This allows killer T cells to recognize the tumor cell as abnormal. NK cells also kill tumorous cells in a similar way, especially if the tumor cells have fewer MHC class I molecules on their surface than normal; this is a common phenomenon with tumors. Sometimes antibodies are generated against tumor cells allowing for their destruction by the complement system.

Clearly, some tumors evade the immune system and go on to become cancers. Tumor cells often have a reduced number of MHC class I molecules on their surface, thus avoiding detection by killer T cells. Some tumor cells also release products that inhibit the immune response; for example by secreting the cytokine TGF-β, which suppresses the activity of macrophages and lymphocytes. In addition, immunological tolerance may develop against tumor antigens, so the immune system no longer attacks the tumor cells.

Paradoxically, macrophages can promote tumor growth when tumor cells send out cytokines that attract macrophages, which then generate cytokines and growth factors that nurture tumor development. In addition, a combination of hypoxia in the tumor and a cytokine produced by macrophages induces tumor cells to decrease production of a protein that blocks metastasis and thereby assists spread of cancer cells.

Physiological Regulation

Hormones can act as immunomodulators, altering the sensitivity of the immune system. For example, female sex hormones are known immunostimulators of both adaptive and innate immune responses. Some autoimmune diseases such as lupus erythematosus strike women preferentially, and their onset often coincides with puberty. By contrast, male sex hormones such astestosterone seem to be immunosuppressive. Other hormones appear to regulate the immune system as well, most notably prolactin, growth hormone and vitamin D.

When a T-cell encounters a foreign pathogen, it extends a vitamin D receptor. This is essentially a signaling device that allows the T-cell to bind to the active form of vitamin D, the steroid hormonecalcitriol. T-cells have a symbiotic relationship with vitamin D. Not only does the T-cell extend a vitamin D receptor, in essence asking to bind to the steroid hormone version of vitamin D, calcitriol, but the T-cell expresses the gene CYP27B1, which is the gene responsible for converting the pre-hormone version of vitamin D, calcidiol into the steroid hormone version, calcitriol. Only after binding to calcitriol can T-cells perform their intended function. Other immune system cells that are known to express CYP27B1 and thus activate vitamin D calcidiol, are dendritic cells,keratinocytes and macrophages.

It is conjectured that a progressive decline in hormone levels with age is partially responsible for weakened immune responses in aging individuals. Conversely, some hormones are regulated by the immune system, notably thyroid hormone activity. The age-related decline in immune function is also related to dropping vitamin D levels in the elderly. As people age, two things happen that negatively affect their vitamin D levels. First, they stay indoors more due to decreased activity levels. This means that they get less sun and therefore produce less cholecalciferol viaUVB radiation. Second, as a person ages the skin becomes less adept at producing vitamin D.

The immune system is affected by sleep and rest, and sleep deprivation is detrimental to immune function. Complex feedback loops involving cytokines, such as interleukin-1 and tumor necrosis factor-α produced in response to infection, appear to also play a role in the regulation of non-rapid eye movement (REM) sleep. Thus the immune response to infection may result in changes to the sleep cycle, including an increase in slow-wave sleep relative to REM sleep.

Nutrition and Diet

Overnutrition is associated with diseases such as diabetes and obesity, which are known to affect immune function. More moderate malnutrition, as well as certain specific trace mineral and nutrient deficiencies, can also compromise the immune response. Foods rich in certain fatty acids may foster a healthy immune system. Likewise, fetal undernourishment can cause a lifelong impairment of the immune system.

Manipulation In medicine

The immune response can be manipulated to suppress unwanted responses resulting from autoimmunity, allergy, and transplant rejection, and to stimulate protective responses against pathogens that largely elude the immune system. Immunosuppressive drugs are used to control autoimmune disorders or inflammation when excessive tissue damage occurs, and to prevent transplant rejection after an organ transplant.

Anti-inflammatory drugs are often used to control the effects of inflammation. Glucocorticoids are the most powerful of these drugs; however, these drugs can have many undesirable side effects, such as central obesity, hyperglycemia, osteoporosis, and their use must be tightly controlled. Lower doses of anti-inflammatory drugs are often used in conjunction with cytotoxic or immunosuppressive drugs such as methotrexate or azathioprine. Cytotoxic drugsinhibit the immune response by killing dividing cells such as activated T cells. However, the killing is indiscriminate and other constantly dividing cells and their organs are affected, which causes toxic side effects. Immunosuppressive drugs such as ciclosporin prevent T cells from responding to signals correctly by inhibiting signal transduction pathways.

Larger drugs (>500 Da) can provoke a neutralizing immune response, particularly if the drugs are administered repeatedly, or in larger doses. This limits the effectiveness of drugs based on larger peptides and proteins (which are typically larger than 6000 Da). In some cases, the drug itself is not immunogenic, but may be co-administered with an immunogenic compound, as is sometimes the case for Taxol. Computational methods have been developed to predict the immunogenicity of peptides and proteins, which are particularly useful in designing therapeutic antibodies, assessing likely virulence of mutations in viral coat particles, and validation of proposed peptide-based drug treatments.

Early techniques relied mainly on the observation that hydrophilic amino acids are overrepresented in epitope regions than hydrophobic amino acids;however, more recent developments rely on machine learning techniques using databases of existing known epitopes, usually on well-studied virus proteins, as a training set. A publicly accessible database has been established for the cataloguing of epitopes from pathogens known to be recognizable by B cells. The emerging field of bioinformatics-based studies of immunogenicity is referred to as *immunoinformatics*. Immunoproteomics is the study of large sets of proteins (proteomics) involved in the immune response.

Manipulation by Pathogens

The success of any pathogen depends on its ability to elude host immune responses. Therefore, pathogens evolved several methods that allow them to successfully infect a host, while evading detection or destruction by the immune system. Bacteria often overcome physical barriers by secreting enzymes that digest the barrier, for example, by using a type II secretion system. Alternatively, using a type III secretion system, they may insert a hollow tube into the host cell, providing a direct route for proteins to move from the pathogen to the host. These proteins are often used to shut down host defences.

An evasion strategy used by several pathogens to avoid the innate immune system is to hide within the cells of their host (also called intracellular pathogenesis). Here, a pathogen spends most of its life-cycle inside host cells, where it is shielded from direct contact with immune cells, antibodies and complement. Some examples of intracellular pathogens include viruses, the food poisoning bacterium *Salmonella* and the eukaryotic parasites that cause malaria (*Plasmodium falciparum*) and leishmaniasis (*Leishmania spp.*). Other bacteria, such as *Mycobacterium tuberculosis*, live inside a protective capsule that prevents lysis by complement.

Many pathogens secrete compounds that diminish or misdirect the host's immune response. Some bacteria form biofilms to protect themselves from the cells and proteins of the immune system. Such biofilms are present in many successful infections, *e.g.*, the chronic *Pseudomonas aeruginosa* and *Burkholderia cenocepacia* infections characteristic of cystic fibrosis. Other bacteria generate surface proteins that bind to antibodies, rendering them ineffective; examples include *Streptococcus* (protein G), *Staphylococcus aureus* (protein A), and *Peptostreptococcus magnus* (protein L).

The mechanisms used to evade the adaptive immune system are more complicated. The simplest approach is to rapidly change non-essential epitopes (amino acids and/or sugars) on the surface of the pathogen, while keeping essential epitopes concealed. This is called antigenic variation. An example is HIV, which mutates rapidly, so the proteins on its viral envelope that are essential for entry into its host target cell are constantly changing. These frequent changes in antigens may explain the failures of vaccines directed at this virus.

The parasite *Trypanosoma brucei* uses a similar strategy, constantly switching one type of surface protein for another, allowing it to stay one step ahead of the antibody response. Masking antigens with host molecules is another common strategy for avoiding detection by the immune system. In HIV, the envelope that covers the virion is formed from the outermost membrane of the host cell; such "self-cloaked" viruses make it difficult for the immune system to identify them as "non-self" structures.

VACCINATION APPLICATION OF IMMUNOLOGY

Vaccination is the most widespread application of immunology. It aims to artificially induce immunological memory to protect against primary infections by established pathogens. In designing a vaccine, it is important to take the pathogen's route of infection and its mechanism of pathogenicity into account. Symptoms of diphtheria and tetanus are caused exclusively by bacterial toxins. Consequently, it is of prime importance that these toxins be inactivated; going after the bacteria themselves is secondary. The polyvalent vaccine for babies starting at the age of two months therefore contains inactivated toxins, so-called toxoids, to generate neutralizing antibodies. In case of infection, no harm is done, as the antibody-coated toxins cannot bind to their cellular receptors. For polio, it is necessary to catch the virus before it enters the CNS. The virus enters the body via the enteral pathway, first replicating in intestinal epithelial cells, then spreading via the blood. Two ways of immunization have been successfully developed.

In the vaccine developed by Jonas Salk, inactivated polio virus is injected, inducing neutralizing antibodies which prevent the virus from reaching the CNS. In contrast, oral live-attenuated polio vaccine, developed a few years later by Albert Sabin, induces local immunity in the gut. Secretory IgA in the intestinal lumen prevents the virus from infecting enteric cells. Following immunization, attenuated virus can be spread to contacts of the vaccinee, resulting in protection of additional individuals.

Live-attenuated polio vaccine is easy to administer (no needles required, etc.) and cheap to produce, but it has one drawback: one of the three mutated virus strains included very rarely reverts to a pathogenic virus, causing vaccine-associated paralytic poliomyelitis (VAPP) in about one in a million newly vaccinated persons. In many countries having eradicated indigenous polio, this risk is higher than that from imported wild polio infections. Therefore most developed countries, including Austria, switched back to inactivated vaccine a few years ago. Oral vaccination remains the method of choice in countries with ongoing wild poliovirus circulation and lower vaccination rates. Here, the larger reduction in numbers of poliomyelitis obtained by the simpler immunization protocol outweigh the small number of VAPP cases. Inevitably, vaccinations entail certain risks and therefore tend to cause highly emotional debates, especially among parents nervous about their kids' wellbeing. In deciding for or against a specific vaccination, it is imperative to quantify the risks of either decision. Let's consider measles as an example. 'Measles are a harmless children's illness', some parents argue, and were easily overcome before the advent of vaccination.

Therefore, the risk of vaccinating a healthy child would outweigh the benefit of preventing measles. From an individual adult's experience, this sounds plausible. But do the data support this view? Measles vaccine, part of MMR (measles, mumps, rubella) is a live-attenuated vaccine with two goals: induction of CD8+ T-memory cells and induction of neutralizing IgG. A small risk exists: many children develop a fever, some develop postvaccinal measles, a markedly attenuated form with a slight skin rash. A complication of encephalitis in extremely rare cases cannot be completely excluded, but if it exists, it certainly affects fewer than one in a million vaccinees (with events of this rarity, it is hard to establish causality).

On the other hand, risks are much higher if a non-vaccinated person attracts measles. The most frequent complication is *otitis media*, which is very painful. Viral pneumonia, for which no causal therapy exists, occurs in one of 200 cases. Encephalitis due to the virus occurs with a frequency between 1:1000 and 1:5000. Mortality associated with encephalitis is about 15 per cent, and lasting neurologic defects are common in those who overcome the disease. An extremely rare complication, subacute sclerosing panencephalitis, which manifests itself many years after the acute infection, is universally fatal. As a concrete illustration of the risks incurred by non-vaccinated persons serves a limited outbreak documented in the Netherlands in 1999: About 2300 cases (almost exclusively in families opposing vaccination) were brought to the attention of authorities. Three children died.

Fifty-three had to be admitted to the hospital, of which 30 suffered from pneumonia, 4 from encephalitis and 19 from other complications. 130 people were treated for pneumonia at home, 152 for *otitis media*. Ethically not unproblematic, as long as only few people refuse to be vaccinated from fear of side effects, these individuals profit in two ways: they don't incur any potential risk from vaccination, but are nevertheless protected by herd immunity due to the vaccination of the vast majority of their contacts. As soon as the fraction of people opposing vaccination exceeds a certain threshold, however, relative risk is reversed, as exemplified in the Dutch measles outbreak. Back to methodological aspects of immunization. Vaccination against hepatitis B virus, of paramount importance for medical personnel, relies on induction of neutralizing antibodies, which prevent the virus from entering liver cells. In this case, the vaccine consists exclusively of the envelope protein of the virus, HBs-antigen, that is produced by recombinant DNA technology and self-assembles to empty viral envelopes.

This excludes any potential for the emergence of a pathogenic virus by mutation. The majority of vaccines against viral diseases contain attenuated live viruses. If we intend to induce CD8+ T memory cells, against, *e.g.*, the measles virus, we will not succeed by using inactivated material: for a strong CD8+ T cell response, viral peptides have to be produced in the cell and presented on MHC-I. The virus used for immunization has to be able to replicate, yet must not be dangerous. Attenuation of a human virus can be achieved by repeatedly passaging the original virus on animal cells, *e.g.* ape cells. By mutation and selection, the virus over time adapts to the monkey cells. For example, it may change its surface protein to better interact with its receptor on the ape cell.

When used back in humans as a vaccine, it will have trouble replicating in human cells and only do so very slowly. Today, using recombinant DNA-technology, attenuating mutations can be generated directly without lengthy animal passaging. For vaccines against bacterial infections, where the goal is to induce antibodies, the tendency is to reduce complexity.

In the early days of vaccination, there was no other way than to use easy to produce, but biologically messy preparations of inactivated bacteria. Inevitably, these caused high rates of unwanted effects, which were partly responsible for the lingering reservations about vaccination in collective memory. To minimize the potential for side effects and complications, modern vaccines aim to use the lowest number of defined antigen molecules possible. These vaccine molecules sometimes look strange to the untrained eye. Remember T cell help, required to "release the safety catch" from B cells to prevent production of unnecessary and potentially dangerous antibodies. Many pathogenic bacteria, *e.g.*, *Haemophilus influenzae* and *Streptococcus pneumoniae* are capsulated, making them invisible to neutrophils. Vaccine-induced antibodies against capsular polysaccharides can solve this problem by efficient opsonization.

But when the bacterial polysaccharides are purified and injected, especially in children, inadequate amounts of antibody are produced. Why? T cell help is missing! T cell help is contingent on the B cell presenting an antigen-derived peptide on MHC-II, and in the case of pure polysaccharide antigens, the B cell has nothing to present.

The solution is a trick: take the polysaccharide and couple some polypeptide to it. This protein doesn't even have to be derived from *H. influenzae*. In contrast, it may be even better to use a protein that for sure has already generated TH2 cells in the children, for example tetanus toxoid. So, the "conjugated" vaccine against *H. influenzae* consists of a polysaccharide from *H. influenzae* coupled to the toxoid from *Clostridium tetani*. The B cell with a B cell receptor binding the polysaccharide will internalize the whole conjugate into its endosomal pathway and present peptides from the toxoid on MHC II. Lots of TH2 cells recognizing these peptides are around, since the child has been repeatedly immunized with tetanus toxoid as part of the polyvalent vaccination against diphtheria, pertussis, tetanus etc. So, the anti-tetanus TH2 cell gives help to the anti-*Haemophilus* B cell. Strange?- It works!

Still, a vaccine molecule optimized along these lies by itself frequently fails to elicit a satisfactory immune response. Another aspect to consider in immunizations is the requirement for costimulation. Dendritic cells activate naive T cells only when expressing B7. This, in turn, depends on dendritic cell activation via pattern recognition receptors (PRRs) by pathogen-associated molecular patterns (PAMPs). Old immunization protocols used additives, termed adjuvants, that included bacterial PAMPs. The classical adjuvant for immunization of laboratory animals was *complete Freund's adjuvant*, consisting of inactivated *Mycobacterium tuberculosis* in mineral oil. While frequently causing side effects, the old human vaccines containing inactivated bacteria included their own adjuvants, as many of their components activated PRRs. Modern human vaccines contain adjuvants that are less prone to cause side effects. The most frequent is "alum", particles of aluminum salts, which directly activate NOD-like receptors and the inflammasome, thereby inducing expression of costimulatory molecules.

How about tuberculosis, the bacterium hiding in macrophages, where antibodies are of little use? The French vaccine pioneers A. Calmette and C. Guérin grew*Mycobacterium bovis* for years on glycerin-bile-potato media (BCG-Bacille Calmette Guérin). This treatment finally attenuated the mycobacterium to an extent that it could be used as an anti-bacterial live vaccine. It promotes an early and more intense immune response against *M. tuberculosis* by TH1 memory cells. However, a protective effect is found only in 60-80 per cent of those immunized, is only relative, and is of limited duration. In addition, it prevents easy diagnosis of tuberculosis by the Mendel-Mantoux skin test, as the immunized test positive. Therefore, most countries have discontinued BCG immunization.

An idea that sounds brilliant but hasn't yet resulted in a working routine protocol is DNA immunization. Plasmids encoding antigens could be injected right into the muscle, which then expresses the encoded proteins. It would even be possible to do that without a needle, shooting the DNA right into the muscle with a "gene gun", a modified air gun. Yet, in spite of positive proof of concept, actual immune responses so far have been too weak to switch to this method.

INADEQUATE DEFENCE

Inadequate defence against pathogens can result from genetic causes, acquired causes (foremost acquired immunodeficiency syndrome –AIDS— by HIV) or from escape strategies developed by pathogens during their co-evolution with humans.

Primary Immunodeficiency Diseases

The majority of primary immunodeficiency's are rare diseases, that are instructive for the contribution of individual parts of the human immune system to overall defence. Depending on the genes concerned, the following functions may be impaired:

- T- and B cell function: severe combined immunodeficiency (SCID)
- global or partial B cell response
- phagocytosis
- complement functions

In addition, the immune system is affected in a number of more complex syndromes. Here, only a select few primary immunodeficiencies are mentioned that should illustrate certain aspects of immune system functioning.

SCID

Severe combined immunodeficiency (SCID) is caused by several genetic defects, *e.g.*, by a deficiency of RAG proteins. If neither immunoglobulin genes nor T cell receptor genes are rearranged, the result is a total loss of adaptive immunity. Only a few patients with defective RAG proteins have been described; more frequent causes for SCID are defects that primarily concern T cells. These patients' inability to produce antibodies underscores the importance of T cell help for immunoglobulin production.

Autosomal recessive deficiencies of two enzymes in purine metabolism, ADA and PNP, cause problems in T cell development. Adenosine deaminase (ADA) deaminates (deoxy-) adenosine to (deoxy-) inosine. Purine nucleoside phosphorylase (PNP) cleaves (deoxy-) inosine and (deoxy-) guanosine, resulting in ribose-1-phosphate plus base. Both defects lead to an accumulation of dAMP/dATP. High concentrations of dAMP/dATP cause substrate-inhibition of the enzyme ribonucleotide reductase, necessary for reducing ribonucleotides to their deoxy-forms.

The resulting lack of dCTP, dGTP, and dTTP impairs synthesis of DNA. Why this is deleterious for T cells, but tolerable for other cells is not entirely clear. Maybe this effect is most pronounced in the thymus, as apoptotic death of more than 95 per cent of thymocytes results in locally increased concentrations of dAMP/dATP due to breakdown of DNA. ADA deficiency is successfully treated by infusion of PEG-ADA. Obviously, this only works extracellularly, but intracellular concentrations are rapidly equilibrated by nucleoside transporters. ADA deficiency was the first disease where gene therapy was attempted. A functioning version of the gene was first introduced into T cells, later into hematopoietic stem cells. Expression of the enzyme was successful in part of the cells, but mostly that part was too small to cure immunodeficiency.

So far, gene therapy was most successful in attempts to cure another form of the disease, X-linked SCID. The disease got some public awareness from the "bubble boy", a little boy who was kept alive by isolation in a pathogen-free plastic bubble; he died in 1984 in an attempt to cure his disease by a bone marrow transplant. In X-linked SCID, T cells fail to develop due to a missing common γ-chain of interleukin receptors for IL 2, IL 4, IL 7, IL 9 and IL 15. For gene therapy, a sound copy of this X-chromosomal gene was introduced into stem cells of affected boys by a retroviral vector. The boys successfully developed T cells and responded favourably to typical immunizations against diphtheria, tetanus and polio. Initial euphoria quickly subsided, however, when two of the boys developed T cell leukemia. Further investigations indicated that the retroviral vector in both cases had inserted near the proto-oncogene LMO2, resulting in its activation. Overexpression of the encoded protein had caused leukemia. The trials were halted.

Immunoglobulin deficiency

An X-chromosomally inherited disease also exists at the B cell level: X-linked or Bruton's agammaglobulinemia. Missing in affected boys is Bruton's tyrosine kinase (BTK), a kinase necessary for B cell maturation. As a quality control step in pre-B cells, the product of a rearranged heavy chain is brought to the surface together with a temporary, "surrogate" light chain. This *ersatz*-immunoglobulin then signals via BTK, indicating successful rearrangement of a heavy chain, so that the cell now initiates light chain rearrangement. If no BTK signal is detected, it is assumed that heavy chain rearrangement failed (wrong reading frame on both alleles, or similar problems), making the cell useless; the cell undergoes apoptosis. A defect in BTK thus results in apoptosis of all pre-B cells and a general lack of immunoglobulins. The affected boys suffer from recurrent infections with pyogenic bacteria such as *Streptococcus pneumoniae*.

A third X-linked disease is hyper-IgM syndrome. Here, normal numbers of B and T cells combine with high serum levels of T cell-independent IgM but a lack of other immunoglobulin isotypes. The defective molecule is CD40-ligand, required for TH2 cells to help B cells, as well as for TH1 cells to activate macrophages. Without T cell help, class switch mostly doesn't occur. Children suffer from recurrent infections with extracellular bacteria, as well as with the parasite *Pneumocystis jirovecii* that is otherwise easily cleared by activated macrophages. A range of additional causes for class switch problems exist. One of them is hyper IgM syndrome type 2, which is caused by a deficiency of the enzyme AID. Both class switch recombination and somatic hypermutation are initiated by this enzyme, which deaminates cytosine to form uracil. Uracil is removed from DNA by the enzyme UNG (uracil-N-glycosylase) followed by additional steps resulting in double strand breaks in the so called switch regions of the immunoglobulin heavy chain genes (described in section 2.5). This is necessary to switch a B cell's immunoglobulin production from IgM to IgG or another isotype. Accordingly, with a deficiency in AID, class switch is severely impaired, resulting in a lack of IgG and IgA associated with normal or high IgM.

The most frequent form of immunoglobulin deficiency, at 1:800, is selective IgA deficiency. As symptoms of affected children tend to be mild (all kids are sick from time to time...), the disease is underdiagnosed. More severely affected children suffer from recurrent mucosal infections such as otitis media, paranasal sinusitis and bronchitis, as well as pneumonia and intestinal infections. Allergy and autoimmune phenomena are increased. After repeated transfusions, a tendency to produce anti-IgA antibodies may become critical. The genetic basis of IgA deficiency is insufficiently understood, but some progress has recently been made.

Selective IgA deficiency might be a marginal form of another disease entity, common variable immunodeficiency (CVID), as both forms sometimes are found in different members of the same families. CVID is less frequent (approximately 1:25,000) and genetically heterogeneous. CVID is characterized by recurrent infections of respiratory or gastrointestinal tracts starting not before age three, but in most patients only during the second or third decade of life. Characteristically, responses to vaccinations are weak or lacking altogether. Lab work shows hypogammaglobulinemia with low IgG and IgA, but frequently normal IgM levels. A few genetic defects resulting in CVID have been elucidated, each accounting for only a small fraction of total patients. They concern transmembrane proteins that (in addition to CD40-ligand-CD40 contact) are required for germinal center processes including class switch and somatic hypermutation, which in turn are necessary for generation of memory B cells. CVID-causing defects were found in genes encoding ICOS, TACI and CD19. Intriguingly, in some families with TACI deficiency, homozygous members had CVID, while selective IgA deficiency was found in heterozygous members. TACI is a member of the TNF receptor superfamily (TNFRSF13B) and functions as a trimer. Heterozygous TACI deficiency would thus result in a strongly diminished number of functional trimers.

Defects in phagocytosis and complement

Cooperation between antibodies, complement and phagocytes is essential to eliminate pyogenic bacteria that, for their polysaccharide capsule, are not readily recognized by neutrophils. The significance of this cooperation is underscored by the fact that deficiencies of either of these components result in severe infections with this type of pathogens.

Several aspects of the complex processes of chemotaxis and phagocytosis can be affected by genetic defects. A deficiency of surface molecules such as integrins or the carbohydrate ligand of selectins prevents leukocytes from adhering to the endothelial vessel wall in inflamed tissue. Lack of an enzyme necessary to produce reactive oxygen species means pathogens are phagocytosed, but not killed. Examples are chronic granulomatous disease (deficiency of NADPH oxidase) or myeloperoxidase (MPO) deficiency. Chediak-Higashi syndrome is caused by the deficiency of a vesicle transport protein, so that phagosomes fail to fuse with lysosomes.

Symptoms of complement deficiencies depend on their location in the complement cascade. Defects in alternative or lectin pathways predispose to infections with pyogenic bacteria. Deficiencies in components C1, C2 or C4 result in impaired clearance of immune complexes, leading to type III diseases (explained in section 5.1). Defects in the membrane attack complex (C5-C9) predispose to severe infections with *Neisseria meningitidis*.

HIV/ AIDS

By the spread of human immunodeficiency virus (HIV), AIDS has become a common disease. Two virus types exist: HIV-1 can be found around the globe, HIV-2 mainly in West Africa. Both seem to have jumped the species barrier form non-human primates to humans in Africa during the 20th century.

The problem of this disease is that HIV infection targets and kills CD4 T cells, over time depleting these cells that are main and center to the functioning of the immune system. Also dendritic cells, macrophages and several cell types of the central nervous system are infected. The CD4 molecule itself is the most important receptor; in addition, infection requires a chemokine receptor, either CCR5 or CXCR4. A defective CCR5 haplotype exists, CCR5-Δ32, that cannot be used by the virus to enter the cell, making homozygotes resistant to the most frequent strains. About 1 per cent of Caucasian populations are homozygous, while the haplotype is far less common in African and Asian populations.

HIV is transmitted by body fluids, primarily during sexual intercourse. Other routes of infection are by contaminated needles or blood transfusions and from an infected mother to her child before or during childbirth or by breast feeding. The virus particle docks via its gp120 envelope protein to CD4 and the chemokine receptor, fuses its membrane with that of the cell and enters its capsid containing its RNA genome, reverse transcriptase and other enzymes into the cell. Using reverse transcriptase, the virus transcribes its single stranded RNA genome into cDNA and inserts this copy into a host cell chromosome with the help of integrase. The integrated cDNA is called provirus. In this state, the virus can remain latent and unassailable for years. The viral genome consists of retrovirus-typical long terminal repeats (LTRs) flanking the usual gag-, pol-, env- and six additional smaller genes. Virus activation is induced by transcription factor NFκB, in parallel and by the same mechanism as T cell, dendritic cell and macrophage activation. Several transcripts are made and spliced, giving rise to the different viral components. Some of its proteins are synthesized as polyprotein precursors that are subsequently cleaved to their final form by viral protease. After all components have been produced in sufficient quantities, they are packaged by self-assembly and leave the cell by budding.

Three mechanisms contribute to destroying infected CD4 T cells:

- cytotoxic CD8 T cells doing their normal job of killing virus factories
- direct cytopathic effects of the virus
- an increased propensity of activated T cells to enter apoptosis

In the absence of treatment, the disease typically develops in three phases:

Acute HIV infection during the first few weeks, characterized by fever, lymphadenopathy, pharyngitis and aphthae (not rhinitis). Obviously, these symptoms are very unspecific. Differential diagnosis has to take into account many potential causes, *e.g.* Epstein-Barr-Virus (EBV) infection (mononucleosis or kissing disease). At this time, a diagnosis can only be established by PCR, as antibodies appear only after several weeks or months: 6 months after infection, 99 per cent are antibody-positive.

Asymptomatic latent infection. The duration of this phase depends on several factors, *e.g.*, age, nutrition and other infections. In young people with a good standard of living, this phase can last ten and more years. Diagnosis is mostly established by positive Western blot following less specific ELISA screening tests. At the end of this phase, infections become more frequent.

AIDS phase. The onset of the complete clinical picture of AIDS depends on the number of remaining CD4 T cells. Normally, this is 500-1000 CD4 T cells per cubic millimeter (or μl) of blood. When this number falls below a critical threshold of 200, adaptive immunity is so weak that the patient starts to suffer from opportunistic infections with, *e.g.*, *Candida albicans* (esophagitis), *Pneumocystis jirovecii* (pneumonia), cytomegalovirus, herpes zoster (shingles) etc. In the event that a previous infection with tuberculosis was not completely eliminated, the TH1-dependent granuloma walls now start to crumble, giving rise to an acute flare-up. Another possibility is Kaposi's sarcoma, which is caused in endothelial cells by another virus from the herpes group, human herpes virus type 8 (HHV8). In the end, the patient succumbs to one of these infections.

There is neither a vaccine nor a cure for HIV, yet efficient therapy has nevertheless been developed in the form of HAART (highly active antiretroviral therapy). The line of attack is to inhibit enzymes necessary for virus replication, such as reverse transcriptase (RT) and protease. Nucleoside analogue RT inhibitors lead to incorporation of "wrong" nucleotides into the growing cDNA, blocking RT progress, while non-nucleoside inhibitors block RT by other means. A range of protease inhibitors is used; a virus strain may develop resistance by point mutations in its protease gene. Detection of these mutations by sequence analysis is a means to rationally adjust therapy. As a third principle, virus entry inhibitors may be used. The drug cocktail is effective but frequently causes unwanted side effects including mitochondrial dysfunction resulting in myopathy or pancreatitis or lipodystrophy (esthetically displeasing changes in the distribution of subcutaneous fat).

Under optimal conditions, HAART is able to suppress virus load to extremely low levels, sharply reducing morbidity and mortality. Yet, it is not able to eliminate the virus, and therefore has to be taken for the rest of the patient's life. This is not a question of popping two pills a day; therapy protocol is complex, requiring the patient to take medications at exact time points distributed over the entire day. If the protocol is not exactly adhered to, the virus gets breathing space to replicate. This promotes resistance: in contrast to DNA-dependent DNA polymerases with proofreading function, reverse transcriptase lacks proofreading, leading to frequent misincorporations. If this is paired with intermittent selective pressure by therapy, resistant strains will emerge rapidly. Enzymes modified by point mutations cease being inhibited by the drugs, making therapy ineffective.

Anti-HIV therapy is extraordinarily expensive, as all drugs have been newly developed and are patent-protected. The countries needing these medications most, especially in sub-Saharan Africa, are the ones least able to pay for them. Despite some programmes to equip these countries at reduced prices, this discrepancy remains largely unsolved.

CHARACTERISTICS OF THE IMMUNE SYSTEM

OVERVIEW OF THE IMMUNE SYSTEM

We are constantly being exposed to infectious agents and yet, in most cases, we are able to resist these infections. It is our immune system that enables us to resist infections. The immune system is composed of two major subdivisions, the innate or non-specific immune system and the adaptive or specific immune system. The innate immune system is our first line of defence against invading organisms while the adaptive immune system acts as a second line of defence and also affords protection against re-exposure to the same pathogen. Each of the major subdivisions of the immune system has both cellular and humoral components by which they carry out their protective function. In addition, the innate immune system also has anatomical features that function as barriers to infection. Although these two arms of the immune system have distinct functions, there is interplay between these systems (*i.e.*, components of the innate immune system influence the adaptive immune system and vice versa).

Although the innate and adaptive immune systems both function to protect against invading organisms, they differ in a number of ways. The adaptive immune system requires some time to react to an invading organism, whereas the innate immune system includes defences that, for the most part, are constitutively present and ready to be mobilized upon infection. Second, the adaptive immune system is antigen specific and reacts only with the organism that induced the response. In contrast, the innate system is not antigen specific and reacts equally well to a variety of organisms. Finally, the adaptive immune system demonstrates immunological memory. It "remembers" that it has encountered an invading organism and reacts more rapidly on subsequent exposure to the same organism. In contrast, the innate immune system does not demonstrate immunological memory.

All cells of the immune system have their origin in the bone marrow and they include myeloid (neutrophils, basophils, eosinpophils, macrophages and dendritic cells) and lymphoid (B lymphocyte, T lymphocyte and Natural Killer) cells, which differentiate along distinct pathways. The myeloid progenitor (stem) cell in the bone marrow gives rise to erythrocytes, platelets, neutrophils, monocytes/macrophages and dendritic cells whereas the lymphoid progenitor (stem) cell gives rise to the NK, T cells and B cells. For T cell development the precursor T cells must migrate to the thymus where they undergo differentiation into two distinct types of T cells, the CD4+ T helper cell and the CD8+ pre-cytotoxic T cell. Two types of T helper cells are produced in the thymus the TH1 cells, which help the CD8+ pre-cytotoxic cells to differentiate into cytotoxic T cells, and TH2 cells, which help B cells, differentiate into plasma cells, which secrete antibodies.

The main function of the immune system is self/non-self discrimination. This ability to distinguish between self and non-self is necessary to protect the organism from invading pathogens and to eliminate modified or altered cells (*e.g.* malignant cells). Since pathogens may replicate intracellularly (viruses and some bacteria and parasites) or extracellularly (most bacteria, fungi and parasites), different components of the immune system have evolved to protect against these different types of pathogens. It is important to remember that infection with an organism does not necessarily mean diseases, since the immune system in most cases will be able to eliminate the infection before disease occurs.

Disease occurs only when the bolus of infection is high, when the virulence of the invading organism is great or when immunity is compromised. Although the immune system, for the most part, has beneficial effects, there can be detrimental effects as well. During inflammation, which is the response to an invading organism, there may be local discomfort and collateral damage to healthy tissue as a result of the toxic products produced by the immune response. In addition, in some cases the immune response can be directed towards self tissues resulting in autoimmune disease.

ANTIGENS

An antigen is a foreign substance that can elicit a specific immune response. Most antigens are proteins, but some are polysaccharides, nucleoproteins, or glycoproteins. Each antigen has several epitopes (antigenic determinants), or antigenic determinants. Hapten: a small molecules can acts as an antigen only if it binds to a larger protein molecule.

GENERATING ANTIBODY DIVERSITY

The diversity of B cell receptors is sufficient to recognize epitopes on any pathogen we are likely to encounter in our life time.

B-cell diversity is generated by recombining epitopes on any pathogen we are likely to encounter in our life time. B-cell diversity is generated by recombining bits of DNA in our genome to generate 100 millions different antibody genes.

Cells and Tissues of the Immune System

Lymphocytes develop from lymphoid stem cells in the bone marrow. Lymphocytes differenciate into B cells in the bone marrow or into T cells in the thymus. Subsequent differentiatoion of T cells produces four different kinds of cells.

- Cytotoxic (killer) T cells
- Delay-hypersensitivity T cells
- Helper T cells
- Regulatory T cells.

Natural killer cells (NK cells), non B, non T cells, which non-specifically kill cancer cells and cells infected with virus without having to utilize the specific immune responses. By releasing cytotoxic molecules to create holes in the target's cell membrane, leading to lysis.Other molecules enter the target cell and fragment DNA, causing apoptosis(programmed cell death). NK cells are also affected by interferons.

DUAL NATURE OF THE IMMUNE SYETEM

The dual roles of the immune system consist of humoral immunity, which is carried out mainly by antibodies produced by B cells and plasma cells, and cell mediated immunity, which is carried out mainly by certain T cells.

General Properties of Immune Responses

When our first line of defence is breached and our innate immune system fails to control an infection, our adaptive immune system is activated.

Recognition

Major Histocompatibility Complex

MHC Class 1: receptors on all cells, identify as self, present antigen for systemic. Recognized by CD8 Cytotoxic T cells.

MHC Class 2: leukocytes only, intercelluar communication. Recognized by CD4 Helper T cells.

MHC Class 3: all protein produces as listed above.

Self: Class1 receptors on Neutrophils/Macrophage must match

Non-self: Class 2 receptors do not matchà phagocytosis

Recognition of self versus non-self

Embryos contain many different lymphocytes, each genetically programmed to recognize a particular antigen and make antibodies to destroy it. A lymphocyte divides repeatedly to produce a clone.

According to the clonal selection theory, B cells recognize specific epitopes on antigens according to the particular antibody present on the B cell plasma membrane.

When a B cell detects an antigen with which it can react, it binds to the antigen, engulfs it, process it, displays a peptide fragment as MHC class II to T_H2 cells, and divides many times. Clone of genetically identical B cells, which differentiate into many plasma cells and some memory cells, is produced. Tolerance is B or T cells encounters its programmed antigen as part of a normal host substance (self).

Specificity

Immune system fully matures at age 2 to 3. Specificityrefers to the ability of immune responses to respond to and distinguish among different antigens and epitopes. Cross-reaction, reactions of a particular antibody with very similar antigens.

Heterogeneity (Diversity)

Diversity refers to the ability of immune responses to produce many different antibodies and cell substances on the basis of the different antigens they encounter.

Memory

Ability of T and B cells can recognize substances it has previously encountered- memory cells. Anamnestic (secondary) response is prompt due to recall of memory cells. The power and rapid secondary immune response initiated by memory B cellsacts within few days, sometimes suppressing all symptoms. The action of vaccines depends upon their stimulating the formation of memory B cells.

SPECIFIC IMMUNE RESPONSE

Cell Mediated – involves different cells and their secretory products
Antibody mediated – production, secretion and action of antibodies

HUMORAL IMMUNITY

B-cell activation

Native B cells are fully differentiated B cells that have not yet encountered a complementary antigen; they bear membrane–bound IgM and IgD on their outer surface. Clonal selection begins when native B cells bind to their complementary antibodies: Then they multiply; produce soluble IgM and IgD, and undergo a high rate of mutation in their DNA-encoding region, resulting in affinity maturation. Later, class switching occurs: Various activated B cells begin to make all classes of antibodies. Some members of the clone become short-lived effectors (plasma) cells, which make large quantities of antibody; others become long-lived memory cells, which fight future infections by the same pathogen. Lymphocytes, including interleukins-1,-2,-4,-5, and -6, produced by NK cells help B-cell activation stimulated by most antigens. Some T-independent antigens stimulate B-cell activation without help.

B cells are selected to respond to specific antigens in accordance with the particular antibody present on the B cell membrane prior to encountering an antigen. When a B cell detects an antigen with which it can react, it binds to the antigen (sensitized or activates) and divides many times to produce a clone of many plasma cells and some memory cells. Many B cells require helper T cells to proliferate and differentiate into both plasma and memory B cells. Plasma cells synthesize and release large numbers of antibodies. Memory cells remain in lymphoid tissues ready to respond to subsequent exposure to the same antigen.

Properties of Antibodies (Immunoglobulins)

Antibodies are glycoproteins because carbohydrate groups are attached to them.Structually, antibodies consist of two heavy and two light polypeptide chains, joined by disulfide bonds to form a Y shape. The upper ends of the Y, consists of variable region in both the light and heavy chains, differ from antibody to antibody. These variable regions form the two antigen-binding sites (part of the Fab fragment), which are responsible for the specificity of the antibody. The remaining part of the molecule consists of constant regions (Fc) that are similar in all antibodies of a particular class. The constant region binds to and activates phagocytes and complement.

Class of Immunoglobins

Five classes of immunoglobulins have been identified. Each class has a particular kind of constant region which gives that class its distinguishing properties. IgD, IgE, and IgG are secreted as monomers, IgM as pentamers, and IgA as monomers or dimmers.

IgG

The main class of antibodies found in blood, accounts 20 per cent of all plasma proteins. IgG is produced in large quantities during a secondary response. The antigen-binding sites of IgG attach to antigens on microorganisms and their tissue-binding sites attach to receptors on phagocytic cells. IgG is the only immunoglobulin that can cross the placenta from mother to fetus and provide antibody protection. IgG – monomer, predominant type, specific immune response, transmammary, transplacental.

IgA

Occurs in small amounts in blood and in larger amounts in body secretions such as tears, milk, saliva, mucus and linings of GI tracts. Secretory IgA, which consists of two monomer units held together by a J chain, has an attached secretory component, which protects the IgA from proteolytic enzymes and facilitates its transport. Mucosal surfaces such as in the respiratory, GI tracts are major sites for invasion by pathogens. The main function of IgA is to bind antigens on microorganisms before they invade. It also activates complement, which helps to kill the microorganisms. IgA – monomer (plasma), dimer (mucus/saliva/tears/milk/intestinal secretions), inhibit microbe attachment to epithelia

IgM

IgM is found as a monomer on the surface of B cells and is secreted as a pentamer by plasma cells. IgM consists of five units connected by their tails to a J chain and has 10 peripheral antigen-binding sites. As IgM binds to antigens, it also activates complement and causes microorganisms to clump together. High levels of IgM indicate recent infection or expose to antigen. IgM – monomers (antigen receptor) penerates (plasma), non-specific immune response, blood typing

IgE

IgE has a special affinity for receptors of basophils in blood or mast cells in tissue. It binds to these cells by tissue binding sites, leaving antigen-binding sites free to bind antigens which can develop allergy. When IgE binds antigens, the basophils and mast cells secrete histamine which produce allergy symptoms. IgE are elevated in patients with allergies and worm parasites. IgE – monomer, tonsils, skin, mucus membranes. Stimulates basophils to release histamine

IgD

IgD, monomer, is found mainly on B-cell membranes and function is unknown.Only trace amount.

Primary and Secondary Responses

Primary responses are the immune system's first encounter with foreign antigens. First produce IgM, then IgG. Memory cells remain in lymphoid tissue, ready to respond to subsequent exposure to the same antigen. The primary response of B cells can occur by two mechanisms.

- T-independent antigens - B cells can be activated by binding antigen, proliferating and forming plasma cells.
- T-dependent antigens – B cells becomes an antigen presenting cell, and activate the T helper cell (T_H). The activated T_H cells then secretes lymphokines that further activate the B cell causing it to differentiate and proliferate producing B memory cells and T_H memory cells.

Secondary responses bring fast and efficient destruction of antigens recognized by B and T memory cells. IgM is produced in a smaller quantities and IgG is produced in much larger quantities than in primary response.

Kinds of Antigen-Antibody Reactions

Humoral immunity depends upon the production of antibodies by B cells. Antibodies protect against invading microbes by neutralization, opsonization, and activating complement. Humoral immunity is most effective against bacteria, antigen-antibody reaction result in agglutination (clumping).

- Neutralization of pathogens and toxins by IgA or IgG.
- Opsonization of bacteria by IgG, which is activated by antigen-bound IgM or IgG, produces complement C_3b,a powerful opsonin, they coat microbes so that they can be phagocytized.
- Cell lysed by complement after or directly by IgMs or IgG immune complexes

MONOCLONAL ANTIBODIES

Monoclonal antibodies are antibodies produced in the laboratory from a clone of cultured cells that make one specific antibody to one specific epitope. Specific monoclonal antibodies can be used in some diagnostic tests, and methods to use them in treating infectious diseases and cancer are being developed.

LYMPHOCYTES

Lymphocytes are small, smooth, round leukocytes that lack granules. There are three kinds of leukocytes: B cells, T cells, and natural killer (NK) cells. B cells and T cells are triggered into defensive action when they encounter antigens, which are foreign molecules we lack. B cells respond to antigen by producing antibodies. Cytotoxic T (CD_8) cells respond to antigen by killing our own pathogen-infected cells. Helper T (CD_4) cells respond by stimulating phagocytes and B cells.

Lymphoid Tissues

Primary lymphoid tissues are the bone marrow where blood cells, including lymphocytes, are formed and where B cells differentiate; the thymus is where T cells differentiate. Differentiated B and T cells travel to secondary lymphoid tissues, where they are stored and interact. Secondary lymphoid tissues include lymph nodes, spleen, tonsils, adenoids, appendix, and Peyer's patches. Spleen is the largest lymph organ. Lymph is formed in our tissues as fluid from blood leaks across capillary walls. A system of lymph vessels collects lymph and returns it to th thoracic duct that empties into the heart. Lymphocytes circulate through blood and lymph. Lymphatic vessels and lymph nodes usually become swollen and inflamed during infections that activate an immune response.

THE CELL-MEDIATED IMMUNE REACTION

Cell mediated Response:

Cytotoxic (CD_8) T cells, with the aid of helper (CD_4 or Th cells) T cells, are responsible for cell-mediated immunity.

Activated T helper cells in turn activate other cells and processes clonal expansion of undifferentiated B cells.

B cell differentiation creates memory B and Plasma B

Plasma B synthesize and secrete antibodies which neutralize antigen

Memory T cells

Nature Killer cells

Cytotoxic T cells

Leukokine production of all leukocytes.

Involves T cells, requires presentation of the antigen on the surface of cell with major histocompatibility complex (MHC) proteins by antigen presenting cells.

Antigen Recognition

- All nucleated cells have major MHCI proteins on their surfaces.
- Dendritic cells and macrophages (antigen presenting cells) also have MHCII on their surfaces. They phagocytize pathogens, they digest and present pieces of the foreign peptides on their surface by MHCII proteins to T cells that have the proper antigen receptor.
- T helper (T_H) cells are activated by antigen present by MHCII from antigen-presenting cells.
- Cytotoxic (killer) T (T_C) cells are activated by antigen-presented by MHCI – cells infected by virus, intracellular bacterial pathogens, transformed cancer cells, or foreign tissues (organ transplant).
- Macrophages that have processed an antigen secrete lymphokine interleukin-1 (IL-1), which activates T helper cells, in turn, T help cells secrete lymphokines such as interleukin-2 (IL-2) and gamma interferon.

- IL-1 from macrophages and IL-2 from T helper cells activate B cells to make antibody and other T cells, such as cytotoxic (killer) T (T_C) cells and memory cells.
- T_C cells can be recognized by a CD8 glycoprotein on their membrane. T helper cells can be recognized by a CD4 glycoprotein on their membrane.
- IL-1, Il-2 and gamma interferon together cause undifferentiated cells to become natural killer (NK) cells.

Processed antigens on MHC class II molecules bind with T cell receptors. Next, IL-1 secreted from macrophages and IL-2 secreted from T helper cells activate the T helper cells, which can then differentiate into T_H1 cells and T_H2 cells. Certain pathogenic bacteria can grow in macrophages after they have been phagocytized. T_H1 cells can release γ-interferon, a cytokine that causes such infected macrophages to become resensitized to other T cells – cell-mediated immunity. T_H2 can activated B cell to produce antibody – humoral immunity.

How Killer Cells Kill

T_C and NK cells destroy target cells by releasing the lethal protein perforin. Peforins bores holes in the target cell membranes, so that essential molecules leak out and the cells die.

The Role of activated Macrophages

Certain pathogenic bacteria can grow in macrophages after phagocytosis, such as those that cause tuberculosis, leprosy. The lymphokine macrophage activating factor helps stimulate antimicrobial processes by increasing production of hydrogen peroxideand other enzymes to kill the organismsWhen macrophages fails to kill pathogens, the pathogens are walled off in granulomas.

Superantigens

Such as staphylococcal toxins that cause food poisoning, can bind to MHCII molecules and T cells but does not involve specificity. The superantigens binds to T cells with different specificities, it is polyclonal. This activates T cells at up to 100 times the normal rate and then secrete immense amounts of IL-2.

The excess IL-2 gets to the blood stream, and cause nausea, vomiting, fever, malaise and symptoms of shock.

2

Applied Immune System in Health and Disease

BASIC CONCEPTS IN IMMUNOLOGY

NATURAL IMMUNITY

The immune system's response to antigenic challenge can be categorized as natural (innate) or acquired. Natural immunity provides a first line of defence against infectious agents. It is non-specific in that the response is the same for different bacteria, viruses and other microbes. Repeated infections with the same microbe (*e.g.*, same strain of bacteria) do not improve the innate immune response.

The natural immune system is composed of several defence mechanisms. Skin and mucus membranes serve as mechanical barriers to microbial invasion. Mucus entraps microbes and contains lysozyme and other proteolytic enzymes. Lysozyme is also found in urine and tears. Urine and tears provide a flushing action for the urinary tract and eyes, respectively. Phagocytic cells (*e.g.*, neutrophils, monocytes, macrophages) ingest (phagocytize) bacteria and kill them. Natural killer cells lyse neo-plastic and virally-infected cells. These cells of innate immunity may be considered a second line of defence since the offending agents have penetrated the first line of defence (*e.g.*, skin).

Acquired Immunity

Acquired immunity is the result of a specific immune response to an infectious agent that has penetrated the first line of defence. T cells (thymus-derived) and B cells (bone marrow-derived) are the major lymphocytes involved with acquired immunity. There are subsets of T cells, namely T helper (TH) and cytolytic T (TC) cells. There are also subsets of TH cells, TH1 and TH2. TH1 cells produce cytokines (IL2, IL-12, IFN-γ) that favour cell-mediated immunity, whereas TH2 cells produce cytokines (IL-4, IL-5, IL6, IL-10) that enhance the humoral (antibody) response. B cells have antibodies on their membrane (*i.e.*, surface immunoglobulin or sIg). When the sIg recognizes and binds to a specific antigen such as a bacterial cell (first signal) and a second signal is delivered by a TH2 cell, the B cell may become activated. Upon activation, the B cell will proliferate into a clone of B cells. Different clones develop in response to different antigenic determinants (small parts; 5-7 amino acids, for example) on the antigen*. Some B cells from each clone will become plasma cells that produce antibody that attaches to the antigen (*i.e.*, the antigenic determinants). Bacteria that are coated with antibody are easily phagocytized; thus, the initial phase of the killing process is enhanced. Other B cells from each clone will become memory cells.

Memory cells live for years and become activated very quickly upon exposure to the same strain of bacteria. For most antigenic challenges, TH2 cells are necessary to help B cells become fully activated. An acquired immune response that involves antibody production is referred to as humoral immunity. The humoral immune response is most commonly employed against pyogenic (pus-producing) bacteria, but antibodies are also produced against viruses, tumor antigens, transplanted tissue antigens, yeasts/fungi, and parasites; however, the humoral response is not capable of eliminating the problem in these latter cases.

Cell-mediated immunity is called upon to rid the body of viruses, yeasts/fungi, parasites, tumors, and grafts (*i.e.*, transplanted tissue). **The immune response is not directed against an entire antigen molecule, but rather against small parts of it (5-7 residues, typically amino acids) that serve as antigenic determinants.*

Regarding humoral immunity, a discussion of the different types of antibody molecules produced by humans is necessary to understand some studies that have measured antibody responses to exercise. There are five major classes or isotypes of antibodies. IgG is the most common antibody circulating in peripheral blood, comprising approximately 75 per cent of the total antibody level (about 1,200 mg/dL). IgG is a good opsonin. It also activates complement, a series proteins that ultimately lyse target cells (*e.g.*, bacteria). IgG is the only antibody that crosses the placenta.

Thus, newborns are born with an adult level of IgG, which gradually disappears over the next few months. They start making their own antibody at 2-3 months of age. IgG is the major antibody of the secondary immune response (*i.e.*, the response that occurs upon re-exposure to a specific antigen), also called the anamestic or memory response. IgM is the largest antibody molecule, consisting of five monomeric units (IgG is comprised of a single monomeric unit). It can also activate complement, and it is the major antibody of the primary immune response (*i.e.*, the response that occurs upon the first exposure to a specific antigen). IgA circulates in the peripheral blood and is also found in abundance in secretions (*e.g.*, saliva, mucus, breast milk). Secretory IgA is a first line of defence in that it can bind to infectious agents before they have a chance to attach to and infect host cells. IgE and IgD are found in very low concentrations in peripheral blood. IgE is involved in allergies (Type I hypersensitivity reactions) and certain parasitic (helminth) infections. The role of IgD is unknown, but it is found on the surface of many B cells together with IgM.

Cell-Mediated Immunity

Cell-mediated immunity refers to an acquired immune response in which T cells are the major players. Both TH1 cells and cytolytic T cells (TC cells) are typically activated by the offending antigen (*e.g.*, a virus) and a second signal (interaction of other membrane molecules). The TC cells (also called T cytotoxic cells) lyse the infected cells, tumor cells, etc. As stated previously, viruses, yeasts/fungi, parasites, tumors and grafts typically evoke predominantly a cell-mediated immune response, although antibodies are also produced. A pure cell-mediated immune response (no B cells or antibody involved) is uncommon.

Regardless of whether the acquired immune response is humoral or cell-mediated, the offending antigen is usually presented to T cells by an antigen-presenting cell (APC). More specifically, a peptide fragment of the antigen is presented to T cells. Cells that can act as APCs include macrophages, follicular dendritic cells, B cells, Langerhans cells of the skin, and cytokine-stimulated cells (*e.g.*, activated T cells). The peptide is presented to the T cell via interaction with an MHC class I or class II molecule on the APC and the T cell receptor (TCR) on the T cell. In other words, part of the peptide is bound to an MHC class I or II molecule and another part is bound to the TCR. This serves as one signal.

The second signal may be provided by interaction of other membrane molecules. Interleukin-1 (IL-1) is a cytokine produced by macrophages and other cells that activates TH cells. Interleukin-2 (IL-2) is a cytokine produced by activated T cells that drives the proliferation and differentiation of T cells. Some antigens, such as lipopolysaccharides, are known as T-independent antigens because they can activate B cells directly without

T cell help, but the immune response is weaker and a memory (anamestic) response does not occur. *Note: MHC molecules and TCRs are glycoproteins that are part of the cell membrane. MHC is an acronym for major histocompatibility complex, which is a region on chromsome 6 that codes for these glycoproteins.*

Phagocytosis

The phagocytic system consists of neutrophils, monocytes and macrophages. Monocytes become macrophages when they leave the peripheral blood and enter tissues. These phagocytic cells have membrane receptors (*i.e.*, specific molecules on their cell membrane) that recognize and bind to complement proteins (*e.g.*, C3b) and IgG, a type of antibody. Bacteria that are coated with complement and/or IgG antibody will adhere to the phagocytic cells via these receptors. This process is called opsonization and it makes it much easier for phagocytes to ingest bacteria. Once the bacterial cell is ingested, enzymes and other substances are released into the phagocytic vacuole from cytoplasmic granules fused with the vacuole. Some enzymes serve a digestive function while other enzymes and substances contribute to the killing of the bacterial cell. One means of killing bacteria is by generating oxygen radicals (superoxide radical, hydroxyl radical, singlet oxygen) through the hexose monophosphate shunt (HMS). Glucose-6-phosphate dehydrogenase (G6PD) is a very important enzyme for this pathway in that it connects glycolysis to the HMS. In other words, without G6PD the HMS could not function.

Phagocytes also generate these unstable forms of oxygen in inflammatory conditions other than just bacterial infections. When tissues such as muscle or tendons are damaged, an inflammatory process is typically activated; however, the resulting tissue fragments may be too large for ingestion by phagocytes. The "frustrated" phagocytes release the contents of their cytoplasmic granules in the damaged area. Free oxygen radicals that are generated damage tissue in the area via oxidation. Consequently, ingestion of antioxidants (*e.g.*, bioflavanoids, vitamins A, C, E) may help minimize inflammation. Interestingly, antioxidants have been purported to curtail atherosclerosis by inhibiting the oxidation of LDL.

Complement Proteins

Complement is a series of proteins that normally circulate in the plasma. A number of substances can activate complement, including IgG and IgM. Typically, when the first complement protein is activated, the remaining complement proteins are sequentially activated ultimately leading to lysis of the target cell (*e.g.*, bacterium). Some of the complement proteins serve other biological functions in addition to cell lysis. For example, C5a, C3a and C4a produce smooth muscle contraction, increase vascular permeability, and induce the release of histamine from mast cells and basophils (*i.e.*, they are anaphylatoxins). C5a is also chemotactic; it attracts neutrophils. Some complement proteins serve as opsonins (*e.g.*, C3b, C4b) as phagocytes and other cells have membrane receptors for these proteins. C3 and C4 are commonly measured complement proteins. A deficiency or defect of one or more of the complement proteins is often associated with an increased frequency of infections.

Membrane Marker Terminology

Since studies on exercise and immunology typically use membrane marker terminology to indicate specific cell types, a discussion of the most common membrane markers is necessary. Standardized nomenclature uses the clusters of differentiation (CD) designation for various proteins on the surface of lymphocytes and other immune cells. CD2 is found on all T cells. It is an adhesion molecule that binds to the LFA-3 receptor (CD58) on other cells (*e.g.*, antigen-presenting cells). The T cell receptor (TCR; no CD designation) is also found on all T cells. Structurally, it resembles the antigen-binding region of antibody molecules. As stated previously, it recognizes protein antigens (peptide fragments) as the T cell interacts with an antigen-presenting cell. CD3 consists of four polypeptide chains that are physically associated with the TCR. It appears to transduce activating signals to the cytoplasm of the T cell when antigen binds to the TCR. Helper/inducer T cells are identified by CD4. About two-thirds of peripheral blood T cells express CD4. CD8 is expressed by about one-third of peripheral blood

T cells and identifies these cells as cytolytic T cells. CD4 and CD8 play an important role in antigen presentation in that CD4 T cells will only interact with APCs that present antigen bound to MHC class II molecules, and CD8 T cells interact only with APCs that present antigen bound to MHC class I molecules.

A key membrane marker of B cells is surface immunoglobulin (sIg), which plays a major role in antigen recognition and activation of the immune response. B cells also carry CD19, CD20 and numerous other membrane proteins. CD16 and CD56 are membrane markers found on natural killer cells. It is noteworthy that while a particular membrane marker may be used to identify a specific cell or subset of cells, that marker may be found on other cells as well. Typically two or more markers are used to identify a specific cell. Many membrane markers have been described for several cell types including lymphocytes and their subsets, monocytes, macrophages, neutrophils, endothelial cells, dendritic cells, and erythrocytes.

Cytokines and Cytokine Receptors

Cytokines are proteins made by cells that affect the behaviour of other cells. Cytokines act on specific cytokine receptors on the cells that they affect. Interleukin-1 (IL-1) is produced by macrophages and other cells. It activates T cells and produces fever. Interleukin-2 (IL-2) is produced by T cells and stimulates T cell proliferation. It is also known as T cell growth factor. Interleukin-3 (IL-3) is produced by T cells. It works with colony stimulating factors (CSFs) to stimulate the proliferation and differentiation of hematopoietic cells (*e.g.*, lymphocytes, granulocytes, monocytes, erythrocytes). Interleukin-6 (IL-6) stimulates T and B cell growth and differentiation, acute phase protein production and fever. T cells, macrophages, and endothelial cells produce it.

T cells, NK cells and other leukocytes produce interferons (IFN-α, IFN-β, IFN-γ). Interferons exhibit anti-viral properties, activate macrophages, and increase the expression of MHC molecules. Tumor necrosis factors (TNFs)

are produced primarily by macrophages, T cells, B cells and NK cells. They contribute to the inflammatory response, activate cells, and kill tumor (and other) cells. Transforming growth factor β (TNF-β) is produced by T and B cells, macrophages and other cells. This cytokine suppresses the immune system at the systemic level, but stimulates immune and inflammatory responses at the local level. Colony-stimulating factors promote the growth and differentiation of various cell lines.

EFFECTS OF EXERCISE ON THE IMMUNE SYSTEM

Before discussing the effects of exercise on the immune system, problems with assessing immune function need to be addressed. These issues make interpretation of the findings of studies challenging and may account for some differences among studies evaluating the same or similar immune responses to exercise. To begin with, the type, intensity, frequency, and duration of exercise vary among the different studies. There are also significant differences between animal and human studies. For example, invasive sampling can be performed on animals, whereas human studies typically rely on immune cells obtained from peripheral blood only. Additional differences among studies include age, gender, heredity, diet, life style, and initial fitness level of subjects. There are also different techniques employed for measuring immune parameters and variations in the way in which results are reported. Nonetheless, some generalizations can be made.

HOW EXERCISE BOOSTS THE IMMUNE SYSTEM

When you exercise regularly, there are a number of things that benefit your body. Your heart gets stronger and is able to pump more blood throughout your body when you exercise. Your lungs get better equipped at handling oxygen and dishing it out to the rest of your body. Your muscles also get stronger as you use them more often. Your immune system is no different. Doctors have found that exercise can boost your immune system by providing a boost to the cells in your body that are assigned to attack bacteria. These cells appear to work more slowly in people who don't exercisethan in those that do. As a result, if you exercise, your immune system is better equipped to handle bacteria that could cause you to become sick. Though this boost only lasts for a few hours after you exercise, it's often enough to help keep you healthier than you would be if you didn't exercise.

EXERCISING TOO MUCH CAN HURT YOUR IMMUNE SYSTEM

While it's obviously beneficial to give your immune system a boost by exercising, you also need to be aware of the fact that you could actually hurt your immune system if you don't give your body enough rest. Too much exercise can actually cause your immune system to weaken. It's one of the reasons that you may feel very rundown and weak if you're training for a marathon or doing a lot of exercise during a short window of time. In order to avoid having this effect on your immune system, make sure that you get enough rest for your body.

IMPROVING YOUR IMMUNE SYSTEM BY EXERCISING

The truth is that you don't have to be a super athlete to boost your immune systemthrough exercise. All you need to do is walk for a half hour every day or find time to hit the gym a few times every week. By speeding up the cells in your immune system that fight off bacteria, you can get healthier in no time. Studies have also shown that people who work out often take half as many sick days per year as those that don't work out. Try to incorporate more exercise into your day to help strengthen your immune system over time.

CELL COUNTS

The total white cell count increases during and after a bout of exercise most likely due to demargination (detachment from the endothelial lining). Whether or not increased production and release from the bone marrow occurs may be debatable, although hematologists consistently attribute the increase to demargination. Other sources such as the lung, spleen, and GI tract have also been reported. The increase in the leukocyte count is due primarily to an increase in neutrophils, although lymphocytes and monocytes are increased as well. Exercise intensity, duration and/or fitness level may play a role in the degree of leukocytosis. Both the neutrophil and lymphocyte count are normal in athletes suggesting that training does not alter these cell counts. Some studies have reported decreased numbers of NK cells and monocytes during periods of intense training. Mechanisms that may be involved with exercise-induced leukocytosis include increased catecholamines, which increase cardiac output and modify adhesion molecules, and alterations in cytokine levels that influence the expression of adhesion molecules.

Cell Function

Conflicting results have been reported on neutrophil function, which may be due to different exercise protocols and the particular function being measured. Brief high intensity, prolonged submaximal and intense exercise have been reported to increase oxidative burst activity in neutrophils, an indication of enhanced microbicidal activity. Various exercises have induced increased neutrophil activation as inferred by degranulation. A number of neutrophil functions at rest and after exercise tend to be lower in athletes compared to nonathletes. On the other hand, some studies have reported no change or an increase in certain functions (*e.g.*, adhesion) in response to moderate training, whereas heavy training tends to decrease neutrophil function.

Studies on the effects of exercise on lymphocyte function have also produced inconsistent results; however, MacKinnon states that acute exercise and exercise training may activate lymphocytes. It is not known if this is due to selective recruitment of activated cells into the circulation or because cells are activated during exercise or both. MacKinnon cites studies that suggest both brief and very prolonged intense exercise induce activation of T cells.

Lymphocyte proliferation may be stimulated or not affected by brief moderate exercise, whereas intense or prolonged exercise may suppress proliferative responses. Studies noted by Shephard depict a similar pattern, although there are too many contradictory results to reach any firm conclusions. NK cells typically show increased cytolytic activity during brief and prolonged exercise, but a consistent postexercise pattern has not emerged from the data, although prolonged exercise appears to produce postexercise suppression of NK cytolytic activity.

The increased NK activity during exercise may by due simply to an increased number of NK cells in the circulation. Although there are some inconsistencies among studies that evaluated lymphocyte function in response to training, most studies have reported no difference in lymphocyte activity between athletes and nonathletes suggesting that training does not alter lymphocyte function.

T cell function and B cell function have also been assessed via cytokine production and antibody production, respectively. Cytokine and antibody responses to exercise are discussed in the next section. Studies of monocyte/ macrophage function have produced disparate results for both acute exercise and training effects. Despite the inconsistent studies, it is feasible that moderate exercise may have a beneficial effect on macrophage function, while exhaustive exercise may have a suppressive effect.

Cytokines

MacKinnon discusses several issues concerning the significance of cytokine changes in response to exercise. Cytokines are normally present at extremely low concentrations and are rapidly cleared from the blood and other body compartments. Although the pro-inflammatory cytokines (IL-1, IL-6) are released during and after exercise, the responses appear to be subtle and have not been consistently observed. Furthermore, interpretation of changes in cytokine levels is difficult due to the large number of cytokines and their diverse actions.

Vigourous and prolonged exercise or eccentric exercises typically produce an inflammatory reaction. Urinary excretion of IL-1β, IL-6, and IFN-γ has been noted following prolonged exercise. Interestingly, these four cytokines were chronically elevated in the urine of trained versus untrained persons. Pedersen has proposed a model to explain the possible relationship between cytokines and muscle damage. He suggests that eccentric exercise damages muscle leading to necrosis and inflammation. Inflammatory cytokines are produced which augment the inflammatory response. Neutrophils accumulate in the muscle followed by macrophages. Cytokines induce the macrophages to produce prostaglandins (*e.g.*, PGE2), which bring about muscle pain.

In contrast, Malm suggests that cells do not migrate to skeletal muscle after exercise. He also reports that muscle adaptation to exercise may occur in a non-inflammatory fashion.

The immune system may affect skeletal muscle adaptation via interactions between leukocyte and endothelial cell adhesion molecules and release of cytokines and growth factors. Additionally, Malm indicates that moderate exercise enhances a

TH1-type cytokine response, which should boost protection against viral infection, while strenuous exercise augments TH2 cytokines and, thus, promotes protection against bacterial infection. Clearly, more research is needed to determine the cytokine response to exercise.

IMMUNOGLOBULINS (ANTIBODIES)

Both MacKinnon and Shephard cite studies that report substantial decreases in salivary IgA after intense and/or prolonged exercise, but little or no effect after moderate exercise. Generally, serum immunoglobulins either do not change or increase slightly after various types of exercise. Both salivary and serum immunoglobulins either do not change or increase after moderate training, but decrease with intense training. While MacKinnon notes that athletes undergoing intense training can still mount an appropriate serum antibody response, Shephard observes that decreases in salivary IgA have been associated with an increased prevalence of upper respiratory tract infections (URTIs).

Pedersen has proposed an open window hypothesis to at least partly explain the increased incidence of URTIs in elite athletes. The hypothesis asserts that the immune system is enhanced during moderate and severe exercise, but suppressed following intense long-duration exercise. The immunosuppression includes a decreased number of lymphocytes, decreased natural killer cell cytotoxicity, and decreased secretory IgA levels in mucosa. The period of immunosuppression following intense long-duration exercise is referred to as the "open window." It is during this time that infectious microbes, particularly viruses, may take advantage of the opportunity to establish an infection. This window of opportunity may be longer and more pronounced in elite athletes. Pedersen also proposes a potential benefit of this period of immunosuppression. If tissue damage results from the intense exercise, the immune system could be exposed to new antigens. The immunosuppression may serve to prevent autoimmune reactions.

Overtraining

Overtraining involves physiological, psychological, and immunological factors. This discussion will focus on the immune factors, particularly the reactions to tissue injury and the similarity of these reactions to sepsis. The information from this section is derived from Shephard. A single bout of exhaustive exercise, especially eccentric exercise, can cause an inflammatory reaction in the active muscle, which resembles the process of sepsis. The affected muscle is infiltrated by neutrophils followed by macrophages. Free radicals (unstable forms of oxygen) accumulate as the neutrophils and macrophages are activated.

Inflammatory cytokines and acute phase reactants are released. Complement and the coagulation and fibrinolytic pathways are activated. Given these inflammatory events, icing the affected muscle and ingestion of antioxidants (bioflavanoids, vitamins A, C, and E) should help control the inflammation and, consequently, reduce muscle soreness.

Icing will slow the delivery of neutrophils and monocytes/macrophages to the site by reducing blood flow. It will also slow enzyme reactions that proceed optimally at body temperature, thus slowing the entire inflammatory process. Antioxidants will counteract the oxygen radicals. Since antioxidants must be at the site to be effective, ingestion must occur prior to the initiation of exercise and should continue throughout the training period (*i.e.*, daily dosages). While these measures will help control inflammation, they will not prevent the many symptoms associated with overtraining, nor is it likely that muscle soreness can be entirely prevented during extreme training periods.

EFFECTS OF EXERCISE ON THE IMMUNE SYSTEM IN THE ELDERLY POPULATION

Immune function of humans and most animals declines with age. Impaired immune function in ageing, 'immunosenescence', is of importance, not just in terms of protection against infectious diseases, but in several age-associated diseases. Increasing numbers of old citizens have formed the basis of a growing interest in ageing research worldwide in order to discover ways of reducing disability and enhancing independence in human ageing.

Physical exercise training is known to increase functional ability in elderly humans by improving muscle function and is important in the prevention of age-associated diseases, such as type II diabetes, atherosclerosis, hypertension and osteoporosis. It is well known that physical exercise influences the immune system.

However, relatively little is known about the effects of exercise on the senescent immune system. During exercise, leucocytes are recruited to the peripheral blood, resulting in increased concentrations of neutrophils, lymphocytes and monocytes. The increased lymphocyte concentration is caused by recruitment of all lymphocyte subsets (NK, T and B cells). Strenuous exercise, but not moderate exercise, is followed by decreased concentrations of lymphocytes and impaired cellular-mediated immunity.

Increased levels of adrenalin, and to a lesser degree noradrenalin, are believed to be the main responsible factors for recruitment of lymphocytes during acute exercise. Catecholamines, together with growth hormones, may mediate the acute effects on neutrophils, whereas cortisol exerts its effect within a time lag of at least 2 h. It has previously been pointed out that, given that a number of age-related changes occur in many physiological systems (*e.g.* neuroendocrine), it would be of value to learn the extent to which both acute and chronic exercise influence immune function in the elderly.

These considerations form the basis for raising the questions of whether it is possible to reverse, restore and modulate immune function in ageing and whether physical exercise provides a tool, in isolation or combined with other methods, to affect the process of immunosenescence. Most long-term studies suggest that moderate exercise training exerts little effect on immune function in healthy populations, but it is possible, however, that moderate exercise training beneficially influences immune function in other groups, such as the elderly.

Can elderly humans thus exercise to make their immune system fitter or is moderate to severe exercise deleterious to the aged cellular immune system? Exercise has also been suggested as a prototype for studying the effects of stress factors on the cellular immune system, because several other physical stressors, such as burns, surgery, acute myocardial infarction and hyperthermia, induce similar changes.

Studies of interactions between an acute bout of exercise and immune function may be a useful and ethically acceptable tool to investigate cell trafficking, immune mobilization/deficiency and the acute phase response during physical stress situations in relation to human ageing. The purpose of the present review is to summarize what is current knowledge regarding human immunosenescence, its clinical relevance and the effects of acute stress and physical exercise training on immune function in relation to ageing.

AGEING AND IMMUNE FUNCTION

Operationally, ageing is the process of growing older starting at birth, whereas senescence is the process of somatic deterioration at older age. Most parts of the immune system show pronounced changes in relation to ageing. It is unclear whether these changes represent dysfunction/ dysregulation of the immune system or whether they represent a complex and continuous remodelling of immune parameters during ageing. However, human immunosenescence has been suggested to be the consequence of the continuous exposure to antigenic stress occurring throughout life.

T Lsymphocytes

The lymphocyte count in blood is decreased in elderly humans due to decreased numbers of T lymphocytes. The integrity of the T-cell compartment during ageing has been subject to intensive research. Proliferation of T lymphocytes is essential for the capability of rapid clonal expansion, which constitutes the first step in an adaptive immune response. T-cell proliferation tends to decline with donor age, whether measured *in vitro* in mitogen-stimulated cultures or *in vivo* as delayed-type hypersensitivity responses (DTH). Mitogens, such as PHA, stimulate mainly proliferation of virgin $CD4^+$ cells, whereas recall antigens mainly cause activation of memory cells. Elderly people have increased percentages of memory cells and decreased percentages of virgin cells within T lymphocytes and poor PHA-induced proliferative responses are positively correlated with decreased numbers of virgin $CD4^+$ cells in 174 81-year-old humans.

CD28 expression has an important role in costimulatory events that occur along with engagement of the T-cell antigen receptor. With regard to ageing, downregulation of CD28 has consistently been described, especially on $CD8^+$ cells. $CD28^-CD8^+$ cells represent oligoclonal expanded cells with short telomeres, decreased proliferative potentials and high cytotoxic activities. Accordingly, ageing is associated with an increased number of differentiated effector cells and a decreased presence of immunologically naïve cells. This supports the hypothesis that elderly humans are especially vulnerable to the introduction of new pathogens, whereas it is more unclear whether or not the immunological response to recall antigens is preserved.

Decreased numbers of T lymphocytes together with shifts in the phenotype have traditionally been ascribed to thymic involution causing a decline in the infusion of new virgin T cells accompanied by the continued antigen-driven conversion of virgin to memory cells throughout life. Thymic involution starts during the first year of postnatal life with a reduction of approximately 3 per cent per year until middle age and 1 per cent per year for the rest of life. Furthermore, the aged thymic microenvironment has a decreased capacity to support thymocyte differentiation and intrinsic changes in stem cells have also been detected.

Decreased T-cell proliferation associated with ageing has been linked to the so-called Hayflick limit, which describes the phenomenon that all normal somatic cells can only undergo a finite and predictable number of divisions in tissue culture before reaching an irreversible state of growth arrest. Telomeres are the repetitive DNA sequences at the end of eucaryotic chromosomes and they may be the molecular basis for a mitotic clock. The ends of linear chromosomes cannot be fully replicated during each round of cell division, the so-called 'end replication problem'. Thus, somatic cells lose telomeric DNA with age *in vivo* and during proliferation *in vitro* and the mean length of telomeric terminal restriction fragments (TRF) can be used as a measure of replicative history and proliferative potentials of cells. The mean length of TRF declines with age in lymphocytes *in vivo* as well as *in vitro*. Furthermore, memory cells have shorter TRF than virgin cells.

Although T cells with the surface characteristics of memory cells increase with age, it is still unclear whether the function of these cells is impaired by ageing. Increased apoptosis due to enhanced expression of death receptors have been described. Alterations in the homeostasis of the cytokine network may result in inefficient or inappropriate immune responses by the elderly. Increased incidences of infections, reappearance of latent viral infections and autoimmune phenomena in elderly humans have formed the basis for the hypothesis that ageing involves a shift in the balance between Th1/Tc1 lymphocytes, characterized by a cytokine profile dominated by IL-2 and IFN-γ, and Th2/Tc2 lymphocytes, characterized by IL-4 and IL-5 production, towards dominance of type 2 cytokine responses. However, data in this area is controversial.

The B cell Repertoire

Specific antibody responses in humans to virtually all vaccines decrease with age but, despite these defects, neither the level of serum immunoglobulins nor the number of Ig-secreting B cells decline with age. This reflects that age-associated changes in humoral immunity include shifts in antibody specificities from foreign to autoantigens, in antibody affinities from high to low and in the antibody idiotypic repertoire. Consistent with these changes, levels of serum autoantibodies and monoclonal immunoglobulins are increased in elderly humans.

Many of the changes in B-cell function can be traced to an impaired capacity of T cells to support isotype switching and somatic mutation in the periphery and the generation of a diverse B cell repertoire from bone marrow B cell precursors.

Natural Killer Cells

Natural killer cells play a critical role in the innate immune response against infections and tumours, which are seen with increasing incidence during ageing. Furthermore, NK cells secrete immunoregulatory cytokines and chemokines promoting downstream Th1-mediated responses against infections. Most studies have reported increased percentages of NK cells within blood mononuclear cells (BMNC) and increased or unaltered concentrations in the blood.

Furthermore, there is a general consensus that NK cells from elderly humans show decreased cytotoxic capacity on a 'per cell' basis. It has been suggested that increased concentrations of NK cells in the blood compensate for the decreased cytotoxicity per NK cell. Middle-aged humans have decreased

NK cell activity compared to young controls, whereas centenarians have activity in the range of the young group. This has formed the basis of the hypothesis that a well-preserved NK cell activity can help in becoming a centenarian.

Ageing and Inflammatory Activity

Healthy elderly humans show low-grade inflammatory activity in the blood *in vivo*including increased number of neutrophils and high circulating levels of TNF-α, IL-6 cytokine antagonists, such as IL-1 receptor antagonist (IL-1RA) and soluble TNF receptors, and acute phase proteins. Low-grade chronic inflammatory activity may induce lymphocyte activation and cause accelerated immunosenescence.

In support of this hypothesis, poor IL-2 production *ex vivo* is correlated with high plasma levels of TNF-α and IL-1RA in elderly humans. Interleukin-1RA is known to inhibit IL-2 production and T-cell proliferation *in vitro*. Low-grade inflammatory activity in plasma is associated with age-related diseases such as Alzheimer's disease, atherosclerosis and type II diabetes. Interleukin-6 is positively correlated to functional disability, as well as to self-rated health in elderly humans.

Tumour necrosis factor-α is associated with obesity as well as with cachexia. Furthermore, TNF-α is known to affect lipid metabolism. In accordance with this, plasma TNF-α has been correlated with high concentrations of triglycerides and a low high-density lipoprotein/total cholesterol ratio, which are known as risk factors of atherogenesis and thromboembolic complications, in 130 humans aged 81 years.

The Clinical Relevance of Immunosenescence

Elderly humans show increased morbidity and mortality from infectious diseases. Thus, age-associated increases have been reported with regard to the incidence of community-acquired pneumonia, herpes zoster infections and bacteremia caused by *Escherichia coli* and *Streptococcus pneumoniae*. Furthermore, in elderly humans the relative mortality rate from pneumonia, pyelonephritis, infective endocarditis, bacterial meningitis, tuberculosis, sepsis, cholecystitis and appendicitis is increased compared with young adults. A causal relationship between immunosenescence and increased risk of infections remains to be demonstrated.

However, it is well documented in several cohorts that immune function predicts mortality risk: Low $CD4^+$ cell counts and/or low NK cell number predicts high all-cause mortality risk and appears to be related to malignancies. Poor DTH response *in vivo*, lack of responses to mitogens *in vitro* and high circulating levels of TNF-α, IL-6 and C-reactive protein (CRP) have also been related to high mortality risk. Low NK cell activity has been associated with a history of severe infections and with death caused by infections.

THE FREE RADICAL THEORY OF AGEING

Nutrition is of special interest in elderly subjects, because the age-related immune deficiency may be aggravated in malnourished individuals. Nutritional supplementation may in theory partly revert immunosenescence. In support of this hypothesis, supplementation with a modest physiological amount of micronutrients results in higher numbers of certain T-cell subsets and NK cells, enhanced proliferation response to mitogen, increased IL-2 production, higher antibody response and NK cell activity and decreased risk of infection.

Most focus has been on the free radical theory of ageing, which suggests that ageing is linked to injury of DNA by superoxide anions and other reactive oxygen species formed during normal cellular oxygen metabolism in the mitochondria, the respiratory burst of phagocytes, hyperoxia and arachidonic acid metabolism. DNA damage and mutation may result in a failure of T cells to proliferate caused by DNA damage-mediated cell cycle arrest, decreased rates of proliferation as a result of selection *in vivo* against cells carrying certain mutations and increased apoptosis triggered by critical levels of DNA damage. With advance of ageing, demand for anti-oxidants appears to increase. In elderly humans, β-carotene supplementation has been shown to increase NK cell activity, whereas data is controversial regarding the effect on T cell-mediated immunity. Vitamin E supplementation has been shown to enhance the lymphocyte proliferative response, DTH and IL-2 production. However, besides being an anti-oxidant, vitamin E may act through inhibition of prostaglandin E_2 (PGE_2) production.

EXERCISE

Physical exercise increases the consumption of oxygen, which in turn increases the generation of reactive oxygen species. However, enduring moderate physical exercise, but not acute strenuous exercise, enhances the production of anti-oxidant products such as superoxide dismutase and catalase. Regular, moderate exercise combined with other methods, such as dietary manipulation, may thus be beneficial for immune functions in the elderly. Furthermore, moderate exercise has been suggested to reverse immunosenescence by increasing the production of endocrine hormones, which may contribute to less accumulation of autoreactive immune cells by enhancing the programmed cell death. Exercise may also affect body composition and the lipid metabolism, which may result in decreased inflammatory activity.

Ageing, Acute Exercise and Lymphocytes

Acute exercise models allow the study of leucocyte recruitment, cell function and immune depression during an acute stress situation in young versus old humans. It is assumed that lymphocytes in the blood only constitute 2 per cent of the total pool in the body. Accordingly, cell redistribution from tissue to blood during exercise also offers the opportunity to investigate the composition of lymphocytes originating from other compartments of the body during rest in elderly versus young humans.

To our knowledge, only three studies have studied the recruitment of T lymphocytes in relation to human ageing. Ceddia *et al.* have studied leucocyte recruitment and T-lymphocyte function in 33 elderly humans (65.3 ± 0.8 years) and 14 young controls (22.4 ± 0.7 years) in response to a bout of maximal exercise. The elderly group responded similarly to the young with an exercise-induced leucocytosis, but the magnitude of the increase was lower. Furthermore, the older group had an attenuated exercise-induced leucocytosis. In the immediate post-exercise samples, the $CD3^+$ cell number was increased to a similar extent in the two age groups but the old recruited fewer $CD4^+$ cells and more $CD8^+$ cells to the blood, although it is unclear if this difference was significant. Approximately equal proportions of memory ($CD45R0^+$) and virgin ($CD45RA^+$) $CD8^+$cells were recruited regardless of age, whereas exercise induced a significant increase in the percentage of $CD4^+$ memory cells and a significant decrease in the percentage of $CD4^+$ virgin cells in older subjects when compared with that of young subjects.

Bruunsgaard *et al.* have studied the effect of an acute bout of maximal bicycle exercise in 10 elderly (76–80 years) and 10 young (19–31 years) humans. In accordance with the study by Ceddia *et al.*, the elderly group recruited a significantly lower total number of leucocytes but an equal number of T lymphocytes compared with the young controls. In both the elderly and young humans, immediate increases in the numbers of $CD8^+$ and $CD4^+$ cells could be ascribed to cells with an increased replicative history reflected in cells with shorter mean TRF lengths within BMNC and $CD8^+$ cells for the young group and within $CD4^+$ cells for the old group.

Furthermore, both young and elderly humans showed increased percentages of $CD28^-$ cells ($CD4^+$ and $CD8^+$ cells) and memory cells ($CD8^+$ cells). This suggests that the mobilization of $CD4^+$ and $CD8^+$ cells during acute exercise is not due to a repopulation by newly generated cells, but is mainly a redistribution of previously activated cells with an increased replicative history than cells isolated from the blood at rest.

With regard to age-related differences in T-lymphocyte mobilization, young humans showed a more pronounced increase in the proportion of memory cells within $CD8^+$ cells (resulting in a more pronounced decrease in virgin cells) in response to exercise whereas there were no age-related differences in the changes between pre-exercise and post-exercise levels with regard to the proportions of memory/virgin cells within $CD4^+$ cells and the expression of CD28 and the mean TRF length within $CD4^+$ and $CD8^+$ cells. The reason for the discrepancy between this study and that by Ceddia *et al.* with regard to changes in the proportions of memory/virgin cells immediately after exercise may be due to these subsets being defined differently in the two studies, making direct comparisons difficult. Thus, in our study virgin cells were defined as $CD62L^+CD45R0^-$ cells and memory cells were defined as the sum of $CD45R0^+$ cells and $CD45R0^-CD62L^-$ cells. The latter subset represents revertant/ intermediate cells. This division was based on the fact that within the $CD45RA^+$ cell compartment there is also a subset which shows characteristics of activated cells with regard to cytokine production and effector functions. Furthermore, $CD45R0^+$ T cells are able to revert to the CD45RA phenotype. Thus, 'true' virgin T cells are not defined by CD45 isoforms alone. Reduced CD62L expression changes the homing of virgin cells from lymphoid to non-lymphoid tissues and has been proposed as a marker of 'memory'. Thus, 'true' virgin T cells coexpress CD62L and CD45RA and show distinct functions from $CD62L^-$ $CD45RA^+$ cells.

Mazzeo *et al.* have studied six young (26 ± 3 years) and nine old men (69 ± 5 years) at rest and immediately after 20 min of submaximal exercise at 50 per cent peak work capacity. Consistent with the two previous mentioned studies, the exercise-induced increases in $CD4^+$ and $CD8^+$ cells were similar across age groups. Thus, the main finding of these studies is that elderly subjects have a preserved ability to recruit T lymphocytes in response to exercise.

Mazzeo *et al.* and Ceddia *et al.* have also studied mitogen induced proliferative responses of BMNC before and after the acute bout of exercise. Mazzeo *et al.* have found that proliferative responsiveness to PHA increases significantly in young subjects; however, for old subjects this response does not differ significantly from resting values. The interpretation of these data is difficult, because it is consensus that mitogenic responsiveness decreases in relation to exercise due to the decreased percentage of $CD4^+$ cells and due to the fact that mainly cells with an increased replicative history are recruited during exercise. Ceddia *et al.* have reported reduced Con A-induced proliferation on a per $CD3^+$ cell basis when measured immediately after exercise in the young but not in the old.

With regard to recruitment and function of NK cells in response to an acute bout of exercise, Fiatarone *et al.* have studied eight young (30 ± 1 years) and nine elderly (71 ± 1 years) women before and after maximal bicycle exercise. The elderly group was found to have a preserved ability to recruit $CD16^+$ NK cells and they increased their NK cell activity in response to exercise at least as effectively as the young controls.

In accordance with this, Woods *et al.* have reported that elderly humans increase NK cytotoxicity to the same extent as young subjects and show preserved ability to recruit $CD56^+$ NK cells. Preserved ability to recruit $CD56^+$ NK cells in ageing has been confirmed by Mazzeo *et al.* Crist *et al.* have studied NK cell cytotoxicity in response to maximal treadmill exercise in seven elderly women (73 ± 1 years) who had participated in a 16-week-long programme of physical exercise training versus seven age- and gender-matched non-exercising controls (71 ± 2 years). The trained group showed a significantly greater increase in cytotoxic activity.

The Inflammatory Response During Eccentric Exercise Models

Eccentric exercise is when force is generated by the muscles as they lengthen. Eccentric exercise is used to induce experimental muscle damage. Eccentric exercise models make it possible to apply a quantifiable and reproducible inflammatory stimulus in order to study the magnitude of the acute phase response in relation to ageing. However, few studies have emphasized this aspect.

Cannon *et al.* have studied 21 male volunteers representing two ranges of age (22–29 and 55–74 years) who ran downhill on an inclined treadmill to accentuate damaging eccentric muscular contractions. The subject groups were further divided into a double-blind placebo-controlled protocol, which examined the influence of 48 days of dietary vitamin E supplementation before the exercise. All subjects were monitored for 12 days after exercise for changes in circulating leucocytes, superoxide release from neutrophils, lipid peroxidation and efflux of the intramuscular enzyme creatine kinase (CK) into the circulation. Among those receiving the placebo, the young subjects responded to exercise with a significantly greater neutrophilia and higher plasma CK concentrations than the elderly subjects.

Dietary supplementation with vitamin E tended to eliminate the differences between the two age groups, primarily by increasing the responses of the elderly group. In a later study of 12 elderly humans (aged 61–72 years) and nine young controls (aged 20–32 years) neutrophil mobilization has again been reported to be diminished in the older group in relation to eccentric exercise. In the same study, elderly humans were found not to show neutrophil degranulation, assessed by elastase concentrations in plasma, in contrast to young controls. Supplementation with fish oil increased the response in the old to similar levels to the young controls.

Ageing, Training and Immune Function

Woods *et al.* have studied the effects of 6 months of moderate aerobic exercise on T lymphocyte and NK cell function. Sedentary elderly humans (65 ± 0.8 years) were randomly assigned to a three times/week exercise intervention group (n = 14) or a flexibility/toning control group (n = 15).After 6 months, there were no intervention-induced changes in total white blood cell, neutrophil, lymphocyte, monocyte, eosinophil or basophil blood counts. Furthermore, the percentage of $CD3^+$, $CD4^+$ and $CD8^+$ cells remained unchanged. The exercise group tended to show increased proliferative responses to Con A compared with the control group. No significant changes were found with regard to NK cell cytolysis. Accordingly, 6 months of supervised exercise training did not cause major changes in immune function in elderly humans. In accordance with this conclusion, Rall *et al.* have failed to detect changes in BMNC subsets, IL-1β and TNF-α production after LPS or *Staph epidermidis* stimulation, PGE_2 production, lymphocyte proliferation or DTH in eight healthy elderly people (65–80 years) who performed progressive resistance strength training twice/week for 12 weeks compared with six healthy elderly controls.

Nieman *et al.* have studied the immune systems of 12 highly conditioned elderly women aged 65–84 years who exhibited superior NK cell cytotoxicity and PHA-induced proliferative responses despite no differences in circulating levels of lymphocyte subpopulations compared with 32 sedentary, healthy elderly women (67–85 years).

The sedentary women were randomized to either a walking or calisthenic group for 12 weeks. The intervention group exercised for 30–40 min 5 days/week. Exercise did not result in any improvement of NK cell activity or T-cell function. The incidence of upper respiratory tract infection was lowest in the highly conditioned group and highest in the calisthenic control group with the walking group in an intermediate position.

Shinkai *et al.* have studied immune function in 17 elderly recreational runners (63.8 ± 3.3 years) who reported running or jogging an average of 56 ± 23 min/day, 4.7 ± 1.9 days/week covering a weekly distance of 5–75 km. They had maintained this level of exercise for 17.2 ± 6.1 years. Immune function was compared with 19 elderly sedentary men (65.8 ± 3.5 years) and 16 young sedentary medical students (23.6 ± 1.6 years). The active elderly subjects demonstrated significantly greater mitogen-induced proliferative responses and increased production of IL-2, IFN-γ and IL-4. There was no difference in circulating counts of immunocompetent cells.

Rincon *et al.* have studied the effect of exercise training on NK cell activity in six frail elderly men aged 70 years or above who did not suffer from serious medical problems or receive immune-altering drugs. After 3 months of exercise intervention three times per week, NK cell cytotoxicity significantly decreased compared with seven controls having no intervention. This suggests possible adverse effects on NK cell cytotoxicity in the very frail elderly.

Animal Studies

In a study of six young versus six aged horses, exercise caused a significant decrease in the lymphoproliferative response of the young animals, but not the old. This is in accordance with the human study by Ceddia *et al.* In contrast, old as well as young male BALB/c mice have shown decreased PHA proliferative responses immediately after they had performed swimming until exhaustion. In the same study, an increased PHA-induced proliferative response was found in both age groups after the animals had performed 90 min of moderate swimming each day for a total of 20 days. Ferrández and De la Fuente have used the same mouse model for testing exercise-induced changes in antibody dependent cellular cytotoxicity (ADCC) and NK cell activity. Acute physical exercise induced increased ADCC in the old, but not in young animals, whereas no changes in NK cell activity were detected. Exercise training improved both types of cytotoxicity.

Fifteen weeks of endurance training (treadmill running) increased Con A-induced IL-2 production and proliferative responses in old Fischer 344 rats, but not in young and middle-aged animals. In contrast, Pahlavani *et al.* have detected no effect in the same parameters after 6 months of swimming exercise in old exercised animals compared to sedentary control rats.

There was no difference in the antigen-specific antibody response in old rats compared to non-exercised old and young controls in a study by Barnes *et al.* Lu *et al.* have reported increased IFN-γ- and LPS-stimulated macrophage cytolysis in both young and senescent inbred male BALB/CByJNia mice after 16 weeks of treadmill running, but the exercise effect was larger in young mice.

THE EFFECTS OF EXERCISE ON THE HORMONAL AND IMMUNE SYSTEMS

The Immune Response to Exercise in Health

Leucocytosis, which appears to be mediated initially by catecholamines and at later stages by cortisol, occurs during exercise. This leucocytosis is due to neutrophilia and the recruitment of B and T cells to the peripheral blood. After acute moderate exercise, there is a fall in the ratio of $CD4^+$ (helper) to $CD8^+$ (cytotoxic/suppressor) T cells and a rise in natural killer (NK) cell activity. The fall in CD4/CD8 ratio is mainly due to an increase in the number of $CD8^+$ T cells. The change in the lymphocyte subsets is transient, basal levels usually being reached again within 1.5h, while the neutrophil count remains elevated for a longer period. The rise in NK cell activity is short – lived, levels falling to below normal within 2h. The post–exercise suppression of NK cell activity is mediated by prostaglandins, as this effect can be reversed by the administration of indomethacin.

During and following exercise, there is a rise in the proinflammatory cytokines interleukin (IL) IL-1β, IL-6 and tumour necrosis factor. The level of IL-2 (T-cell growth factor) falls immediately after exercise, but has been found to be elevated 24h afterwards. Cytokine release is thought to be due in part to micromuscular damage caused by exercise.

Healthy individuals who take regular amounts of moderate exercise show no change in basal immune parameters. In contrast, athletes who undergo long-term repetitive intensive training (*e.g.* marathon training) have lower resting levels of immunoglobulins and circulating lymphocytes and reduced lymphocyte responsiveness.

The Immune Response to Exercise in RA

Regular exercise appears to have little effect on the resting immune state in RA patients. An 8 – week bicycle exercise programme carried out by patients with RA demonstrated an increase in the lymphoproliferative response during the acute phase of exercise. However, all immune changes were temporary and no significant difference could be found in the resting levels of blood mononuclear cell populations, NK cell activity, IL-1 and IL-6. The control group in this study was another group of RA patients in which training was prohibited, so no conclusions can be drawn on how the immune response of RA patients compares with that of a group of healthy individuals undergoing the same training regimen.

The Hormonal Response to Exercise in Health

The immune and hormonal systems have close inter]regulatory links. IL-1β, in particular, has a powerful effect on the endocrine system and glucose homeostasis. This cytokine acts at the hypothalamic level, causing the secretion of corticotrophin]releasing hormone (CRH). CRH induces the release of adrenocorticotrophic hormone (ACTH) from the anterior pituitary gland, which in turn stimulates adrenal cortisol secretion. IL-6 has been shown to stimulate the release of prolactin (PRL).

Exercise increases the production and catabolism of cortisol. The level rises transiently during exercise of both moderate and severe intensity, and falls rapidly to the basal level or below within a few hours of completion of the exercise. There is a rise of similar proportions in both fit and unfit individuals when exercising to exhaustion. For a given amount of exercise, there is a greater rise in the unfit. The magnitude of the rise in cortisol declines as training continues and subjects improve their fitness.

Regular moderate training has no significant effect on the basal levels of glucocorticoids. However, it is reported that highly trained endurance athletes have a raised basal level of cortisol and a reduced level of testosterone. The catabolic potential of this hormonal state has not been shown to have an adverse effect on the athletes' performance.

The anterior pituitary hormones and growth hormone show marked increases in plasma levels in response to physical exercise, often by as much as 230 and 2000 per cent respectively. The magnitude of the PRL release appears to depend on exercise intensity.

Cortisol and Prolactin Secretion in RA

Glucocorticoids have an immunosuppressive effect and play an important role in the treatment of RA. Endogenous secretion of glucocorticoids appears to have an anti – inflammatory effect and disease activity throughout a 24-h cycle appears to correlate closely with the serum level of cortisol. In RA there appears to be a loss of the normal diurnal variation in the cortisol level, the more abnormal circadian rhythms being associated with patients with highly active disease.

PRL is a proinflammatory peptide and its presence is essential for the development of a number of experimental autoimmune diseases. For example, rats that are depleted of PRL by hypophysectomy or bromocriptine treatment only develop adjuvant arthritis when the PRL is replaced by injection. PRL induces IL-2 receptor expression on splenocytes and is essential for the proliferation of T lymphocytes in response to IL-2. The PRL level bears some relation to disease activity and the timing of disease onset in RA. The development of RA for the first time and a flare of disease are associated with the post-partum period, when the PRL level is at its greatest, suggesting that the proinflammatory properties of PRL may play a role in disease pathogenesis.

In response to major surgery, RA patients show a minimal and insignificant rise in cortisol level, despite a larger than normal rise in IL – 1â. In contrast, patients with osteoarthritis (OA) and chronic osteomyelitis showed large cortisol rises in the immediate postoperative period, suggesting that chronic inflammation was not the cause of suppression of the hypothalamic–pituitary–adrenal (HPA) axis in RA. Patients with RA and healthy individuals showed similar cortisol responses to infusion of CRH, suggesting that the defect lies at the hypothalamic level, with a failure to secrete CRH.

RA patients showed a significantly greater increase in PRL after surgery compared with the other two groups. A more recent report failed to show significant increases in cortisol and PRL in OA and RA patients after surgery. It has been suggested that cytokines may activate the HPA axis via the prostaglandin pathway, with the consequence that non-steroidal anti-inflammatory drug (NSAID) therapy may have an inhibitory effect on CRH release.

The Clinical Effects of Exercise in Healthy Individuals

Regular and moderate amounts of exercise appear to enhance immunity and reduce the number of infectious episodes that an individual suffers. The incidence of upper respiratory tract infection was studied in two groups of sedentary obese women, and was found to be significantly lower in the group who took up regular exercise than in the group that remained inactive.

The degree of immune enhancement appears to rise as an individual increases the regularity and intensity of training. However, there does appear to be a point at which training becomes so intense that exercise starts to have a negative effect on the immune system. Excessive training in marathon runners (defined as running >97km per week) was associated with an increased risk of an infectious episode.

The Clinical Effects of Exercise in RA

Anecdotal opinion was that dynamic exercise was harmful to patients with RA as it was thought to cause further damage to affected joints. These thoughts have been disproved, and one study even found that the number of swollen joints decreased by 35 per cent when training was carried out in the muscles over the affected joints, whilst another group found that there was an improvement in the progression of X-ray destruction.

However, a more recent, randomized study comparing the effect of regular exercise in a group of RA patients who trained regularly with its effect in a sedentary group failed to detect any significant difference in the rate of radiological joint progression. There were also no significant changes in erythrocyte sedimentation rate, haemoglobin, joint count, pain score, early morning stiffness (EMS), health assessment questionnaire (HAQ) score and medicine cost.

Exercise was reported to have a favourable effect on general health, improving the well – being of patients and their ability to perform normal activities of daily living. Considerable improvement in aerobic capacity, the time taken to walk 50 feet (15.2m), depression and anxiety were observed in patients who were participating in regular aerobic exercise, but no significant difference in the disease activity was seen, as measured by the number of active joints, duration of EMS and grip strength.

There have been a number of reviews on the therapeutic effects of exercise in RA patients, all of which conclude that there is no adverse effect on disease activity or radiological joint destruction. It has been suggested that aerobic is superior to non – aerobic exercise and that dynamic exercise, requiring muscle work, appears to be better than static or isometric exercise. For example, a recent systematic review of six randomized controlled trials analysing the effects of dynamic exercise on patients with RA concluded that exercise improves physical capacity but has no adverse effects on pain or disease activity. Four of the six studies reviewed showed that there was an improvement in functional ability, but the changes were small and one study even reported a decrease in the HAQ score in patients who had exercised. None of the six trials reported any significant change in acute – phase reactants or joint inflammation. There is evidence that exercising an inflamed joint results in a hypoxic–reperfusion injury leading to the generation of reactive oxygen species (ROS). ROS are potent oxidizing agents which may react with IgG, leading to the oxidization of rheumatoid factor and hyaluron and resulting in fragmentation products that may subsequently alter immune function and consequently cause further joint damage.

Discussion

Dynamic exercise in RA patients has no adverse effect on the long – term outlook with regard to disease activity and radiological joint destruction. Healthy individuals who undertake regular exercise, particularly if it is intense, show a degree of immune enhancement that in theory could have an adverse effect on RA disease activity, but this has not been borne out by all the recent literature. The possible reasons for this are threefold.

First, regular exercise of the type described above has no significant effect on the resting immune state of RA patients. Secondly, RA patients may have a degree of immune paralysis compared with healthy individuals. Finally, the level of exercise undertaken by an average patient may be insufficient to have any significant clinical effect on the immune system. During exercise a lymphoproliferative response does occur and it could have clinical consequences; however, there is a rapid return to the basal state, so any joint pain and stiffness is likely to be short-lived.

Although a small number of studies have suggested that regular exercise has a beneficial effect on disease activity, the great majority of reports do not support these findings. If regular training was to have a favourable effect on disease activity, exercise would be expected to have an immunosuppressive effect. Severe endurance training like that described above may well induce immunosuppression and potentially has a therapeutic effect on disease activity; however, this degree of exercise is clearly not going to be possible in RA patients.

There appears to be no literature on the PRL and cortisol responses of RA patients to exercise and how they compare with those of healthy individuals. Any study of this nature would be difficult to control satisfactorily, as there will be marked differences between the two groups in aerobic capacity and the ability to carry out exercise. The mechanisms by which cortisol and PRL vary during exercise are likely to be mediated in part by the cytokines IL-1β and IL-6, both of which increase during exercise. At the hypothalamic level, a possible insensitivity to IL-1β has been described in RA. Whether this is due to the disease itself or the use of NSAIDs remains to be tested, but both anti – inflammatory medication and corticosteroids are likely to have a further effect on the feedback mechanisms and impair the normal HPA axis response to exercise.

Exercising RA patients, particularly those on NSAIDs or corticosteroids, may well lead to a subnormal cortisol response. Given the greater metabolic rate that occurs during exercise—and hence the catabolism of cortisol—a possible fall in cortisol level is likely. However, a comparative study with healthy individuals in which the effects of high – intensity training for 6 weeks on circulating levels of CRH were evaluated found that, although the starting levels of CRH were significantly lower in RA, a small but significant increase in CRH was observed in the patient group. This increase was not seen in healthy individuals; but the resting levels of CRH in RA after training remained lower than those observed in healthy individuals. The reason for the difference between the two groups is likely to be the greater increase in IL-1β in RA. Further studies are needed to determine whether this small increase in CRH is sufficient to avoid a fall in cortisol in response to high – intensity exercise.

INFECTIOUS DISEASE

The relationship between exercise and susceptibility to infection involves several factors, including the type of infection, the quality and quantity of exercise, and the timing of exercise relative to the course of the disease process. Regular moderate exercise enhances immune function, while prolonged intense exercise can suppress immune function. The effect of moderate versus intense prolonged exercise on specific immune parameters (cell number and function, antibodies) has been described above.

After reviewing several human and animal studies, Pedersen provided the following conclusions regarding exercise and infectious disease:

- Exercise or training prior to inoculation of an infectious agent (especially viruses) tends to reduce susceptibility to infectious disease.
- Moderate exercise training during an infection does not affect the outcome of the disease.
- Exhaustive exercise during an infection generally enhances the severity of the infection. This is likely related to exercise-associated immunosuppression (*i.e.*, open window hypothesis).
- The nature of the infectious microbes and the site of infection may play a role.

The higher incidence of upper respiratory tract infections after intense exercise may be due in part to suppression of natural immunity and possibly direct suppression of the secretory immune system by the cold and dry air effects on the local mucosa. Moderate exercise enhances the immune system; intense exercise suppresses the immune response.

EXERCISE-INDUCED ASTHMA

Shephard provides a definition of exercise-induced bronchospasm as a decrease in forced expiratory volume of at least 10 per cent. It typically develops within 5 to10 minutes after starting to exercise and may resolve in 30 to 90 minutes of rest or while still exercising. The usual trigger appears to be inhalation of cold, dry air via the mouth. Mucosal drying may trigger the release of pharmacologic mediators from mast cells, which bring about the bronchospasm. The mediators include histamine, leukotrienes, kinins, serotonin, prostaglandins, thromboxanes, and cytokines. They produce vasodilation, increased vascular permeability, smooth muscle contraction, and activate other cells. Following the bronchospasm a refractory period develops which lasts for several hours. During this period bronchospasm is not easily provoked, possibly due to inhibitory prostaglandins. There is little known about the effects of training on bronchospasm, but improved fitness should decrease the ventilatory effort needed for exercise and should reduce the degree of cooling and drying of the bronchial mucosa. Prophylaxis involves avoiding of known allergens before exercise, wearing a facemask in cold weather to humidify air and treating respiratory infections promptly. The main treatment is an aerosolized β-2 agonist, which inhibits smooth muscle contraction and mediator release. Unfortunately for sufferers, β-2 agonists are banned in many athletic competitions. Antihistamines, calcium channel blockers and other drugs may also be effective.

CANCER

The role of the immune system in preventing and fighting cancer is not entirely clear. The immune system may be involved primarily in malignancies of viral origin. Viral antigens are the most immunogenic molecules on tumors. An immune response that protects against (oncogenic) viral infections may be the primary manner in which the immune system protects against cancer.

Generally, moderate regular exercise seems to decrease the risk of colon cancer and possibly breast cancer and cancer of the female reproductive tract. Possible immune mechanisms for cancer protection that result from training include increases in the number and/or activity of macrophages and natural killer cells and their regulatory cytokines.

There are a number of secondary effects of exercise that may also help protect against cancer. A healthy lifestyle tends to be adopted by those who exercise regularly.

Transit of food through the intestines is likely increased by exercise, which would decrease exposure to carcinogens. Exercise tends to decrease body fat and obesity has been associated with an increased cancer risk. Improved circulation may facilitate interaction of immune cells with tumors.

HUMAN BODY AND IMMUNE SYSTEM

The human body has the capacity to protect itself against pathogens, some toxins and cancer cells through the immune system.

NON-SPECIFIC DEFENCES

In animals, there are two types of defences against foreign invaders: specific and non-specific. Specific immune responses can distinguish among different invaders. The response is different for each invader. With non-specific defences, the protection is always the same, no matter what the invader may be. Whereas only vertebrates have specific immune responses, all animals have some type of non-specific defence. Examples of non-specific defences include physical barriers, protein defences, cellular defences, inflammation, and fever.

Barriers

One way for an organism to defend itself against invasion is through barriers that separate the organism from its environment. Physical barriers such as the skin and mucous membranes mechanically regulate what enters the body.

Secretions provide protection at the barrier as well. Mucus, for example, can trap potential invaders. Also, skin secretions are slightly acidic, inhibiting bacterial growth. Many body secretions (such as mucus, tears, and saliva) contain an enzyme called lysozyme that destroys bacteria.

Proteins

There are proteins that protect the body non-specifically. Complement proteins are found in the blood. When they bind to an invader, they stimulate inflammation, phagocytosis, and destruction of the invader's membrane. Although complement proteins may bind to an invader directly, they are most effective when they bind to antibodies that are attached to an invader. Antibodies are part of the body's specific immune response.

Some immune cells and cells that are infected with viruses produce another set of proteins called interferons. Interferons send a warning to nearby cells. They help prevent infection by stimulating the production of antiviral proteins. Interferons also stimulate natural killer cells and macrophages.

Cellular Defences

Natural killer cells and macrophages are examples of non-specific cellular defences. Natural killer cells are a class of lymphocytes that recognize abnormal cells (such as cancerous cells or virus-infected cells), attach to them, and release chemicals that destroy them. Macrophages, neutrophils, and eosinophils are examples of phagocytes.

In their attempt to defend the body, some phagocytes stay within a tissue and others travel freely throughout the body. However, all phagocytes are attracted to sites of tissue damage.

In a process called phagocytosis, these cells surround debris or a foreign invader, bringing it inside the cell. The phagocyte then uses special enzymes to digest the material. All animals have phagocytes that recognize and eliminate foreign invaders. For example, if a piece of one sponge is transplanted to a sponge from another colony, phagocytes in the sponges will attack and destroy each other.

The same response can be observed in earthworms, arthropods, starfish, and all vertebrates. Scientist Elie Metchnikoff observed this process in starfish. A coloured scanning electron micrograph of a macrophage engulfing a parasite of the *Leishmania* genus. To defend the body, macrophages will surround a foreign invader, bring it inside the cell, then use enzymes to digest the material.

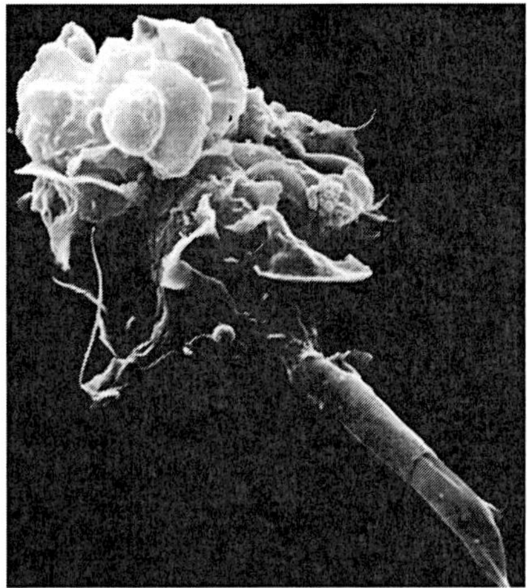

In vertebrates, some phagocytes are also important in stimulating specific immune responses. Additionally, phagocytosis is stimulated when the invaders are coated with antibodies. Consequently, phagocytes (like complement proteins) represent an important link between non-specific and specific immunity.

Inflammation

Infection, mechanical force, chemicals, and extreme heat or cold can damage tissues, causing the non-specific process of inflammation. The goal of inflammation is to clean up the damage and start the repair process. Inflammation begins when damaged tissues release chemical messengers such as histamine, prostaglandins, and leukotrienes. These chemicals cause nearby blood vessels to expand and become more leaky, allowing more blood flow to the damaged area. These chemicals also attract white blood cells (such as phagocytes) to the site to remove debris and foreign invaders. The results of these activities are easily observed when the skin is inflamed: swelling, redness, heat, and pain.

Fever

Another non-specific protection against infection is the development of a fever. Either the invader or the response to an invader causes a part of the brain called the hypothalamus to increase the body temperature. Fevers may increase body metabolism, speeding up the repair process. Fevers may also slow down the reproduction of some bacteria and viruses. Whether the mechanism is as complex as fever and inflammation or as simple as physical barriers and phagocytosis, all non-specific defences provide the body with general protection against foreign invaders.

NON-SPECIFIC RESPONSES - THE SECOND LINE OF DEFENCE

- Non-specific responses are generalized responses to pathogen infection - they do not target a specific cell type
- The non-specific response consist of some WBC's and plasma proteins
- Phagocytes - cells which "eat" foreign material to destroy them
  - Phagocytes are formed from stem cells in bone marrow (stem cells are undifferentiated WBC's)
    a. Neutrophil - phagocytize bacteria
    b. Eosinophils - secrete enzymes to kill parasitic worms among other pathogins
- Macrophage - "big eaters" phagocytize just about anything

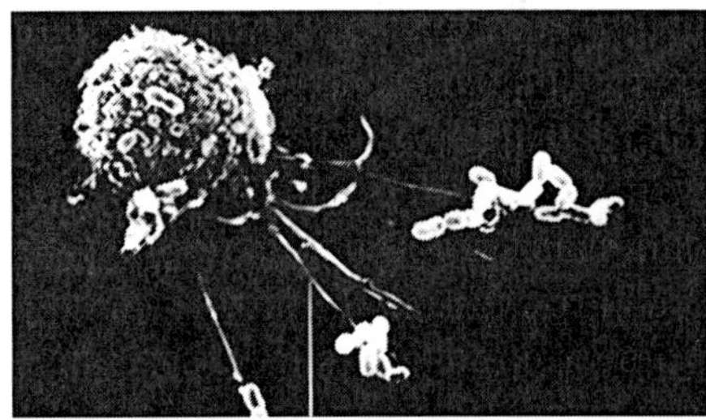

Fig. Macrophage Destroying Bacterial Cells

- Non-phagocytic leucocytes -
  - Basophil - contain granules of toxic chemicals that can digest foreign microorganisms. These are cells involved in an allergic response
  - Mast Cells - similar to basophils, mast cells contain a variety of inflammatory chemicals including histamine and seratonin. Cause blood vessels near wound to constrict.
- Complement proteins - plasma proteins which have a role in non-specific and specific defences

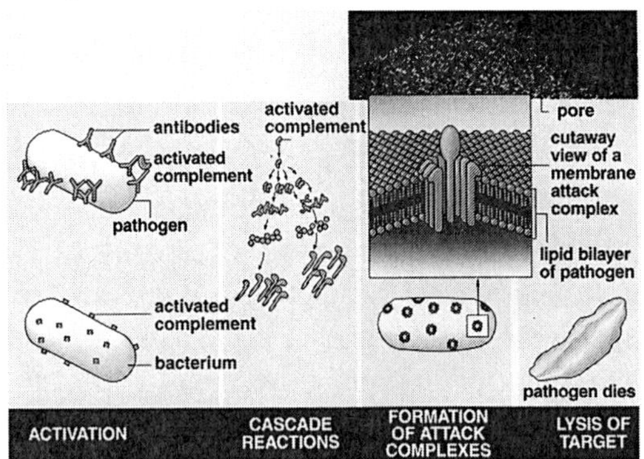

  - Form a cascade effect - if only a few are activated, they will trigger others to become active in great numbers

a. Some punch holes in bacterial walls (forms holes where cellular components leak out)
b. Some promote inflammation
c. Concentration gradients attract phagocytes to irritated or damaged tissue
d. Encourage phagocytosis in phagocytes (promotes "eating")
e. Some bind to the surface of invading organisms

- Chemokines - create a chemical gradient to attract neutrophils and other leucocytes to the wound site
- Inflammation

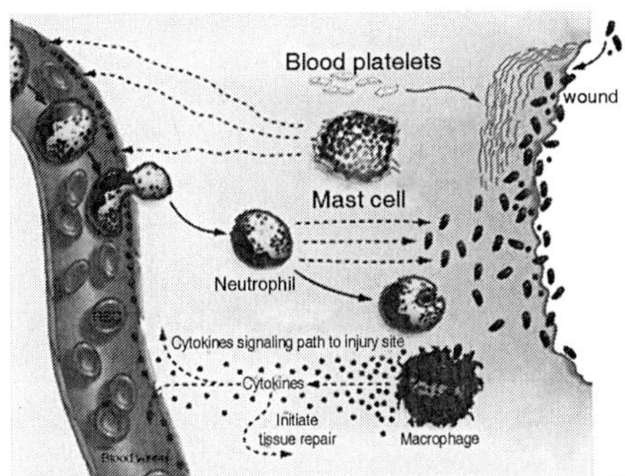

  - Causes localized redness, swelling, heat, and pain
  - Changes in capillary wall structure allow interstitial fluid and WBC's to leak out in tissue
  - Promotes macrophage (phagocytic WBC's) activity
  - Macrophages secrete Interleukins (communication proteins among WBC's)
    a. Interleukin-1: increases body temperature (*i.e.* causes a fever)
    b. This enhances the WBC's ability to protect the body
    c. Causes drowsiness - reduces the body's energy usage and stress

The Immune System (Specific Responses) - the Third Line of Defence

- Called into action when non-specific methods are not enough and infection becomes widespread

Types of cells involved in the immune system:

- Macrophages - engulf foreign objects
  - Inform T lymphocytes at a specific antigen is present
- Helper T cells - produce and secrete chemicals which promote large numbers of effector and memory cells
- Cytotoxic T cells - T lymphocytes that eliminate infected body cells and tumor cells
- B cells - produce antibodies (secrete them in the blood or position them on their cell surfaces)

Each type of virus, bacteria, or other foreign body has molecular markers which make it unique

- Host lymphocytes (*i.e.* those in your body) can recognize *self* proteins (*i.e.* those which are not foreign)
- When a *non-self* (foreign) body is detected, mitotic activity in B and T lymphocytes is stimulated
  - While mitosis is occurring, the daughter populations become subdivided
    a. Effector cells - when fully differentiated, they will seek and destroy foreign
    b. Memory cells - become dormant, but can be triggered to rapid mitosis if pathogen encountered again

Thus, immunological specificity and memory involve three events:

1. Recognition of a specific invader
2. Repeated cell divisions that form huge lymphocyte populations
3. Differentiation into subpopulations of effector and memory cells
   - Antigen - a non-self marker that triggers the formation of lymphocyte armies
   - Antibodies - molecules which bind to antigens and are recognized by lymphocytes

Antigen-presenting cell - a macrophage which digests a foreign cell, but leaves the antigens intact. It then binds these antigens to MHC molecules on its cell membrane. The antigen-MHC complexes are noticed by certain lymphocytes (*recognition*) which promotes cell division (*repeated cell divisions*)

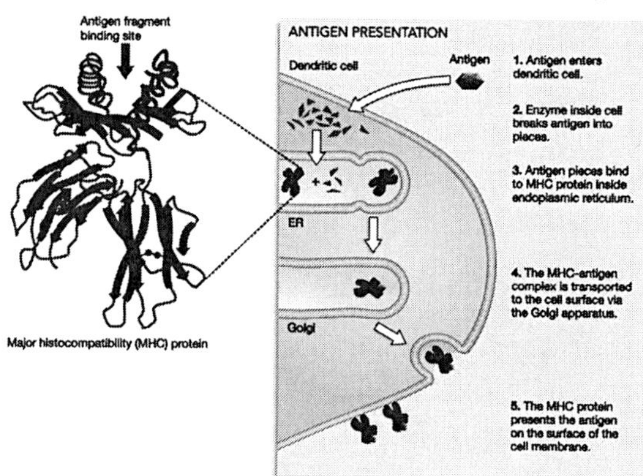

MOLECULAR CUES THAT STIMULATE LYPMPHOCYTES TO CREATE AN IMMUNE RESPONSE

T Cells (Helper T Cells and Cytotoxic T Cells)

- T cells arise from stem cells in the bone marrow - they then travel to the thymus where the differentiate and mature. At maturity, they acquire receptors for self markers (MHC molecules) and for antigen-specific receptors. They are then released into the blood as "virgin" T cells.

- T cells ignore other cells with MHC molecules and they ignore free-floating antigens. However, they will bind with a antigen-presenting macrophage (a macrophage possessing a MHC-antigen complex). This binding promotes rapid cell division and differentiation into effector and memory cells (all with receptors for the antigen)
- Effector helper T cells secrete interlukins (stimulate both T and B cells to divide and differentiate)
- Effector cytotoxic T cells recognize infected cells with the MHC-antigen complex. They then destroy the cell with perforans (enzymes which perforate the cell membrane, allowing cytoplasm to leak out) and other toxins which attack organelles and DNA

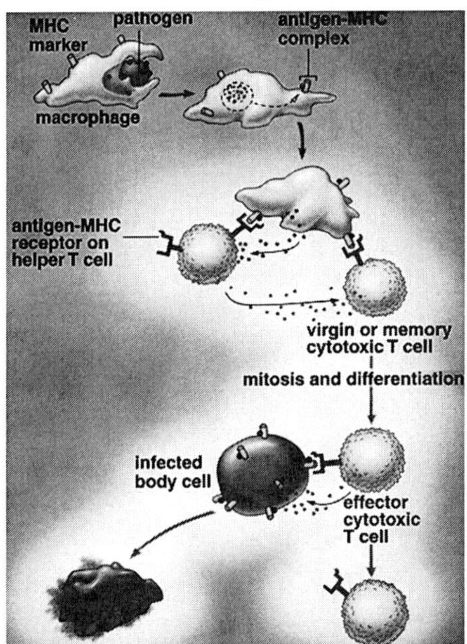

Fig. Cell-mediated immune response

B Cells and Antibodies

- B cells also arise from stem cells in the bone marrow. As they develop and mature, they start synthesizing a single type of antibody
- Antibodies are proteins which recognize antigens
- The virgin B cell produces antibodies which move to the cell surface and stick out
- The B cell floats in the blood - when it encounters the specific antigen it becomes primed for replication

- The B cell must receive an interleukin signal from a helper T cell which has already become activated by a macrophage with a MHC-antigen complex. This promotes *rapid cell division.*
- The B cell population then differentiates into effector and memory B cells
- The effector B cells then produce a staggering amount of free-floating antibodies
  - When these free-floating antibodies encounter an antigen, they tag it for destruction by phagocytes and complementary proteins
  - These types of responses are only good for extracellular toxins and pathogens - they cannot detect pathogens or toxins located inside of a cell

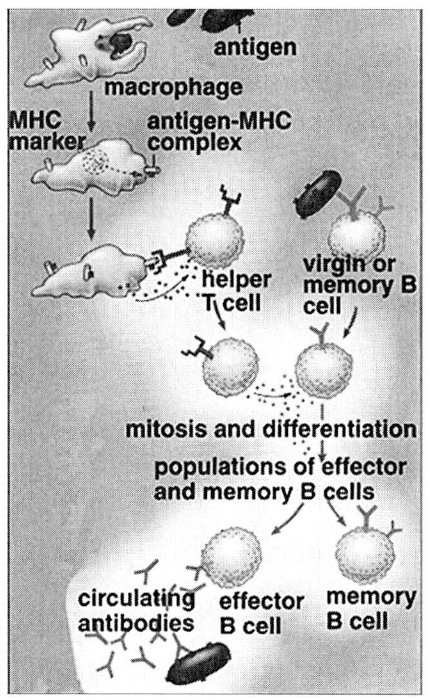

Fig. Antibody-mediated immune response

Physical and Chemical Defences

Epithelial cells on the body surface and cavity linings form a physical barrier and produce secretions that defend against infection. The body's first lines of defence against microbes are the barriers offered by surfaces exposed to the external environment. Very few microorganisms can penetrate the intact skin, and the various skin glands and tear glands all secrete antimicrobial chemicals. The mucus secreted by the epithelial linings of the respiratory and upper gastrointestinal tracts also contains antimicrobial chemicals, but more importantly, mucus is sticky. Particles that adhere to it are prevented from entering the blood. They are either swept by ciliary action up into the pharynx and then swallowed (as occurs in the upper respiratory tract) or phagocytised by macrophages in the various linings.

Other specialised surface defences are the hairs at the entrance to the nose, the cough and sneeze reflexes, and the acid secretions of the stomach and uterus, which kill microbes.

Finally, a major defence against infection is the many relatively innocuous microbes normally found on the skin and other linings exposed to the external environment. Through a variety of mechanisms, these microbes suppress the growth of other potentially more dangerous ones.

Inflammatory Response

Release of histamine by mast cells causes vasodilation and increased capillary permeability. The increased blood flow and the secretion of cytokines result in the accumulation of phagocytes and the delivery of antimicrobial proteins and clotting elements to the site of infection. Inflammation is the body's local response to infection or injury. The functions of inflammation are to destroy or inactivate foreign invaders and to set the stage for tissue repair. The steps and cells involved are detailed below:

Mast Cells

Mast cells are part of a group of cells called leukocytes (white blood cells) that are found in almost all tissues and organs. Once activated, mast cells produce large quantities of histamine. Histamine dilates the surrounding capillaries and increases their permeability.

Vasodilation and Increased Capillary Permeability

Vasodilation results in increased blood flow to the site of infection (accounting for the redness and heat associated with inflammation). The increased blood flow brings an increased number of leukocytes and proteins to the area. Increased permeability allows plasma proteins to gain entry from the blood to the site of infection.

Secretion of Cytokines

The leukocytes that arrive at the site of infection secrete cytokines, which act as chemoattractants (chemotaxins). Chemotaxins stimulate the movement of phagocytes to the infected area.

Phagocytosis

Phagocytes arrive and begin to rid the area of bacteria. The phagocyte engulfs the bacterium in a process known as endocytosis. The bacterium is contained within an intracellular vesicle. The vesicle fuses with a lysosome and powerful enzymes digest the bacterium. The end products are then used by the cell or released by exocytosis.

Complement

Complement proteins are activated in response to infection. Activation of the first protein results in activation of a second protein and so on in a cascade. The complement system consists of at least 30 distinct proteins and is extremely complex. Activation of the complement system amplifies the immune response – complement proteins can help to kill the microbe, stimulate vasodilation, increase permeability and aid phagocytosis.

Tissue Repair

The final stage of inflammation is tissue repair. Platelets form a plug to seal off the site of injury and clotting elements trigger the coagulation cascade, which strengthens the platelet plug. Finally, remodelling takes place as the healing process winds down. The final repair may be imperfect – this results in a scar.

NON-SPECIFIC CELLULAR RESPONSES

A variety of specialised white blood cells provide protection against pathogens. Phagocytes recognise surface antigen molecules on pathogens and destroy them by phagocytosis. Natural killer (NK) cells induce the pathogen to produce self-destructive DNA enzymes in apoptosis. Phagocytes and NK cells release cytokines, which stimulate the specific immune response.

On rare occasions pathogens break through the host's physical and chemical defence mechanisms. The pathogen can then invade host tissues and begin to colonise and infect the host. It is at this point the immune system must become mobilised. The starting point for immunity (whether it is specific, non-specific, humoral or cell-mediated) is contact of a pathogen with a phagocyte. The primary function of a phagocyte is to engulf and destroy pathogens and digest their remains.

Phagocytes

Phagocytes are found in the blood and in the tissues and they are motile. The phagoctyte recognises antigens on the surface of the pathogen, to which it then adheres. The membrane of the phagocyte engulfs the pathogen and pinches off to form an intracellular vesicle. This vesicle then fuses with a lysosome (a granular inclusion containing bactericidal substances such as lysozyme, hydrogen peroxide, proteases, phosphatases, nucleases and lipases). The toxic substances inside the lysosome are capable of killing and digesting the engulfed pathogen. Following digestion of the pathogen, the phagocyte releases a number of inflammatory mediators, some of which include cytokines. This results in a positive feedback loop, the cytokines recruiting more phagocytes to the area.

Natural Killer Cells

NK cells bind to virus-infected and cancer cells without specific recognition and kill them directly. They participate in antibody-dependent cellular cytotoxicity. NK cells constitute a distinct class of lymphocytes. Their major targets are virus-infected cells and cancer cells. They attack and kill these cells directly. NK cells are not specific – they are able to attack cells without any recognition of the specific pathogen involved. NK cells recognise 'normal' cells through their expression of Major Histocompatibility Complex (MHC) class 1 proteins.

They recognise foreign cells by the *absence* of these proteins. The exact nature of NK cells and their method of action is unknown. However, it is known that they kill cells by releasing small cytoplasmic granules of proteins called perforin and granzyme that cause the target cell to die by apoptosis (programmed cell death). The perforin is released in close proximity to the target cell and forms pores in the cell membrane, allowing granzymes to enter the cell.

The granzymes stimulate the cell to produce enzymes that degrade the DNA of the cell, inducing apoptosis. As well as their role in non-specific immunity, phagocytes and NK cells also help to initiate the specific immune response. Following their action against the pathogen they secrete interleukins – cytokines that serve to stimulate the specific immune response through the activation of T cells.

SPECIFIC CELLULAR DEFENCES

Immune Defence against Bacterial Pathogens: Innate Immunity

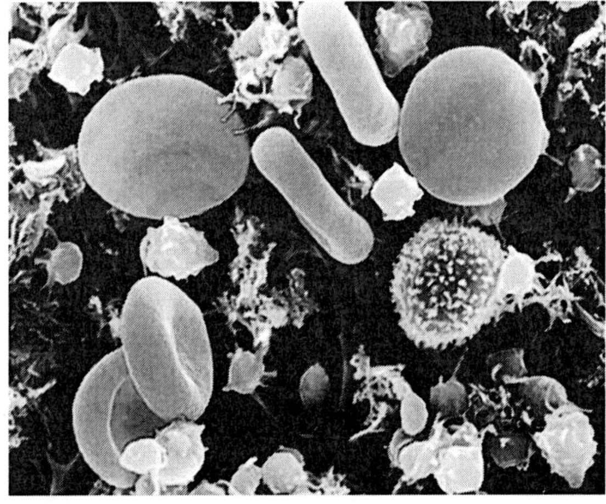

Fig. Human blood contains most cellular and non-cellular factors that participate in host immunity to bacterial pathogens.

Host Defence Mechanisms

Humans are in continuous associations with microorganisms, including those that readily colonize the body surfaces. It is relatively rare that these microorganisms cause damage to their host. In part, this is due to the effectiveness of the host defence mechanisms, which restrict invasion by normal flora (some of which may be potential pathogens), and which defend against non--indigenous microorganisms that are overt pathogens.

The outcome of an interaction between a human host and a microbe, whether it is a component of the normal flora or an exogenous pathogen, depends on specific properties inherent to both the host and the microbe. Sometimes, the host tolerates colonization by a parasite but restricts it to regions of the body where it can do no harm (*e.g. Staphylococcus aureus* on the nasal membranes or *Streptococcus pneumoniae* in the upper respiratory tract). If the parasiteinvades (*i.e.*, breaches an anatomical barrier or progresses beyond the point of colonization), an infection is said to have occurred. If, as a result of infection, pathological harm to the host becomes evident, this is called an infectious disease.

The healthy animal defends itself against pathogens different stages. The host defences may be of such a degree that infection can be prevented entirely. Or, if infection does occur, the defences may stop the process before disease is apparent. At other times, the defences that are necessary to defeat a pathogen may not be effective until infectious disease is well into progress. The host defence mechanisms are mediated by the immune system. For our purposes, the term immunity refers to the relative state of resistance of the host to infectious disease.

I will adopt the nomenclature used by my colleagues at University of South Carolina School of Medicine Microbiology and Immunology On-line to draw lines between the "types of immunity", particularly as it relates to to innate immunity and adaptive immunity.

The immune system is composed of two major subdivisions, the b>innate or non-specific immune system and the adaptive or specific immune system. The innate immune system is a primary defence mechanism against invading organisms, while the adaptive immune system acts as a second line of defence. Both aspects of the immune system have cellular and humoral components by which they carry out their protective functions.

In addition, there is interplay between these two systems, *i.e.*, cells or components of the innate immune system influence the adaptive immune system and vice versa. The innate and adaptive immune systems differ in several ways. The adaptive immune system requires some time to react to an invading organism, whereas the innate immune system includes defences that, for the most part, are constitutively present and mobilized immediately upon infection. Additionally, the adaptive immune system is antigen specific and reacts only with the organism that induced the response. The innate system is not antigen specific and reacts similarly to a variety of organisms. Finally, the adaptive immune system exhibits an immunological memory. It "remembers" that it has encountered an invading organism and reacts more rapidly on subsequent exposure to the same organism. The innate immune system does not exhibit a memory response.

Cellular defence. This term is used to distinguish whether an immune response is mediated by a particular type of cell, as opposed to a non- cellular defence which does not involve a specifically programmed cell. As stated above, a variety of tissue cells are involved in innate and adaptive immunity, hence the term cellular defence. These include neutrophils and macrophages, which are involved in phagocytosis, basophils and mast cells, which are involved in inflammation, and B cells and T cells which account for antibody mediated immunity and cell mediated immunity, respectively.

All these cells have their origin in the bone marrow. Myeloid progenitor (stem) cells in the bone marrow give rise to neutrophils, eosinophils, basophils, monocytes and dendritic cells, while lymphoid progenitor (stem) cells give rise to T cells and B cells. Macrophages and dendritic cells, which play a key role in innate and adaptive immunity, are derived from monocytes; and mast cells, which are fixed in tissues, develop from the same precrusor cell as circulating basophils.

B cells are produced in bone marrow and released into the blood and lymphatic systems. B-cells can develop into plasma cells that secrete antibodies. Precursor T cells undergo differentiation in the thymus into two distinct types of T cells, $CD4^+$ T helper cells, and the $CD8^+$ cytotoxic T cells. Macrophages and dendritic cells function as one of several bridges between innate immunity and adaptive immunity, since they present antigens to immunocompetent T-cells, which initiates an immunological response.

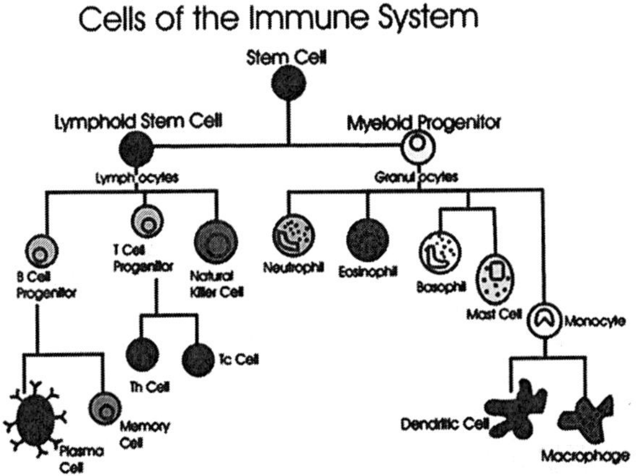

Fig. Development of cells that participate in immunity.

Innate Immunity

Innate Immunity is a form of non- specific host defence against invading bacteria. It is natural or "innate" to the host, depending, in part, on genetics. Innate defence mechanisms are contitutive to the host, meaning they are continually ready to respond to invasion and do not require a period of time for induction.

The most important components of innate immunity are anatomical barriers, intact normal flora, tissue bactericides including complement, and ability to undergo inflammatory and phagocytic responses.

Innate immunity provides the first line of defence against invading bacteria. The skin and mucous membranes provide physical and chemical barriers to infection. The normal bacterial flora antagonize colonization of body surfaces by non-indigenous bacteria. The internal tissues invariably contain bactericidal substances.

The most noteworthy antibacterial substance is the enzyme lysozyme, which is present in mucus and all bodily tissues and secretions. If these barriers are penetrated, the body contains cells that respond rapidly to the presence of the invader.

These cells include macrophages and neutrophils that engulf foreign organisms and kill them. Bacterial invasion is also challenged by the activation of complement in blood and tissues and the incitement of an inflammatory process which has the tendency to focus both the innate and adaptive immune defences on the site of invasion.

Categories of Innate or Non-specific Immunity

The first four categories are generally considered non- cellular defences. Inflammation and Phagocytosis are forms of cellular defence.

- Differences in susceptibility to certain pathogens
- Anatomical defence
- Tissue bactericides, including complement
- Microbial antagonism
- Inflammation (ability to undergo an inflammatory response)
- Phagocytosis

Differences in Susceptibility of Animal Hosts to Microbial Pathogens (Natural Immunity)

Natural immunity or resistance is based on the genetics of the host. There are two aspects:

1. Resistance among all members of a species, called species resistance and
2. Resistance within members of the same animal species, calledindividual resistance.

Species Resistance

Certain animals are naturally resistant or non- susceptible to certain pathogens. Certain pathogens infect only humans, not lower animals, *e.g.* syphilis, gonorrhea, measles, poliomyelitis. On the other hand, certain pathogens (*e.g.* canine distemper virus) do not infect humans. *Shigella* infects humans and baboons but not chimpanzees. Little information is available to explain these absolute differences in susceptibility to a pathogen but it could be due to:

Absence of specific tissue or cellular receptors for attachment (colonization) by the pathogen. For example, different strains of enterotoxigenic *E. coli,* defined by different fimbrial antigens, colonize human infants, calves and piglets by recognizing species-specific carbohydrate receptors on enterocytes in the gastrointestinal tract.

Temperature of the host and ability of pathogen to grow. For example, birds do not normally become infected with mammalian strains of *Mycobacterium tuberculosis* because these strains cannot grow at the high body temperature of birds. The anthrax bacillus (*Bacillus anthracis*) will not grow in the cold-blooded frog (unless the frog is maintained at 37°).

Lack of the exact nutritional requirements to support the growth of the pathogen. Naturally-requiring purine-dependent strains of *Salmonella typhi* grow only in hosts supplying purines. Mice and rats lack this growth factor in blood and pur^{-} strains are avirulent. By injecting purines into these animals, such that the growth factor requirement for the bacterium is satisfied, the organisms prove virulent. Lack of a target site for a microbial toxin. Most toxins produced by bacterial cells exert their toxic activity only after binding to susceptible cells or tissues in an animal.

Certain animals may lack an appropriate target cell or specific type of cell receptor for the toxin to bind to and may therefore be non-susceptible to the activity of the toxin. For example, injection of diphtheria toxin fails to kill the rat. The unchanged toxin is excreted in the urine. If a sample of the rat urine (or pure diphtheria toxin) is injected into the guinea pig, it dies of typical lesions caused by diphtheria toxin.

Individual Resistance

There are many reasons why individuals of the same animal species may exhibit greater or lesser susceptibility to the same ineffective agent. Age. Usually this relates to the development and status of the immunological system which varies with age. It may also be associated with changes in normal flora coincidental to developmental changes in the animal. Sex. Usually this is linked to the presence and/or development of the sex organs. For example, mastitis and infectious diseases leading to abortion will obviously occur only in the female; orchitis would occur only in males. It could also be due to anatomical structure related to sex (bladder infections are 14-times more common in females than males), and possibly the effects of sex hormones on infections. Stress. Stress is a complex of different factors that apparently has a real influence on health.

Undue exertion, shock, change in environment, climatic change, nervous or muscular fatigue, etc. are factors known to contribute to increases in susceptibility to infection. The best explanation is that in time of stress the output of cortisone from the adrenal cortex is increased. This suppresses the inflammatory processes of the host and the overall effect may be harmful. There are also a number of relationships between stress-related hormones and the functioning of the immune defences.

Diet, malnutrition. Infections may be linked with vitamin and protein deficiencies, and this might explain partly why many infectious diseases are more prevalent and infant mortality rates are highest in parts of the world where malnourishment is a problem. Also, overfed and obese animals are more susceptible to infection. Diets high in sucrose predispose individuals to dental caries.

Intercurrent disease or trauma. The normal defences of an animal are impaired by organic diseases such as leukemia, Hodgkin's disease, diabetes, AIDS, etc. Frequently, inflammatory or immune responses are delayed or suppressed. Colds or influenza may predispose an individual to pneumonia. Smoking tobacco predisposes to infections of the respiratory tract. Burned tissue is readily infected by *Pseudomonas aeruginosa.*

Therapy against other diseases. Modern therapeutic procedures used in some diseases can render an individual more susceptible to infection. Under these conditions not only pathogens, but organisms of the normal flora and non-pathogens in the host's environment, may be able to initiate infection. Examples of therapeutic procedures that reduce the efficiency of the host's defences are treatment with corticosteroids, cytotoxic drugs, antibiotics, or irradiation.

Anatomical Defences

The structural integrity of the body surfaces, *i.e.*, the skin and mucous membranes, forms an effective barrier to initial lodgment or penetration by microorganisms. The skin is a very effective barrier to bacterium, so that no bacterium by itself is known to be able to penetrate unbroken skin. Of course, a puncture, cut or scrape in the skin could introduce infectious bacteria.

The mucous membranes are more vulnerable to penetration by infectious bacteria but still pose a formidable barrier of mucus and antimicrobial substances. The anatomical defences are associated with all other aspects of non-cellular immunity, including individual resistance, mechanical resistance, chemical resistance and resistance established by the normal flora.

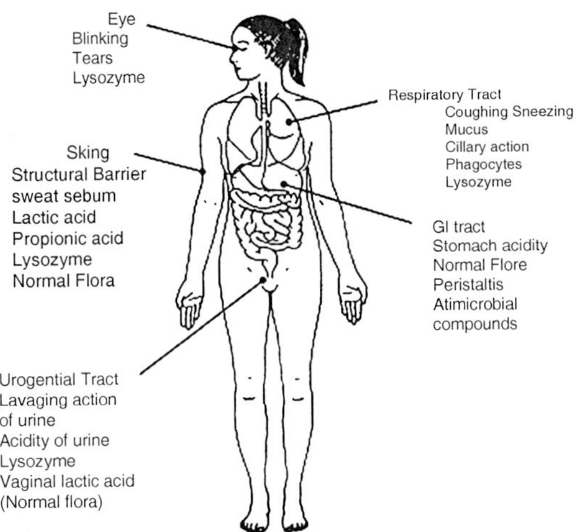

Fig. Anatomical defences associated with tissue surfaces

Skin. The intact surface of the healthy epidermis seems to be rarely if ever penetrated by bacteria. If the integrity of the epidermis is broken (by the bite of an insect, needle stick, abrasion, cut, etc.) invasive microbes may enter. The normal flora of the skin, which metabolize substances secreted onto the skin, produce end products (*e.g.* fatty acids) that discourage the colonization of skin by potential pathogens. Perspiration contains lysozyme and other antimicrobial substances.

Mucous membranes. Many are heavily colonized with bacteria in whose moist secretions they survive. These normal flora are restricted from entry and usually occupy any attachment sites that might otherwise be used by pathogens.

The normal flora established on mucous membranes may antagonize non-indigenous species by other means, as well. Typically, mucus contains a number of types of anti-microbial compounds, including lysozyme and secretory antibodies (IgA). Sometimes phagocytes patrol mucosal surfaces (*e.g.* in the lower respiratory tract). Nonetheless, most infectious agents impinge on the skin or mucous membranes of the oral cavity, respiratory tract, GI tract or urogenital tract, and from these sites most infections occur. Damage to the epithelial cells caused by toxic products of these bacteria may play a role.

Respiratory tract. Fine hairs and baffles of the nares (nasal membranes) entrap bacteria which are inhaled. Those which pass may stick to mucosal surfaces of the trachea or be swept upward by the ciliated epithelium of the lower respiratory tract. Coughing and sneezing also eliminate bacteria. The lower respiratory tract (lung) is well protected by mucus, lysozyme, secretory antibody, and phagocytosis.

Mouth, stomach and intestinal tract. Microorganisms entering by the oral route, more than any other, have to compete with the well-adapted normal flora of the mouth and intestine. Most organisms that are swallowed are destroyed by acid and various secretions of the stomach. Alkaline pH of the lower intestine can discourage other organisms. The peristaltic action of the intestine ultimately flushes out organisms which have not succeeded in colonization. Bile salts and lysozyme are present, which kill or inhibit many types of bacteria.

Urogenital Tract. The flushing mechanisms of sterile urine and the acidity of urine maintain the bladder and most of the urethra free of microorganisms. The vaginal epithelium of the female maintains a high population of Doderlein's bacillus (*Lactobacillus acidophilus*) whose acidic end products of metabolism (lactic acid) prevent colonization by most other types of microorganisms including potentially-pathogenic yeast (*Candida albicans*). Eyes (Conjunctiva). The conjunctiva of the eye is remarkably free of most microorganisms. Blinking mechanically removes microbes, the lavaging action of tears washes the surface of the eye, and lachrymal secretions (tears) contain relatively large amounts of lysozyme.

Microbial Antagonism

This refers to the protection of the surfaces afforded by an intact normal flora in a healthy animal, and it has already been mentioned in several contexts (See The Bacterial Flora of Humans). There are three main ways that the normal flora protect the surfaces where they are colonized:

Competition with non-indigenous species for binding (colonization) sites. The normal flora are highly-adapted to the tissues of their host. That is why they are there. Specific antagonism against non-indigenous species. Members of the normal flora may produce very specific proteins called bacteriocins which kill or inhibit other (usually closely-related) species of bacteria.

Immune Surveillance

A range of types of white blood cell constantly circulate, monitoring the tissues. If tissues become damaged or invaded, a variety of cells release cytokines, which recruit specific white blood cells to the site of infection or tissue damage. Leukocytes (white blood cells) are the most numerous cells of the immune system.

They are produced in the bone marrow and use the blood to transport themselves around the body – they are constantly on the lookout for microbes, pathogens, antigens etc. Leukocytes can leave the circulatory system and enter the tissues, where they function.

If the tissues become damaged or invaded, leukocytes are capable of secreting over 100 different protein messengers known collectively as cytokines. Cytokines regulate host cell growth and function in both specific and non-specific defences. Secretion of cytokines can trigger a number of responses. Some cytokines are chemokines (chemoattractants). Once secreted these chemokines attract phagocytes (non-specific) and T cells (specific) to the site of injury. This stimulates an inflammatory response as well as an immune response.

CLONAL SELECTION THEORY

The body has a vast array of lymphocytes, each with a single type of membrane receptor specific for one antigen. When a receptor is activated by the binding of an antigen, the lymphocyte repeatedly divides, resulting in a clonal population of lymphocytes.

Clonal selection theory states that each antigen-reactive B cell or T cell has only a single type of antigen-specific receptor on its surface. When stimulated by interaction with a specific antigen, each cell is capable of dividing, making a copy of itself. The antigen-driven B and T cells continue to divide, resulting in multiple copies (or clones). Because of the infinite variety of antigens available, a large number of antigen-reactive cells are available in the body and each cell is capable of expanding into an antigen-reactive clone. However, antigen-reactive cells must avoid interactions and subsequent immune reactions with *self*-antigens in the host.

T AND B LYMPHOCYTES

Lymphocytes respond specifically to antigens on foreign cells, cells infected by pathogens and toxins released by pathogens. Lymphocytes are the essential cells in specific immune defences. Lymphocytes must recognise the specific foreign matter to be attacked. *Any* foreign molecule that can trigger a specific immune response against itself or the cell bearing it is termed an antigen.

T Lymphocytes

One group of T lymphocytes destroy infected cells by inducing apoptosis. Another group of T lymphocytes secrete cytokines that activate B lymphocytes and phagocytes. T lymphocytes mature in the thymus. T cells consist of two major subsets: cytotoxic T cells and helper T cells.

Cytotoxic T cells are attack cells. They travel to the location of their target, bind to them via antigens on the target and, following activation, they directly kill the target via secreted chemicals. Responses mediated by cytotoxic T cells are directed against the body's own cells, where these have become cancerous or infected.

There are several mechanisms of target cell killing by activated cytotoxic T cells. One of the most important is by apoptosis. Apoptosis is programmed cell death – the infected cell is instructed to kill itself. Within the infected cell, endogenous enzymes are activated that break down the cell nucleus and its DNA, as well as other cell organelles. Importantly, the cell membrane is not destroyed, so when the cell dies its contents are not dispersed. Instead the cell sends out chemical messengers that attract neighbouring phagocytic cells to engulf and digest the dying cell. Helper T cells facilitate the activation of both B cells and cytotoxic T cells. Helper T cells must combine with an antigen and become activated. Once activated they secrete cytokines that act on B cells and cytotoxic T cells that have also bound to antigens. B cells and cytotoxic T cells cannot function properly unless they are stimulated by cytokines produced by helper T cells.

B lymphocytes

Each B lymphocyte clone produces a specific antibody molecule that will recognise a specific antigen surface molecule on a pathogen or a toxin. Antigen–antibody complexes may inactivate a pathogen or toxin or render it more susceptible to phagocytosis. In other cases the antigen–antibody complex stimulates a response that results in cell lysis.

B cells mature in the bone marrow. All new generations of B cells are derived from and are identical to their parent cells – hence they are all clones. On activation, B cells differentiate into plasma cells, which secrete antibodies. The antibodies combine with a specific antigen and guide an attack that eliminates the antigens or the cells bearing them. The antibodies bind to the antigen on the surface of the cell, but they do not directly kill the cell. Instead, they link the target cell to the actual killing mechanism.

Antibodies can act as opsonins – they can link a phagocyte to an antigen, which then triggers phagocytosis. In other cases, antibodies can activate the classical complement pathway. This results in the production of chemicals that make the cell membrane 'leaky', causing cell lysis. Antibody-mediated responses are the major defence against bacteria, viruses and other microbes in the extracellular fluid, and against toxic molecules.

Recognition of Self and non-self

T lymphocytes have specific surface proteins that allow them to distinguish between the surface molecules of the body's own cells and cells with foreign molecules on their surface. Failure in regulation of the immune system leads to an immune response to self cells (autoimmune disease). Allergy is a hypersensitive response to an antigen that is normally harmless.

While T cells are maturing, their antigen receptors are tested for potential self-reactivity. For the most part, T lymphocytes bearing receptors for molecules already present in the body are either rendered non-functional or are destroyed by apoptosis – thus the body *normally* has no mature lymphocytes that react against self components. The immune system exhibits self-tolerance. Failure of self-tolerance can lead to autoimmune disease.

Major histocompatibility complex (MHC) are molecules that mark body cells as 'self'. T lymphocytes have specific receptors that can recognise MHC and therefore recognise cells that belong to the body. Sometimes the body loses tolerance for self, this then leads to autoimmune disease. Autoimmune disease is caused by an inappropriate immune attack triggered by the body's own proteins acting as antigens. The immune attack, mediated by auto-antibodies and self-reactive T cells, is directed specifically against the body's own cells that contain these proteins. Allergy refers to diseases in which immune responses to environmental antigens cause inflammation and damage to the body itself. Antigens that cause allergies are called allergens. Most allergens are relatively or completely harmless: it is the immune response to them that causes damage. Allergy is a result of the immune system going wrong.

Antigen-presenting Cells

When pathogens infect tissue, some phagocytes capture the pathogen and display fragments of its antigens on their surface. These antigen-presenting cells activate the production of clones of T lymphocytes, which move to the site of infection under the direction of cytokines. B lymphocytes activated by antigen-presenting cells and T lymphocytes produce clones of B lymphocytes that secrete antibodies into the lymph and blood, from where they make their way to the infected area.

After a microbe or other non-cellular antigen has been phagocytosed by a macrophage it is partially broken down into smaller fragments. These fragments bind to MHC class II proteins, which are then transported to and displayed on the plasma membrane. The antigen fragments are presented to T lymphocytes (antigen presentation). The antigenic binding of the antigen presenting cell (APC) to the T lymphocyte causes the T lymphocyte to proliferate and differentiate into a clone of activated helper T cells. These secrete cytokines, which recruit more lymphocytes to the area of infection. The arriving lymphocytes secrete more cytokines which stimulate B lymphocytes to produce large quantities B lymphocyte clones, which produce antibodies that are then secreted into the lymph and blood, making their way to the infected area.

Memory Cells (Immunological Memory)

Some T and B lymphocytes produced in response to antigens by clonal selection survive long term as memory cells. A secondary exposure to the same antigen rapidly gives rise to a new clone of lymphocytes, producing a rapid and greater immunological response.

Once a lymphocyte is activated to divide and differentiate it forms two clones of cells. One clone contains a large number of effector cells – short-lived cells that combat the antigen. The other clone consists of memory cells, long-lived cells bearing receptors specific for the same antigen. This antigen-driven cloning of lymphocytes is called clonal selection. The primary immune response (the first time the body is exposed to an antigen) takes 10–17 days from initial exposure until selected lymphocytes generate the maximum effector cell response. During this time the effected individual may become ill. On re-exposure to the same antigen some time later, it takes only 2–7 days to produce a response of greater magnitude and which lasts for a prolonged period of time – this is the secondary immune response.

Memory cells are poised to proliferate and differentiate rapidly when they meet the same antigen. The antibodies produced during the secondary immune response have a greater affinity for the antigen compared to those produced in the primary immune response.

IMMUNOLOGY IN ALLERGIC DISEASE

Allergy represents an exaggerated immunologic response to an otherwise innocuous agent, which causes harm to the host. The inciting agent is known as the allergen. There are four types of hypersensitivity reactions, which were originally characterized by Gell and Combs.

- *Type I:* Immediate IgE mediated hypersensitivity causes rapid degranulation of mast cells with pro-inflammatory cytokines. IgE binds to mast cells via a high affinity Fc receptor. Characterized by early phase, within minutes, and late phase, hours after initial response. Examples include allergic rhinitis, food allergy, and allergic or atopic asthma.
- *Type II:* Antibody mediated, in which antibodies bind to cells and causes damage or impairment of function. Examples include transfusion reactions, hemolytic anemias, hyperacute graft rejection Myasthenia Gravis and Goodpasture's syndrome.
- *Type III:* Immune complex mediated occurs when IgG or IgM binds with antigens, and the complexes are deposited in tissues, especially small vessels. Once in the tissues, damage occurs secondary to complement activation. Examples include serum sickness, glomerulonephritis, and arthritis.
- *Type IV:* T-cell mediated (delayed hypersensitivity), on first exposure, T cell is sensitized. On subsequent exposures, the allergen is detected on the surface of target cells and these cells are lysed by T cells. Examples include contact dermatitis, granulomatous diseases.

Allergic diseases important to the otolaryngologist are allergic rhinitis and food allergy, both of these are IgE mediated (type I). Early phase ranges from a minimal wheal and flare reaction to anaphylaxis. The response is characterized by vasodilation, vascular leakage, smooth muscle spasm and glandular secretions. These changes occur within 5 to 30 minutes and tend to subside within 60 minutes. Late phase reactions occur 2 to 8 hours after initial exposure and last for several days. Migration of eosinophils, neutrophils, basophils, and CD4+ T cells occurs and mucosal tissue damage also occurs.

CELLS IMPORTANT FOR ALLERGIC RESPONSE

B cells are the only lymphocytes that can produce antibodies. They mature in the bone marrow, and are responsible for humoral immunity. They produce IgA, IgD, IgE, IgG and IgM antibodies. IgA is a dimer that is predominantly found in secretions. IgD is produced by naïve B cells, and may be involved in antigen-induced lymphocyte proliferation.

IgE is found in immediate hypersensitivity and helminthic infections. IgG is the major antibody of secondary responses. It is active against viruses, bacteria, and fungi, the only immunoglobulin that crosses the placenta, and fixes complement by the classic pathway. IgM is a pentamer and the predominant antibody in the early immune response. Naïve B cells produce IgM and IgD, and undergo isotype class switching under the influence of T cells (T_H2) and certain antigens.

T cells travel from the bone marrow and mature in the thymus. They recognize peptide fragments of foreign proteins bound to self-major histocompatibilty complex (MHC) in other cells in the body. T helper cells (CD4+) recognize antigens found on MHC class II molecules on antigen presenting cells. TH1 cells are involved in phagocyte mediated defences against intracellular microbial infections. TH2 cells secrete IL-4, IL-5, IL-9, IL-10, and IL-13. TH2 cells down regulate TH1 cells, and induce B cell isotype switching. Catalytic T lymphocytes (CD8+) recognize antigens on MHC I molecules. Antigen presenting cells include monocytes, macrophages, dendritic cells, and B cells. Process antigens and present peptides on their cell surface via MHC molecules that activate T cells.

Mast Cells and Basophils are the major effector of type I mediated hypersensitivity. IgE cross-links these cells causing rapid degranulation of their contents. Activation of these cells leads to release of chemokines by three different pathways. 1) immediate release of histamine, heparin, proteases, and TNF alpha. This leads to vasodilatation and leaky vessels, as well as changes in the endothelium that allows migration other inflammatory cells. 2) enzymatic modification of arachidonic acid into prostaglandins and leukotrienes, within 1 or 2 hours. 3) Synthesis and secretion of IL-3, IL-4, IL-5, and GM-CSF, which recruit other inflammatory cells and are responsible for the late phase of an allergy attack.

ALLERGIC CASCADE

The immune system is very specific and goal oriented. Although you may beallergic to a number of substances, allergic reactions are directed at specific allergens. For example, you may be allergic to Bermuda grass, but not oysters. At times, however, two or more foreign substances might appear similar in nature to the immune system, which may mistake one for the other and react to both. For example, if you are allergic to birch trees, your immune system may also react to apples or other fruits, which it mistakes for birch pollen. These cross-reactions occur because of similar allergens that are produced by a variety of plants. The allergic response, however, is by no means vague or ill-defined. It is a definite, vigourous attack aimed, unfortunately, at harmless agents. The end result is well-defined symptoms and disorders.

The deeper our understanding of the intricate nature of the allergic reaction, the more likely we are to find more effective treatments. We need to look more closely at the chain of events from the initial response to allergens to the many symptoms that may result. Although misguided, it is an efficient, well-orchestrated, and potentially explosive sequence of cellular and chemical interactions. This is the so-called "allergic cascade."

The "Players" in the Allergic Cascade

Our body's immune system is designed to constantly be on the lookout for intruders. It has the remarkable ability to distinguish between "self" and "non-self" (foreign substances, which it tirelessly protects us from). Let us look more closely at this complex process. Take for example an exposure to ragweed pollen.

Once in the body, the ragweed pollen is engulfed by the immune system's scouts, the so-called Antigen Preventing Cells or APC's. These APC's slice up the ragweed pollen into small fragments, which then combine with special proteins in the cell, called human leukocyte antigens or HLA's. HLA's function like a guideline to help the body distinguish "self" from "non-self." When combined with the HLAs, the fragments become visible to a key player in the allergic cascade (the lymphocytes), which recognizes them as foreign. This ragweed pollen fragment-HLA combination is exposed on the surface of the APC's in full view of these specialized white blood cells. Before we review details of how the various players in the allergic cascade fulfill their roles, let's note these basic concepts of types of important cells and messenger proteins of the immune reaction:

The term white blood cells or leukocytes is derived from Greek words "leukos" meaning white and "cytes" meaning cells. The white blood cells are essential to the immune system and include the monocytes, macrophages, neutrophils, and lymphocytes. Lymphocytes are white blood cells that play a key role in both immunity andallergy.

They are divided into two types, the T and B lymphocytes. Each type is responsible for a particular branch of the immune system. It is the duty of the T-lymphocytes to be ready to directly shift into action to attack foreign substances (cell-mediated immunity). Some T-lymphocytes are experts at "killing" (cytotoxic or killer T cells) while others assist the immune response and are termed "helper" cells (TH cells). The TH cells are further divided into TH1 (infection fighters) and TH2 (allergy promoters), depending on the proteins they release. The partners of the T-lymphocytes are the B-lymphocytes. B-lymphocytes are tiny antibody factories that produce antibodies to help destroy foreign substances when stimulated to do so by the TH cells.

Basophils and eosinophils are other white blood cells that play an important role in allergy. T cells often call these cells into action in allergic conditions. Blood levels of eosinophils are commonly elevated in people with asthmaand other allergic diseases. Cytokines are a diverse group of proteins that are released by lymphocytes and macrophages in response to an injury or activation, such as by an allergen. They act as chemical signals that "step up" or "step down" the immune reaction.

Lymphocytes - T's & B's

Lymphocytes are part of the white blood cell family and consist of T and B varieties. Each T lymphocyte, or T cell, is like a specially trained detective. The T cell examines the evidence that is exposed by the APC. When specific T cells come into contact with the ragweed pollen fragment on the APC and recognize it as foreign, an army of specialized T cells called "helper" cells (actually TH2 cells) is activated, thus releasing chemicals (cytokines) that stimulate B lymphocytes. B lymphocytes produce IgE antibodies that bind to the allergens (such as the pollen fragment).

Once the IgE is produced, it specifically recognizes the ragweed pollen and will recognize it on future exposure. The balance between allergy-promoting TH2 cells and infection-fighting TH1 cells has recently been found to be a critical component of our immune system. Whereas allergy reactions involve large numbers of TH2 cells, infections generate an army of TH1 cells, which then release chemicals that help destroy microbes.

Allergy and asthma rates have been increasing in recent decades. One currently favoured theory explaining the increase is that it is a consequence of inadequately "geared up" human immune systems because of the relatively sterilized environment of modern man, possibly due to antibiotics and vaccinations! This has been referred to as the "hygiene hypothesis." What this concept implies is that the immune systems of individuals who have been exposed to sufficient microbes make TH1 cells when stimulated. But, if an individual's immune system is inadequately stimulated to produce TH1 cells by exposure to microbes, it will instead lean towards the allergy-producing system and make TH2 cells. A tendency towards allergic reactions is the result.

Although this appears complicated, an understanding of the different lymphocyte responses is important in treating allergies. Ideally, we would like to respond to ragweed pollen with TH1 lymphocytes and not TH2 lymphocytes, which promote allergic reactions and produce IgE in large amounts. Allergic individuals summon a large number of TH2 cells in response to allergens, whereas non-allergic people do not.

Finally, the tendency to develop allergic conditions (*i.e.*, to develop strong TH2 responses to allergens) is thought to be partially inherited from our parents. At birth, there seems to be a balance between the infection-fighting TH1 cells and the allergy-promoting TH2 cells. Current thinking is that allergy develops after birth when a child is exposed to certain substances in the environment. The immune system is stimulated by these exposures so that the scales are now tipped towards the production of allergy-promoting TH2 cells. They are especially tipped towards allergy promotion in individuals that have inherited the genetic tendency from their parents.

Mast Cells and Basophils

Mast cells and basophils are the next key players in the allergic cascade. They are volatile cells with potentially explosive behaviour. Mast cells reside in tissues while basophils are found in the blood. Each of these cells has over 100,000 receptor sites for IgE, which binds on their surfaces. The binding of IgE to these cells acts like the fuse on a bomb. The cells are now sensitized or primed with the IgE.

When this allergic or sensitized individual is exposed to ragweed pollen again, the IgE is ready to bind to this pollen. When this occurs, the mast cells and basophils are activated and explosively release a number of chemicals that ultimately produce the allergic reaction we can see and feel. Wherever these chemicals are released in the body will display the allergy symptoms. In the ragweed pollen example, when the mast cells are activated in the nose by exposure to the pollen, the release of chemicals will likely result in sneezing, nasal congestion, and a runny nose - the typical symptoms of hay fever. Once sensitized, mast cells and basophils can remain ready to ignite with IgE for months or even years!

Chemical Mediators

Each mast cell and basophil may contain over 1000 tiny packets (granules). Each of these granules holds more than 30 allergy chemicals, called chemical mediators. Many of these chemical mediators are already prepared and are released from the granules as they burst in an allergic response. The most important of these chemical mediators is histamine. Once released into the tissues or blood stream, histamine attaches to histamine receptors (H1 receptors) that are present on the surface of most cells. This attachment results in certain effects on the blood vessels, mucous glands, and bronchial tubes. These effects cause typical allergic symptoms such as swelling, sneezing, and itching of the nose, throat, and roof of the mouth.

Some chemical mediators are not formed until 5 to 30 minutes after activation of the mast cells or basophils. The most prominent of these are the leukotrienes. Leukotriene D4 is 10 times more potent than histamine. Its effects are similar to those of histamine, but leukotriene D4 also attracts other cells to tarea, thereby aggravating the inflammation.

Allergy Facts

- Leukotrienes were initially discovered in 1938 and were called the "slow reacting substances of anaphylaxis (SRS-A)." Forty years later, Samuelsen in Sweden identified them as playing an important role in allergic inflammation.
- Recently, a new family of medicines, called leukotriene modifiers, have been found to be helpful in treating asthma. Examples are Singulair (monlelukast) and Accolate (zafirlukast).

The other group of inflammation-causing chemical mediators that form after mast cell stimulation is the prostaglandins. Prostaglandin D2, in particular, is a very potent contributor to the inflammation of the lung airways (bronchial tubes) in allergic asthma.

What are Cytokines?

Cytokines are small proteins that can either step-up or step-down the immune response. One of the cytokines, interleukin 4 (IL4), is essential for the production of IgE. Interleukin 5 (IL5) and others are important in attracting other cells, particularly eosinophils, which then promote inflammation. This spectrum of cytokines is also released by the TH2 lymphocytes, thus further promoting allergic inflammation.

The "Early Phase" of an Allergic Reaction

We have seen how the first encounter with ragweed pollen sensitizes the body with the help of lymphocytes and results in the IgE coating of the mast cells and basophils. Subsequent exposure results in the immediate release of the chemical mediators that cause the various symptoms of allergy. This process is the "early phase" of the allergic reaction. It can occur within seconds or minutes of exposure to an allergen. This is also known as an immediate hypersensitivity reaction, which in this case is to the ragweed pollen allergen.

In the context of allergy, hypersensitivity refers to a condition in a previously exposed person in which tissue inflammation results from an immune reaction upon re- exposure to an allergen sensitizer.

The "late Phase" of an Allergic Reaction

About 50 per cent of the time, the allergic reaction progresses into a "late phase." This "late phase" occurs about 4 to 6 hours after the exposure. In the late phase reaction, tissues become red and swollen due to the arrival of other cells to the area, including the eosinophils, neutrophils, and lymphocytes. Cytokines that are released by the mast cells and basophils act as tiny messengers to call these other cells to the area of inflammation. Additional cytokines are released by the TH2 lymphocytes and they attract even more of these cells of inflammation.

The eosinophils appear to be particularly troublesome cells of inflammation. Eosinophils evolved to defend the body against parasites, much like IgE. Nevertheless, they are often present in great numbers in the blood of people with allergies. When they arrive at the site of the allergic reaction, they release chemicals that cause damage to the tissues and continue to promote the inflammation. Repeated episodes of this "late phase" reaction contribute to chronic allergic symptoms and make the tissues even more sensitive to subsequent exposure!

The Consequences of the Allergic Cascade

Now that we understand how the allergic reaction develops, let's review the various changes that occur in the body as a result of these early and late phase reactions. When histamine is injected into the skin, a technique used in diagnosing allergies, a reaction that can mimic an allergic reaction occurs. The histamine injection prompts the development of a pale, central swollen area that is caused by fluid leaking out of local blood vessels into the adjacent tissues. This localized reaction is called a "wheal."

A red "flare," which sometimes has a warm feeling due to inflammation, surrounds this "wheal." Itching occurs because histamine irritates the nerve endings in the skin. This early or immediate response peaks at about 15 minutes and fades within 90 minutes. Sometimes, the immediate effects are followed by a late phase reaction that occurs about 4 to 6 hours later and can last up to a day.

Allergens, such as ragweed pollen, react with the tissues lining the inner surfaces (membranes) of the nose and eyes, thereby stimulating mast cells to release chemical mediators, including histamine. The chemical mediators cause a leakage of fluid and the production of mucous, causing a runny nose, itching, and sneezing.

The late reaction also causes the tissues to swell and the nose to become congested. In the lungs, exposure to inhaled allergens causes wheezing, shortness of breath, and coughing within seconds or minutes. These symptoms tend to subside after about an hour. However, after about 4 hours, the late phase reaction can cause a worsening of shortness of breath, wheezing, and coughing. This phase can last for up to 24 hours. The late phase reaction involves an influx of a variety of inflammatory cells to the affected area (eosinophils, neutrophils, lymphocytes, and mast cells) and, if repeated inhalations of allergens cause recurrent reactions, reactions may merge into each other leading to chronic or persistent allergic asthma. Lastly, allergens can be absorbed into the bloodstream and travel to many sites (including the nose, lungs, throat, skin, and digestive tract), causing multiple symptoms that are typical of a severe allergic reaction (anaphylaxis). Blood vessel dilation may occur throughout the body causing a drop in blood pressure and shock. Although rare, this type of anaphylactic reaction can be caused by medications, insect venoms, and foods.

Understanding The Allergic Cascade

How can we put this new understanding of allergic reaction to good use? By looking closely at the complex steps involved in this chain of events, scientists have been able to find new and innovative treatments for common and troublesome allergic illnesses. The most basic, and best, approach to caring for allergies is avoidance of the substances causing them, the allergens. Some allergens such as pet dander, foods, and medications are relatively easy to avoid. However, many other allergens, such as dust mites, molds, and pollens are more difficult to evade. Measures to reduce exposure to them, however, are still essential for the optimal treatment of allergies.

The most convenient approach to the treatment of allergies involves taking various medications. A classic example of an allergic medication is the standard antihistamine. The importance of histamine in allergic disease is illustrated by the effectiveness of antihistamines (medically termed H1 receptor blockers) in preventing certain allergic symptoms. They are effective in curtailing itching, sneezing, and runny nose.

However, the more severe allergic reactions and symptoms of asthma require different treatments. Anti-inflammatory medications, such as steroids and leukotriene antagonists, may be required. Medications that widen the airways through the lungs (bronchial dilators) have also been a mainstay in the treatment of asthma and are particularly useful in controlling the immediate or early phase reaction. Current research is aimed at finding medications that are targeted at specific steps in the allergic cascade.

The last approach to the management of allergies attempts to interfere with the allergic antibody immune response. Allergy shots (immunotherapy) involve desensitizing a patient by injecting increasing amounts of the allergens to which the person is allergic. Over time, the immune system becomes less reactive to these allergens, generates less IgE in response to them, and becomes more tolerant upon re-exposure to them.

EFFECTOR MECHANISMS IN ALLERGIC REACTIONS

Allergic reactions are triggered when allergens cross-link preformed IgE bound to the high-affinity receptor FcåRI on mast cells.Mast cells line the body surfaces and serve to alert the immune system to local infection. Once activated, they induce inflammatory reactions by secreting chemical mediators stored in preformed granules, and by synthesizing leukotrienes and cytokines after activation occurs. In allergy, they provoke very unpleasant reactions to innocuous antigens that are not associated with invading pathogens that need to be expelled. The consequences of IgE-mediated mast-cell activation depend on the dose ofantigen and its route of entry; symptoms range from the irritating sniffles of hay fever when pollen is inhaled, to the life-threatening circulatory collapse that occurs in systemic anaphylaxis (Fig. 12.9). The immediate allergic reaction caused by mast-cell degranulation is followed by a more sustained inflammation, known as the late-phase response. This late response involves the recruitment of other effector cells, notably T_H2 lymphocytes, eosinophils, and basophils, which contribute significantly to the immunopathology of an allergic response.

IgE is Cell-bound and Engages Effector Mechanisms of the Immune System

Most antibodies are found in body fluids and engage effector cells, through receptors specific for the Fc constant regions, only after binding specific antigen through the antibody variable regions. IgE, however, is an exception as it is captured by the high-affinityFcå receptor in the absence of bound antigen. This means that IgE is mostly found fixed in the tissues on mast cells that bear this receptor, as well as on circulating basophils and activated eosinophils. The ligation of cell-bound IgE antibody by specific antigen triggers activation of these cells at the site of antigen entry into the tissues. The release of inflammatory lipid mediators, cytokines, and chemokines at sites of IgE-triggered reactions results in the recruitment of eosinophils and basophils to augment the type I response.

There are two types of IgE-binding Fc receptor. The first, FcåRI, is a high-affinity receptor of the immunoglobulin superfamily that binds IgE on mast cells, basophils, and activated eosinophils. When the cell-bound IgE antibody is cross-linked by a specific antigen, FcåRI transduces an activating signal. High levels of IgE, such as those that exist in subjects with allergic diseases or parasite infections, can result in a marked increase in FcåRI on the surface of mast cells, enhanced sensitivity of such cells to activation by low concentrations of specific antigen, and markedly increased IgE-dependent release of chemical mediators and cytokines.

The second IgE receptor, FcåRII, usually known as CD23, is a C-type lectin and is structurally unrelated to FcåRI; it binds IgE with low affinity. CD23 is present on many different cell types, including B cells, activated T cells, monocytes, eosinophils, platelets,follicular dendritic cells, and some thymic epithelial cells.

This receptor was thought to be crucial for the regulation of IgE antibodylevels; however, knockout mouse strains lacking the CD23 gene show no major abnormality in the development of polyclonal IgE responses. However the CD23 knockout mice have demonstrated a role for CD23 in enhancing the antibody response to a specificantigen in the presence of that same antigen complexed with IgE. This antigen-specific, IgE-mediated enhancement of antibody responses fails to occur in mice lacking the CD23 gene. This demonstrates a role for CD23 on antigen-presenting cells in thecapture of antigen by specific IgE.

Mast Cells Reside in Tissues and Orchestrate Allergic Reactions

Mast cells were described by Ehrlich in the mesentery of rabbits and named *Mastzellen* ('fattened cells'). Like basophils, mast cells contain granules rich in acidic proteoglycans that take up basic dyes. However, in spite of this resemblance, and the similar range of mediators stored in these basophilic granules, mast cells are derived from a different myeloid lineage than basophils and eosinophils. Mast cells are highly specialized cells, and are prominent residents of mucosal and epithelial tissues in the vicinity of small blood vessels and postcapillary venules, where they are well placed to guard against invading pathogens.

Mast cells are also found in subendothelial connective tissue. They home to tissues as agranular cells; their final differentiation, accompanied by granule formation, occurs after they have arrived in the tissues. The major growth factor for mast cells is stem-cell factor (SCF), which acts on the cell-surface receptor c-Kit. Mice with defective c-Kit lack differentiated mast cells and cannot make IgE-mediated inflammatory responses. This shows that such responses depend almost exclusively on mast cells.

Mast cells express FcåRI constitutively on their surface and are activated when antigens cross-link IgE bound to these receptors. Degranulation occurs within seconds, releasing a variety of preformed inflammatory mediators. Among these are histamine—a short-lived vasoactive amine that causes an immediate increase in local blood flow and vessel permeability—and enzymes such as mast-cell chymase, tryptase, and serine esterases. These enzymes can in turn activate matrix metalloproteinases, which break down tissue matrix proteins, causing tissue destruction. Large amounts of tumor necrosis factor (TNF)-á are also released by mast cells after activation. Some comes from stores in mast-cell granules; some is newly synthesized by the activated mast cells themselves. TNF-á activates endothelial cells, causing increased expression of adhesion molecules, which promotes the influx of inflammatory leukocytes and lymphocytes into tissues.

On activation, mast cells synthesize and release chemokines, lipid mediators such as leukotrienes and platelet-activating factor (PAF), and additional cytokines such as IL-4 and IL-13 which perpetuate the T_H2 response. These mediators contribute to both the acute and the chronic inflammatory responses. The lipid mediators, in particular, act rapidly to cause smooth muscle contraction, increased vascular permeability, and mucus secretion, and also induce the influx and activation of leukocytes, which contribute to the late-phase response. The lipid mediators derive from membrane phospholipids, which are cleaved to release the precursor molecule arachidonic acid. This molecule can be modified by two pathways to give rise to prostaglandins, thromboxanes, and leukotrienes. The leukotrienes, especially C4, D4, and E4, are important in sustaining inflammatory responses in the tissues. Many anti-inflammatory drugs are inhibitors of arachidonic acid metabolism. Aspirin, for example, is an inhibitor of the enzyme cyclooxygenase and blocks the production of prostaglandins.

IgE-mediated activation of mast cells thus orchestrates an important inflammatory cascade that is amplified by the recruitment of eosinophils, basophils, and T_H2 lymphocytes. The physiological importance of this reaction is as a defence mechanism against certain types of infection. In allergy, however, the acute and chronic inflammatory reactions triggered by mast-cell activation have important pathophysiological consequences, as seen in the diseases associated with allergic responses to environmental antigens.

Eosinophils are Normally Under Tight Control

Eosinophils are granulocytic leukocytes that originate in bone marrow. They are so called because their granules, which contain arginine-rich basic proteins, are coloured bright orange by the acidic stain eosin. Only very small numbers of these cells are normally present in the circulation; most eosinophils are found in tissues, especially in the connective tissue immediately underneath respiratory, gut, and urogenital epithelium, implying a likely role for these cells in defence against invading organisms. Eosinophils have two kinds of effector function.

First, on activation they release highly toxic granule proteins and free radicals, which can kill microorganisms and parasites but can also cause significant tissue damage in allergic reactions. Second, activation induces the synthesis of chemical mediators such as prostaglandins, leukotrienes, and cytokines, which amplify the inflammatory response by activating epithelial cells, and recruiting and activating more eosinophils and leukocytes.

The activation and degranulation of eosinophils is strictly regulated, as their inappropriate activation would be very harmful to the host. The first level of control acts on the production of eosinophils by the bone marrow. Few eosinophils are produced in the absence of infection or other immune stimulation.

But when T_H2 cells are activated, cytokines such as IL-5 are released that increase the production of eosinophils in the bone marrow and their release into the circulation. However, transgenic animals overexpressing IL-5 have increased numbers of eosinophils (eosinophilia) in the circulation but not in their tissues, indicating that migration of eosinophils from the circulation into tissues is regulated separately, by a second set of controls. The key molecules in this case are CC chemokines. Most of these cause chemotaxis of several types of leukocyte, but two are specific for eosinophils and have been named eotaxin 1 and eotaxin 2.

The eotaxin receptor on eosinophils, CCR3, is a member of the chemokine family of receptors. This receptor also binds the CC chemokines MCP-3, MCP-4, and RANTES, which also induce eosinophil chemotaxis. The eotaxins and these other CC chemokines also activate eosinophils. Identical or similar chemokines also stimulate mast cells and basophils. For example, eotaxin attracts basophils and causes their degranulation, and MCP-1, which binds to CCR2, similarly activates mast cells in both the presence or absence of antigen. MCP-1 can also promote the differentiation of naive T_H0 cells to T_H2 cells; T_H2 cells also carry CCR3 and migrate towards eotaxin. These findings show that families of chemokines, as well as cytokines, can coordinate certain kinds of immune response.

A third set of controls regulates the state of eosinophil activation. In their non-activated state, eosinophils do not express high-affinity IgE receptors and have a high threshold for release of their granule contents. After activation by cytokines and chemokines, this threshold drops, FcåRI is expressed, and the number of Fcã receptors and complement receptors on the cell surface also increases. The eosinophil is now primed to carry out its effector activity, for example degranulation in response to antigen that cross-links specific IgE bound to FcåRI on the eosinophil surface.

The potential of eosinophils to cause tissue injury is illustrated by rare syndromes due to abnormally large numbers of eosinophils in the blood (hypereosinophilia). These syndromes are sometimes seen in association with T-cell lymphomas, in which unregulatedIL-5 secretion drives a marked increase in the numbers of circulating eosinophils. The clinical manifestations of hypereosinophilia are damage to the endocardium and to nerves, leading to heart failure and neuropathy, both thought to be caused by the toxic effects of eosinophil granule proteins.

Eosinophils and Basophils Cause Inflammation

In a local allergic reaction, mast-cell degranulation and T_H2 activation cause eosinophils to accumulate in large numbers and to become activated. Their continued presence is characteristic of chronic allergic inflammation and they are thought to be major contributors to tissue damage.

Basophils are also present at the site of an inflammatory reaction. Basophils share a common stem-cell precursor with eosinophils; growth factors for basophils are very similar to those for eosinophils and include IL-3, IL-5, and GM-CSF. There is evidence for reciprocal control of the maturation of the stem-cell population into basophils or eosinophils. For example, transforming growth factor (TGF)-â in the presence of IL-3 suppresses eosinophil differentiation and enhances that of basophils. Basophils are normally present in very low numbers in the circulation and seem to have a similar role to eosinophils in defence against pathogens. Like eosinophils, they are recruited to the sites of allergic reactions. Basophils express FcåRI on the cell surface and, on activation by cytokines or antigen, they release histamine and IL-4 from the basophilic granules after which they are named.

Eosinophils, mast cells, and basophils can interact with each other. Eosinophil degranulation releases major basic protein, which in turn causes degranulation of mast cells and basophils. This effect is augmented by any of the cytokines that affect eosinophil and basophil growth, differentiation, and activation, such as IL-3, IL-5, and GM-CSF.

An Allergic Reaction is Divided into an Immediate Response

The inflammatory response after IgE-mediated mast-cell activation occurs as an immediate reaction, starting within seconds, and a late reaction, which takes up to 8–12 hours to develop. These reactions can be distinguished clinically. The immediate reaction is due to the activity of histamine, prostaglandins, and other preformed or rapidly synthesized mediators that cause a rapid increase in vascular permeability and the contraction of smooth muscle. The late-phase reaction is caused by the induced synthesis and release of mediators including leukotrienes, chemokines, and cytokines from the activated mast cells.

These recruit other leukocytes, including eosinophils and T_H2 lymphocytes, to the site of inflammation. Although the late-phase reaction is clinically less marked than the immediate response, it is associated with a second phase of smooth muscle contraction, sustained edema, and the development of one of the cardinal features of allergic asthma: airway hyperreactivity to non-specific bronchoconstrictor stimuli such as histamine and methacholine.

The late-phase reaction is an important cause of much serious long-term illness, as for example in chronic asthma. This is because the late reaction induces the recruitment of inflammatory leukocytes, especially eosinophils and T_H2 lymphocytes, to the site of the allergen-triggered mast-cell response. This late response can easily convert into a chronic inflammatory response ifantigen persists and stimulates allergen-specific T_H2 cells, which in turn promote eosinophilia and further IgE production.

The Clinical Effects of Allergic Reactions

When reexposure to allergen triggers an allergic reaction, the effects are focused on the site at which mast-cell degranulation occurs. In the immediate response, the preformed mediators released are short-lived, and their potent effects on blood vessels and smooth muscles are therefore confined to the vicinity of the activated mast cell.

The more sustained effects of the late-phase response are also focused on the site of initial allergen-triggered activation, and the particular anatomy of this site may determine how readily the inflammation can be resolved. Thus, the clinical syndrome produced by an allergic reaction depends critically on three variables: the amount of allergen-specific IgE present; the route by which the allergen is introduced; and the dose of allergen.

If an allergen is introduced directly into the bloodstream or is rapidly absorbed from the gut, the connective tissue mast cells associated with all blood vessels can become activated. This activation causes a very dangerous syndrome called systemic anaphylaxis (Acute Systemic Anaphylaxis, in *Case Studies in Immunology*, see Preface for details). Disseminated mast-cell activation has a variety of potentially fatal effects: the widespread increase in vascular permeability leads to a catastrophic loss of blood pressure; airways constrict, causing difficulty in breathing; and swelling of the epiglottis can cause suffocation.

This potentially fatal syndrome is called anaphylactic shock. It can occur if drugs are administered to people who have IgE specific for that drug, or after an insect bite in individuals allergic to insect venom. Some foods, for example peanuts or brazil nuts, can cause systemic anaphylaxis in susceptible individuals. This syndrome can be rapidly fatal but can usually be controlled by the immediate injection of epinephrine, which relaxes the smooth muscle and inhibits the cardiovascular effects of anaphylaxis.

The most frequent allergic reactions to drugs occur with penicillin and its relatives. In people with IgE antibodies against penicillin, administration of the drug by injection can cause anaphylaxis and even death. Great care should be taken to avoid giving a drug to patients with a past history of allergy to that drug or one that is closely related structurally. Penicillin acts as a hapten; it is a small molecule with a highly reactive â-lactam ring that is crucial for its antibacterial activity.

This ring reacts with amino groups on host proteins to form covalent conjugates. When penicillin is ingested or injected, it forms conjugates with self proteins, and the penicillin-modified self peptides can provoke a T_H2 response in some individuals.

These T_H2 cells then activate penicillin-binding B cells to produce IgE antibody to the penicillin hapten. Thus, penicillin acts both as the B-cell antigen and, by modifying self peptides, as the T-cell antigen.

When penicillin is injected intravenously into an allergic individual, the penicillin-modified proteins can cross-link IgE molecules on the mast cells and cause anaphylaxis.

Allergen Inhalation is Associated with the Development of Rhinitis and Asthma

Inhalation is the most common route of allergen entry. Many people have mild allergies to inhaled antigens, manifesting as sneezing and a runny nose. This is called allergic rhinitis, and results from the activation of mucosal mast cells beneath the nasal epithelium by allergens such as pollens that release their protein contents, which can then diffuse across the mucus membranes of the nasal passages. Allergic rhinitis is characterized by intense itching and sneezing, local edema leading to blocked nasal passages, a nasal discharge, which is typically rich in eosinophils, and irritation of the nose as a result of histamine release.

A similar reaction to airborne allergens deposited on the conjunctiva of the eye is called allergic conjunctivitis. Allergic rhinitis and conjunctivitis are commonly caused by environmental allergens that are only present during certain seasons of the year. For example, hay fever is caused by a variety of allergens, including certain grass and tree pollens. Autumnal symptoms may be caused by weed pollen, such as that of ragweed. These reactions are annoying but cause little lasting damage.

A more serious syndrome is allergic asthma, which is triggered by allergen-induced activation of submucosal mast cells in the lower airways. This leads within seconds to bronchial constriction and increased secretion of fluid and mucus, making breathing more difficult by trapping inhaled air in the lungs. Patients with allergic asthma often need treatment, and asthmatic attacks can be life-threatening.

An important feature of asthma is chronic inflammation of the airways, which is characterized by the continued presence of increased numbers of T_H2 lymphocytes, eosinophils, neutrophils, and other leukocytes.

Although allergic asthma is initially driven by a response to a specific allergen, the subsequent chronic inflammation seems to be perpetuated even in the apparent absence of further exposure to allergen. The airways become characteristically hyperreactive and factors other than reexposure to antigen can trigger asthma attacks. For example, the airways of asthmatics characteristically show hyperresponsiveness to environmental chemical irritants such as cigarette smoke and sulfur dioxide; viral or, to a lesser extent, bacterial respiratory tract infections can exacerbate the disease by inducing a T_H2-dominated local response.

Skin Allergy is Manifest as Urticaria or Chronic Eczema

The same dichotomy between immediate and delayed responses is seen in cutaneous allergic responses. The skin forms an effective barrier to the entry of most allergens but it can be breached by local injection of small amounts of allergen, for example by a stinging insect. The entry of allergen into the epidermis or dermis causes a localized allergic reaction. Local mast-cell activation in the skin leads immediately to a local increase in vascular permeability, which causes extravasation of fluid and swelling. Mast-cell activation also stimulates the release of chemicals from local nerve endings by a nerve axon reflex, causing the vasodilation of surrounding cutaneous blood vessels, which causes redness of the surrounding skin. The resulting skin lesion is called a wheal-and-flare reaction.

About 8 hours later, a more widespread and sustained edematous response appears in some individuals as a consequence of the late-phase response. A disseminated form of the wheal-and-flare reaction, known as urticaria or hives, sometimes appears when ingested allergens enter the bloodstream and reach the skin. Histamine released by mast cells activated by allergen in the skin causes large, itchy, red swellings of the skin.

Allergists take advantage of the immediate response to test for allergy by injecting minute amounts of potential allergens into the epidermal layer of the skin. Although the reaction after the administration of antigen by intraepidermal injection is usually very localized, there is a small risk of inducing systemic anaphylaxis. Another standard test for allergy is to measure levels of IgEantibody specific for a particular allergen in a sandwich ELISA.

Although acute urticaria is commonly caused by allergens, the causes of chronic urticaria, in which the urticarial rash can recur over long periods, are less well understood.

In up to a third of cases, it seems likely that chronic urticaria is an autoimmune disease caused by autoantibodies against the á chain of FcåRI. This is an example of a type II hypersensitivity reaction in which an autoantibody against a cellular receptor triggers cellular activation, in this case causing mast-cell degranulation with resulting urticaria.

A more prolonged inflammatory response is sometimes seen in the skin, most often in atopic children. They develop a persistent skin rash called eczema or atopic dermatitis (Atopic Dermatitis, in *Case Studies in Immunology*, see Preface for details), due to a chronic inflammatory response similar to that seen in the bronchial walls of patients with asthma. The etiology of eczema is not well understood. T_H2 cells and IgE are involved, and it usually clears in adolescence, unlike rhinitis and asthma, which can persist throughout life.

Allergy to Foods Causes Symptoms Limited to the gut and Systemic Reactions

When an allergen is eaten, two types of allergic response are seen. Activation of mucosal mast cells associated with the gastrointestinal tract leads to transepithelial fluid loss and smooth muscle contraction, causing diarrhea and vomiting. For reasons that are not understood, connective tissue mast cells in the dermis and subcutaneous tissues can also be activated after ingestion of allergen, presumably by allergen that has been absorbed into the bloodstream, and this results in urticaria.

Urticaria is a common reaction when penicillin is given orally to a patient who already has penicillin-specific IgE antibodies. Ingestion of food allergens can also lead to the development of generalized anaphylaxis, accompanied by cardiovascular collapse and acute asthmatic symptoms. Certain foods, most importantly peanuts, tree nuts, and shellfish, are particularly associated with this type of life-threatening response.

IgE Production or the Effector Pathways

The approaches to the treatment and prevention of allergy are set out in Fig. 12.18. Two treatments are commonly used in clinical practice—one is desensitization and the other is blockade of the effector pathways. There are also several approaches still in the experimental stage. In desensitization the aim is to shift the antibody response away from one dominated by IgE towards one dominated by IgG; the latter can bind to the allergen and thus prevent it from activating IgE-mediated effector pathways. Patients are injected with escalating doses of allergen, starting with tiny amounts. This injection schedule gradually diverts the IgE-dominated response, driven by T_H2 cells, to one driven by T_H1 cells, with the consequent downregulation of IgE production. Recent evidence shows that desensitization is also associated with a reduction in the numbers of late-phase inflammatory cells at the site of the allergic reaction. A potential complication of the desensitization approach is the risk of inducing IgE-mediated allergic responses.

An alternative, and still experimental, approach to desensitization is vaccination with peptides derived from common allergens. This procedure induces T-cell anergy, which is associated with multiple changes in the T-cell phenotype, including downregulation of cytokine production and reduced expression of the CD3:T-cell receptor complex. IgE-mediated responses are not induced by the peptides because IgE, in contrast to T cells, can only recognize the intact antigen.

A major difficulty with this approach is that an individual's responses to peptides are restricted by their MHC class II alleles; therefore, patients with different MHC class II molecules respond to different allergen-derived peptides. As the human population is outbred and expresses a wide variety of MHC class II alleles, the number of peptides required to treat all allergic individuals might be very large.

Another vaccination strategy that shows promise in experimental models of allergy is the use of oligodeoxynucleotides rich in unmethylated cytosine guanine dinucleotides (CpG) as adjuvants for desensitization regimes. These oligonucleotides mimic bacterial DNA sequences known as CpG motifs and strongly promote T_H1 responses.

The signaling pathways that enhance the IgE response in allergic disease are also potential targets for therapy. Inhibitors of IL-4, IL-5, and IL-13 would be predicted to reduce IgE responses, but redundancy between some of the activities of these cytokines might make this approach difficult to implement in practice. A second approach to manipulating the response is to give cytokines that promote T_H1-type responses. IFN-γ, IFN-α, IL-10, IL-12, and TGF-β have each been shown to reduce IL-4-stimulated IgE synthesis*in vitro*, and IFN-γ and IFN-α have been shown to reduce IgE synthesis *in vivo*. Another target for therapeutic intervention might be the high-affinity IgE receptor. An effective competitor for IgE at this receptor could prevent the binding of IgE to the surfaces of mast cells, basophils, and eosinophils. Candidate competitors include humanized anti-IgE monoclonal antibodies, which bind to IgE and block its binding to the receptor, and modified IgE Fc constructs that bind to the receptor but lack variable regions and thus cannot bind antigen. Yet another approach would be to block the recruitment of eosinophils to sites of allergic inflammation. The eotaxin receptor CCR3 is a potential target for this type of therapy. The production of eosinophils in bone marrow and their exit into the circulation might also be reduced by a blockade of IL-5 action.

The mainstays of therapy at present, however, are drugs that treat the symptoms of allergic disease and limit the inflammatory response. Anaphylactic reactions are treated with epinephrine, which stimulates the reformation of endothelial tight junctions, promotes the relaxation of constricted bronchial smooth muscle, and also stimulates the heart. Inhaled bronchodilators that act on â-adrenergic receptors to relax constricted muscle are also used to relieve acute asthma attacks.

Antihistamines that block the histamine H_1 receptor reduce the urticaria that follows histamine release from mast cells and eosinophils. Relevant H_1 receptors include those on blood vessels that cause increased permeability of the vessel wall, and those on unmyelinated nerve fibres that are thought to mediate the itching sensation.

In chronic allergic disease it is extremely important to treat and prevent the chronic inflammatory tissue injury. Topical or systemic corticosteroids are used to suppress the chronic inflammatory changes seen in asthma, rhinitis, and eczema. However, what is really needed is a means of converting the T-cell response to the allergenic peptide antigen from predominantly T_H2 to predominantly T_H1.

IGE MEDIATED HYPERSENSITIVITY

The pathogenesis of a type I hypersensitivity reaction starts with IgE antibody production, also called the sensitization phase. Antigen is presented by antigen presenting cells to CD4+ Th2 cells. The activated Th2 cells then produces a cluster of cytokines, including IL-3, IL4, IL-5, IL-13 and GM-CSF.

IL-4 is absolutely essential for turning on the IgE –producing B cells and for sustaining the development of Th2 cells. IL-3 and IL-5 promote the survival of eosinophils. IgE antibodies produced by B cells quickly attach to mast cells and basophils. When mast cells and basophils are exposed to antigen again, antigen binds to the IgE antibodies on the surface of these cells. Multivalent antigen causes cross-linking of IgE antibodies, which activates cell degranulation with discharge of preformed mediators and de novo synthesis of mediators. These mediators are responsible for the observed increased vascular permeability, increased mucus secretion, and smooth muscle contraction in the allergic reaction. These mediators also have chemotactic properties. Eosinophils, neutrophils, and monocytes are recruited and release additional waves of mediators. The recruited cells amplify and sustain the inflammatory response without additional exposure to the triggering antigen. This is the late phase reaction.

Allergic Rhinitis

Inflammation of the membrane lining the nose secondary to hypersensitivity to aeroallergens, characterized by rhinorrhea, sneezing, pruritis, congestion, post nasal drip and associated conjunctival, otologic or pharyngeal inflammation. These symptoms can be episodic, seasonal or perennial. Severity ranges from mild, to seriously debilitating with excess days of missed school or work. Risk factors include family history of atopy, serum IgE > 100 IU/ml before age six, higher socioeconomic class, exposure to aeroallergens, presence of positive allergy skin prick test.

It is important to illicit timing, severity, onset, duration, and effect on daily living. Many patients will have an idea of what triggers their symptoms and the seasonality of symptoms. Environmental questions should include home, work school/daycare exposures, and exposure to tobacco. Past nasal trauma, positive family history, current and past treatments, should al be included in history.

Physical exam includes a complete head and neck exam. Special attention is paid to the patient's general appearance. Facial pallor, allergic shiners, nasal crease, mouth breathing, and clubbing of the fingers can signify allergic rhinitis. Examine the eyes for conjunctivitis and Dennie-Morgan lines, accentuated lines or folds below the margin of the inferior eyelid. The nose may reveal polyps, enlarged turbinates, presence of mucus or purulent drainage, septal deviation or blood. The exam of the oropharynx may reveal tonsillar hypertrophy or cobblestoning. The ears must be examined for abnormalities to the middle ear, or tympanic membrane. The neck should be examined for lymphadenopathy and thyroid enlargement. Auscultation of the lungs is necessary to assess for wheezing, or other signs of asthma, and the skin should be examined for eczema, dryness, or dermatographism.

PATHOPHYSIOLOGY OF ALLERGIC RHINITIS

Atopic subjects inherit the propensity to produce IgE-mast cell lymphocyte immune responses. Exposure to low levels of aeroallergens for prolonged periods of time leads to presentation of epitopes being presented to $CD4^+$ cells by APC's. These $CD4^+$ cells then secrete IL-3, IL-4, IL-5, GM-CSF and other cytokines. This promotes proliferation of plasma cells that produce IgE, mast cells, and infiltration of nasal mucosa and eosinophilia.

Early response with continued exposure, IgE coated mast cells infiltrate the nasal mucosa, and are activated when they encounter the allergen. Mast cells release, histamine, heparin, tryptase, kinase, chymase and other chemokines. Arachidonic acid is broken down to prostaglandins and leukotrienes that stimulate leaky vessels and nasal edema, release of mucus, and dilate arteriole-venule anastomoses causing occlusion of nasal air passages. Sensory nerves are stimulated and relay sensations of nasal itching and congestion, and initiate the sneeze reflex.

Late response occurs 2 to 11 hours after initial exposure. Mast cell chemokines affect the endothelium promoting VCAM and E-selectin expression. These molecules allow circulating leukocytes to stick to the endothelium. IL-5 attracts eosinophils, neutrophils, basophils, T cells, and macrophages. Over the course of 4 to 6 hours, these cells release even more chemokines. Eosinophils release major basic protein, eosinophil cationic protein, hypochlorate, and leukotrienes, which cause inflammation and damage seen in chronic allergic reactions.

ALLERGY TESTING

Screening tests should have the following characteristics:

- Be rapid, efficient, and cost effective method to assess allergy.
- Antigens should be representative of what the patient may encounter, and should be geographically based.

Most allergic individuals will react to common antigens via *in vivo* or *in vitro* techniques. Negative result usually requires no additional testing. Positive result requires further testing of other antigens in the group or family. There may be some cross-reactivity, especially with molds. Also, they should test for 12 to 14 antigens, (pollen, mold, weeds, dust mite, animal dander)

Nasal smear used to differentiate allergic rhinitis and NARES, from other forms of rhinitis. Typically find eosinophilia, but its absence does not rule out allergic rhinitis. May find neutrophils in smear as well.

Skin testing is the most widely used form of allergy testing. 2003 AAOA guidelines for allergy testing state:

- The goal of testing is to identify antigens to which patients are symptomatically reactive and to quantify the sensitivity if immunotherapy is planned

- There are a variety of acceptable techniques:
  - Prick testing, intradermal testing, intradermal dilutional testing, and in vitro testing
- Allergy care shall be directed by a trained and competent physician who regularly participates in the care
- Members shall practice in an ethical and fiscally responsible manner

Prick/scratch testing (SPT) is a superficial skin reaction that does not penetrate dermis. It is highly specific, sensitive, convenient and safe. It does require a positive (histamine) and negative (saline) control. Disadvantages include: patient discomfort, intertester variability, and non-standaridized allergen extracts, as well as different interpretation scales.

An example of this is the multitest II. This introduces 6 to 10 antigens plus the positive and negative control using an instrument that scratches the skin. A test is positive if there is a wheal and flare reaction which is greater than or equal to the histamine control.

Intradermal testing (IT) a dilute antigen extract is injected into the dermis, and a superficial wheal forms. After ten minutes, the wheal is measured again to see if there was any progression. If the diameter of the wheal has increased by 2mm or greater, then a positive response has occurred. This causes relatively minimal patient discomfort. Disadvantages include higher risk of anaphylaxis, time intensive and possible false positive.

Intradermal dilutional testing/Set endpoint titration (IDT/SET) Intradermal testing utilizing serial dilutions to quantify degree of sensitivity to specific antigen. Very labour intensive and uncomfortable to patient due to multiple sticks. Wheal measures similar to intradermal testing. 1st dilution that causes a wheal of 2mm, with progression of this wheal by another 2mm (confirmatory wheal). This type of testing is important for determining the initial concentration used for immunotherapy.

Modified quantitative testing (MQT) a hybrid of skin prick and IDT. Skin prick determines an approximate range of sensitivity, followed by a single intradermal test to further identify the level of sensitivity and quantify the allergic response.

In Vitro testing RAST (radioallergosorbent testing) RAST is a radioimmunoassay test developed in the late 60's for the detection of specific serum IgE antibodies. Initial studies demonstrated a 96 per cent efficiency, sensitivity and specificity. The modified RAST is the form now used, introduced by Fadal and Nalebuff in 1977 with the advantages of increased test sensitivity without a loss in specificity.

Soluble allergens bound to solid phase support (paper disc) to create a stable immunosorbent media. The paper disc is incubated with the test sera, specific IgE antibody will bind to the solid phase allergen. The paper disc is then washed to remove all unbound sera and IgE. The disc is then exposed to rabbit anti-human IgE antibodies which are radiolabeled. It interacts with the Fc determinant portion on human IgE bound to the solid phase allergen. The unbound anti-IgE is washed off the disc and the disc is then quantified by a scintillation counter. This test should be used when there are contraindications to skin testing. These include children that can not tolerate skin testing, patients on antihistamines, patients with dermatographism, and those taking beta blockers (may be impossible to treat anaphylaxis).

COMPARING THE TESTS

Efficacy

Gungor et al found that skin prick testing correlates with RAST and SET 81-89 per cent of the time depending on the antigen. Skin prick testing is fast, inexpensive, and has only mild patient discomfort. However, there are false negatives, and this type of testing cannot be performed in patients who are on antihistamines.

Simons et al compared Multitest II (skin prick) to IDT. Found that patients were positive to more antigens with IDT. This may be because IDT is more sensitive or there could be more false positives. However, he did find that multitest II did correlate with the IDT endpoint. In 2006 McKay performed a retrospective chart review of patients with a positive IDT after negative skin prick test.

Certain antigens were more likely to have a positive IDT after negative skin prick (dust mite, cockroach, fulsarium rough marsh elder, and ragweed). He concluded that this could be from glycerin reaction, or true positive due to the increased sensitivity of IDT. In order to know for sure, he recommended nasal provocation testing.

2007 Peltier et al performed a prospective study using five antigens to compare MQT, SPT, and IDT. Found a 77 per cent concordance rate between MQT and IDT, wheal size from SPT is predictive of IDT endpoint, and that MQT is nearly as effective as IDT for starting doses of immunotherapy.

Cost

2003 Shah et al compared multitesting with SET (MQT) versus IDT/SET. Concluded that multitesting is a cost effective screening test. MQT can be used to find the starting doses for immunotherapy and is one third less costly and time consuming then IDT/SET alone. 2006 Seshul et al defends the use of IDT/SET on an overall cost effectiveness. With IDT, the highest dose to safely start immunotherapy is known.

Thus this is the starting dose for immunotherapy. With SPT, he found that it correlated poorly to endpoint titration. This would cause a lower starting dose, with more time and cost to reach the maintenance doses needed for successful immunotherapy.

ADJUVANT TESTING

Nasal Endoscopy allows direct visualization of nasal mucosa. It allows for accurate, site specific nasal smears and is important in ruling out other nasal pathology. Acoustic rhinometry measures cross sectional area and intranasal cavity volume by bouncing sound signals on the nasal structures. Measurements are taken before and after decongestion. Nasal provocation takes this one step further, by introducing an allergen via a metered dose spray, then taking measurements. Cross sectional area 2, corresponds with the anterior border of the inferior turbinate, is the best site for assessing sensitivity to an allergen (Uzzamann et al). This is still an experimental test, but some Allergists have pushed for its use in the evaluation of allergic rhinitis. Dykewicz et al 1998 Joint Task Force on Practice parameters in Allergy, Asthma and Immunology cited that nasal provocation has a role in workplace allergies. Also, it may play a role in deciphering whether IDT has higher sensitivity or higher rate of false positives than SPT.

Treatment

Environmental measures should be taken by all people that suffer from allergic rhinitis. This includes avoidance of specific allergen, dehumidifiers, HEPA filters, special linens, weekly laundering of linens in hot water, frequent cleaning of household furniture, and minimizing carpet. For those with pets, they can consider removing pet from the home, the bedroom, and should wash the pet weekly. Medical treatment is the mainstay of therapy for allergic rhinitis. There are many different classes of medications that can be used alone or in combination.

Nasal saline is an inexpensive treatment that is believed to cleanse the nasal mucosa of allergens.

Mast cell stabilizers such as cromolyn sulfate act by decreasing the release of mast cell contents. It is fairly safe, but must be used four times per day and can not be used as a rescue medication.

Decongestants work by vasoconstriction, which leads to decreased edema and increased nasal patency. Topical therapies such as oxymetazoline and phenylephrine provide quick relief, but can lead to tachyphylaxis and rhinitis medicamentosa with prolonged use. Oral medicines such as pseudoephedrine are also useful, but many over the counter medications are using it less often due to its significant side effects. These side effects include hypertension, tachyarrhythmia, wakefulness, and urinary retention.

Antihistamines decrease symptoms of sneezing, itching, and edema by blocking the H1 receptor. Diphendydramine (benadryl) is the most well known drug in this class. It has H1 receptor blockade, peripheral and central, as well as anticholinergic effects. Its central H1 activity causes sedation, and its anticholinergic effects include dry oral/nasal mucosa, urinary retention, memory impairment, and blurred vision. Due to its side effect profile, second generation antihistamines were developed. Cetirizine, loratidine, desloratidine, and fexofenadine are oral preparations, and azelastine is topical. These are also known as non-sedating antihistamines, and are free of anticholinergic effects.

Leukotriene receptor antagonists block the late phase of the allergic response. Montelukast is approved for seasonal allergic rhinitis and is useful in abating sneezing and nasal congestion. Higher efficacy in patients with Samter's triad because of their increased production of leukotrienes.

Intranasal steroids should be first line therapy for allergic rhinitis. All of the drugs used in the US for allergic rhinitis have a good safety profile, and high efficacy, when used regularly. Many people prefer oral to intranasal medications, or cannot tolerate associated epistaxis or dry mucosa. Also, there are concerns about growth suppression in children, and decreased bone density.

Immunotherapy should be considered for patients with evidence of specific IgE antibodies to clinically relevant allergens. It is an effective treatment for allergic rhinitis, asthma, and hymenoptera stings. The decision to begin immunotherapy depends on the severity of symptoms, and their resistance to environmental and medical interventions. Also, some patients may want to avoid medication side effects, costs, and long term use and are good candidates for immunotherapy. Immunotherapy may also prevent the development of asthma in children with allergic rhinitis.

Successful immunotherapy is associated with a shift from TH2 to TH1 CD4+ cells, immunologic tolerance, increases in allergen-specific IgG blocking antibodies, and variable levels of specific IgE. In order to have successful immunotherapy, the specific allergen must be elucidated and a standardized vaccine should be made. Weekly injections are continued with elevation of allergen dose until a maintenance dose is met. At this time, the injections will need to continue for at least a total of three to five years. With immunotherapy, comes the risk of anaphylaxis. To reduce this risk, an assessment of the patient's general medical condition is necessary, *i.e.* history of asthma. Physicians should be trained in and prepared for treating anaphylaxis.

IMMUNE RESPONSE TO VACCINES

Vaccination evokes an antibody response which is, in turn, a measure of the effectiveness of the vaccine in stimulating B lymphocytes. Antiviral antibodies are classified as IgA, IgM, or IgG and can be measured by various techniques. Some antibody categories (IgA and IgM) are normally more abundant in respiratory and intestinal secretions; others (mainly IgG) are more abundant in the circulatory system.

Vaccines also stimulate T lymphocytes, leading to cell-mediated responses that influence protection. Antibody assays are now routine laboratory procedures, but measuring cellular immunity in vitro usually requires the utilization of complex laboratory techniques. In general, despite the complexities of the immune system, resistance to the vaccine-preventable viral diseases often correlates well with the presence of circulating antiviral antibodies, which are easily measured.

Effectiveness is a key concern with any vaccine. Here the standard for comparison is usually the immunity conferred by the natural disease; an example of an exception is rabies. Both epidemiologic and laboratory methods are used to generate comparative data. Vaccine-induced immunity can be defined by the percentage of recipients protected, the projected duration of protection, and the degree of protection. Most viral vaccines considered effective protect more than 90 per cent of recipients, and the immunity produced appears to be fairly durable, lasting several years or more.

However, vaccines usually do not induce an immunologic response entirely comparable to that seen in the natural disease. Immunity to viral diseases should not be thought of as absolute. Persons immune due to the natural infection, as well as, vaccinees, sometimes experience subclinical reinfection if exposed. Evaluating the protection conferred by a vaccine often involves measuring the frequency and extent to which subclinical reinfection can override vaccine-induced resistance.

Often, upon revaccination or reinfection, a boost in IgG antibodies is observed with little or no detectable IgM response, suggesting prior exposure with antibody priming. Such anamnestic responses may be seen in individuals who lack detectable antibody prior to reexposure. Therefore, the absence of measurable antibody may not mean that an individual is unprotected.

Immune responses to viral vaccines may be influenced by a number of factors related to the vaccine as well as to the host. As already discussed, the

- Magnitude and duration of immunity differ significantly between live and killed vaccines.
- The immune response to vaccines can be enhanced by adding adjuvant substances such as aluminum salts (*e.g.*, hepatitis B vaccine).
- The route of administration of a vaccine can also influence the immunogenicity of some vaccines.
- Also, maternal antibodies acquired transplacentally can interfere with responses to measles, mumps, and rubella (MMR) vaccine, as demonstrated by lower response rates when the vaccine is administered earlier than 15 months of age. In this case, it is thought that the antibodies interfere with the post-vaccination replication of these live vaccine viruses in the host.

VACCINE PRODUCTION

Because viruses are obligate intracellular parasites, all viral vaccines contain substances derived from the cells or living tissues used in virus production. Technical advances have improved production methods. One can think of generations of vaccines:

- Those prepared in the tissues of an inoculated animal are the first generation (*e.g.*, smallpox vaccine from the skin of a calf),
- Products from the inoculation of embryonated eggs are the second generation (*e.g.*, inactivated influenza virus vaccine),
- And tissue culture-propagated vaccines are the third generation (*e.g.*, poliomyelitis, measles, mumps, and rubella vaccines).

The vaccine generation indicates the production methodology, sophistication, and relative purity. Third generation vaccines usually contain the least host protein and other extraneous constituents, but they have been the most difficult to produce. Advances in biotechnology, *i.e.*,

- Recombinant DNA-derived subunit vaccines, now serve as the cornerstone for a fourth generation of vaccines and have led to the development and licensure of a recombinant hepatitis B vaccine. In addition, exciting new technologies such as polynucleotide vaccines are now being tested in animal studies for several viral diseases.

Developing New Vaccines

The past success with developing highly effective viral vaccines has been considerable. To develop a new vaccine, researchers must first identify and then produce the virus (or virus components) in quantity under circumstances acceptable for vaccine preparation. Normally this means production of virus or virus components in cell cultures, embryonated eggs, or tissues of experimental animals or humans, or through nucleic acid recombinant technology.

Finding an acceptable production system can be a problem, especially in developing inactivated viral vaccines, because a high concentration of antigen is needed. As already mentioned, production of specific viral proteins by recombinant DNA procedures is providing a solution to many of these problems. A final consideration is the clinical importance of the virus. Normally, it must cause a disease of some severity and there must be an identifiable at-risk target population before consideration is given to developing a vaccine.

However, there are still important indications for which there is no effective vaccine. From a public health perspective an important example for which there is no effective vaccine available is human immunodeficiency virus type 1 (HIV-1). Some of the challenges for the development of an HIV-1 vaccine include the following:

- The type of immune response required to prevent HIV-1 infection is unknown;
- There is no animal model for AIDS caused by HIV-1;
- There are multiple types or clades of HIV-1 which may require the development of a multivalent vaccine;

- Even within a clade, there is considerable viral antigen variation;
- Some successful traditional approaches to viral vaccines, such as live attenuated viruses, pose considerable potential safety risks to the vaccinee.

Passive Prophylaxis

The use of immunoglobulin preparations remains a mainstay of passive prophylaxis (and occasionally of therapy) for viral illnesses. Passive immunoprophylaxis is most often recommended in one of these situations:

- When exposure has occurred, or is expected to occur very soon, and time does not allow for vaccination and the development of an adequate post-vaccination immune response;
- When no effective vaccine exists;
- When an underlying illness precludes a satisfactory response to vaccination.

Although once derived exclusively from animal sources, most immunoglobulins are now manufactured from human sources. Standard immunoglobulin is produced by pooling plasma obtained from thousands of donors and contains antibodies to a number of common viruses. Specific immunoglobulins are produced from donors with high titers of antibodies to specific viruses, often selected following immunization with the relevant vaccine.

SANITATION AND VECTOR CONTROL

Several early approaches to virus control deserve recognition even though they are less dramatic than vaccination.

- One approach is the avoidance of viral exposure. This is an effective means of preventing the transmission of HIV-1, which is spread through sexual contact and exposure to blood of infected individuals. Blood bank testing, *e.g.*, for hepatitis B surface antigen and for antibodies to HIV-1, HIV-2, HTLV-I, and hepatitis C, also avoids exposure by identifying and discarding blood units contaminated with these infectious agents.
- Control of non-human viral reservoirs is another early, worthwhile approach. Unfortunately, few opportunities exist for practical application. The most notable success was the control, and in some cases, the elimination of rabies in some countries through removal of stray dogs, quarantine of incoming pets, and vaccination of domestic animals.
- Another approach of enormous contemporary and historic importance is vector control. Transmission of viral disease by the bite of an arthropod vector was first demonstrated by Walter Reed and his

associates, with their discovery that yellow fever was transmitted by mosquitoes. At the turn of the century, yellow fever was a disease of major consequence in the Americas and Africa. By immediately applying Reed's discovery, Gorgas mounted the anti-*Aedes aegypti* campaign in Havana that marked the beginning of the conquest of epidemic yellow fever. In dealing with the arthropod-borne diseases such as St. Louis encephalitis, any procedure that reduces vector populations or limits the access of the arthropod to humans has potential value. These procedures include draining swamps, applying insecticide, screening homes, and using insect repellant or protective clothing.

- The last of the older approaches is to improve sanitation. This method is applicable in a limited way to diseases whose epidemiology involves fecal-oral transmission. The well-known link between the discharge of raw sewage into tidal waters, contamination of shellfish, and type A hepatitis is an example of a situation readily reversible by improved sanitary practices.

Antiviral Chemotherapy

Antiviral chemotherapeutic agents can be divided into three categories: virucidal agents, antiviral agents, and immunomodulators.

- Virucidal agents directly inactivate intact viruses. Although some of these agents have clinical usefulness (*e.g.*, topical treatment of warts with podophyllin, which destroys both virus and host tissues), most virucides have no demonstrated therapeutic value.
- Antiviral agents inhibit viral replication at the cellular level, interrupting one or more steps in the life cycle of the virus. These agents have a limited spectrum of activity and, because most of them also interrupt host cell function, they are toxic to various degrees. The emergence of drug resistant viruses may occur during clinical use that further limits the effectiveness of various antivirals. and several are under investigation.
- Immunomodulators such as interferons that alter the host immune responses to infection could, in principle, be protective,

A number of antiviral agents with demonstrated effectiveness are now available (TABLE 51-3). These antiviral agents improve the clinical course of disease, but typically have important limitations especially as therapeutics for chronic or latent infections. For example, the four nucleoside analog drugs now available for the therapy of HIV-1 do not prevent the ultimate worsening of disease.

The concept of a targeted approach is now practical since information concerning the structure and replication of viruses and the spatial configuration and function of their proteins is available. Such data may be useful in identifying specific target sites for antiviral agents.

INTERFERONS: CYTOKINES WITH ANTIVIRAL ACTIVITY

Since the mid-1930s, scientists have recognized that under certain circumstances one virus can interfere with another. In 1957, Isaacs and Lindenman made a dramatic discovery that explained the mechanism of resistance. They found that virus-infected cells can elaborate a protein substance called interferon, which, when added to normal cells in culture, protects them from viral infection. Other microbial agents (such as rickettsiae and bacteria) and natural and synthetic polypeptides were later shown to induce interferon.

There are three types of interferon: alpha, beta and gamma. Interferon alpha is produced by leukocytes, interferon beta is produced predominantly by fibroblasts and interferon gamma is produced by activated lymphocytes. Interferons tend to exhibit species specificity (mouse cell interferon protects mouse cells to a much greater extent than human cells) and are inhibitory to numerous viruses.

For many years it was not possible to obtain sufficient quantities of interferons to conduct major studies. However, recombinant DNA technology and cell culture technology led to the production of adequate supplies of interferons and the subsequent conduct of extensive clinical trials. Although broadly antiviral in some animal models, interferon alpha has proven effective in a limited number of viral illnesses of humans, including chronic hepatitis B and C and refractory condylomata acuminata.

In addition, interferons have been effective in the treatment of other diseases. For instance interferon alpha is effective for hairy cell leukemia and AIDS-related Kaposi's sarcoma in a selected group of individuals; interferon beta for relapsing-remitting multiple sclerosis; and interferon gamma for reducing the frequency and severity of serious infections associated with chronic granulomatous disease.

Identifying New Effective Therapeutics

The improved basic science knowledge base of viruses combined with the urgent need for improved therapeutics, especially for HIV-1, has given considerable impetus to the search for new approaches. Some approaches under investigation that may lead to future approved therapies are described here: Combination Therapy: The use of multiple drugs with different mechanisms of action is being studied as a method of improving clinical effectiveness.

Such combinations may offer advantages over monodrug therapy such as improved antiviral activity, preventing or delaying the development of drug resistance, and use of lower, less toxic doses. Combinations of various antiviral agents have been extensively studied for HIV. In addition, approaches investigated for HIV have included combining a cytokine with one or more antiviral agents. Combination therapy has been effective in the treatment of diseases caused by other infectious agents (*e.g.*, *Mycobacterium tuberculosis* and *Pseudomonas aeruginosa*). Discovering New Drugs: New drugs with novel mechanisms of action are being sought and developed. Some of these have displayed considerable antiviral activity in human clinical trials, *e.g.*, protease inhibitors for HIV-1. Evaluating Available Drugs for New Indications: Interleukin-2, a cytokine currently approved for treating renal cell carcinoma, has shown considerable immunomodulatory activity in some HIV-1 infected patients in early human studies.

MULTIPLICITY OF IMMUNE DEFENCES AND STRESS

Recent studies have revealed a great complexity of host immune defences against viral infections. This complexity arises from the many components of the host immune defences and their interactions with one another.

- The existence of a variety of defences is not surprising in view of the diversity of viruses, hosts, routes of infection, body compartments, cells, and mechanisms of virus multiplication and spread.
- The situation is further complicated by the varying effectiveness of the different host defences during the different phases of the primary viral infection (implantation, spread to target organs, and subsequent recovery of each of the infected tissues), as well as during resistance to reinfection.
- Furthermore, the activated host defences can actually cause disease manifestations. The presence of multiple defences against each infection helps explain why impairment of one or a few defences does not entirely abrogate host resistance to viral infections. Several immune and non-immune host defences may operate to control viral infections or, at times, add to the disease process.

Many of the immune defences against viral invasion are fairly well understood, but the relative effectiveness of each requires additional research. In particular, as this chapter attempts to make clear, humoral and cell-mediated immunity are not independent, but interact intimately to influence the duration and magnitude of each type of immune response.

HUMORAL IMMUNITY: B LYMPHOCYTES

The specific B lymphocytes respond to viral antigen introduced by immunization or infection. Binding of antigen to the cell surface immunoglobulin receptors, followed by interaction of the B cell with macrophages and helper T lymphocytes, causes the B cell to differentiate into clones of antibody-secreting plasma cells, each capable of secreting antigen-specific immunoglobulin of one of five major classes: IgG, IgM, IgA, IgD, and IgE.

ANTIBODY-MEDIATED REACTIONS

Neutralization of virion infectivity: At least three immunoglobulin classes have been demonstrated to exert antiviral activity: IgG, IgM, and IgA. These antibodies can neutralize the infectivity of virtually all known viruses. Antibody binds to the virus extracellularly, either neutralizing it immediately or blocking its interaction with host cells.

Antibody that has bound to virus can block the infection of a cell at one of three steps:

1. Attachment of virus to the cell surface,
2. Penetration of virus into the cell, and
3. Uncoating of virus inside the cell.

The mechanism of viral neutralization involves the binding of antibody to virus coat proteins; this usually alters the viral receptor for the target cell. More rarely, bound antibody may also interfere with penetration or uncoating.

The exact mechanism of neutralization is unclear, but it

- probably involves changes in the steric conformation of the virus surface. These antibody-virus interactions can take place independently of complement.
- Antibody also can neutralize virus by causing aggregation, thus preventing adsorption of virus to cells and decreasing the number of infectious particles.
- Antibody and complement acting together can inactivate certain viruses (in most cases, enveloped viruses). Antibody is most effective against virus in large fluid spaces (*e.g.*, serum) and on moist body surfaces (*e.g.*, the respiratory and gastrointestinal tracts), where the virus is exposed to antibody for a relatively long period before escaping into cells.

Consequently, viruses that spread by viremia are effectively eliminated by low levels of circulating antibody. Much higher levels of antibody are needed to prevent the spread of viruses that do not travel in the blood plasma (such as herpesviruses and rabiesviruses), because these viruses spend only a brief period traversing the small extracellular spaces between cells in solid tissue. Besides binding directly to virus, antibodies may enhance phagocytosis. Three types of antibody interactions with phagocytic cells are seen:

- Direct binding of antibody to the surface of the phagocytic cells (cytophilic antibody),
- Uptake of antigen antibody complexes through the Fc receptor, and
- Uptake of antigen-antibody-complement complexes through the C3b receptor. This phagocytosis of virions may result in inactivation of virus, and in the activation of the phagocytic cell which can lead to cytokine production.

Antibody effects on virus-infected cells: Antibody also can act on virus-infected cells by recognizing virus-specific antigens on the surface of infected cells. Complement can then cause lysis of these cells. This complement-mediated lysis occurs both by the classic and the alternative complement pathways. Antibody-coated infected cells also can be destroyed by various effector cells via ADCC. Alternatively, however, some antibodies can mask viral antigens on the surface of infected cells, thereby removing or covering antigens on the surfaces of these infected cells.

Physical barriers to antibody: Before antibody can combine with and neutralize the virus, it must reach the site of virus replication. Barriers to the distribution of antibody include the cell membrane, which excludes antibody, and anatomic tissue barriers, which limit the distribution of macromolecules into certain organs such as the central nervous system. IgG Antibodies: IgG is the most thoroughly studied antibody class and is responsible for most antiviral activity in serum. IgG antibodies reach infected (inflamed) sites by transduction (leakage) from capillaries.

IgG is particularly protective in generalized viral infections that have a viremic phase (*e.g.*, measles, polio, and hepatitis), perhaps because virions in serum are exposed to antibody. IgG antibodies are transferred passively from mother to offspring through the placenta and usually provide temporary protection against generalized viral infections during the first 6 to 9 months of life. Antibody is most protective when present before infection or during the spread of virus to target organs.

Production and the Roles of Antibody Classes

After immunization or infection with viruses, various classes of antibody appear sequentially. For example,

- During primary infection or immunization, most antigens first elicit IgM (early antibody) responses;
- IgA and IgG responses follow within a few days.
- Reinfection, in contrast, stimulates production mainly of IgG, although some IgM and IgA are generated.
- When the primary antigenic stimulation is in the respiratory or gastrointestinal tract, IgA antibody is predominant, accompanied by some IgM. These antibodies are secreted locally at mucosal surfaces and are important in protecting the host against localized surface viral infections such as the common cold, influenza, and enteric viral infections.
- When viral replication is confined to a mucosal surface, resistance to infection is determined primarily by secretory IgA; serum IgG antibody provides less protection.
- Viral infections that begin on a mucosal surface and then spread hematogenously (*e.g.*, measles, rubella, and polio) can be prevented

at the mucosal stage by local secretory antibody and at the viremic stage by IgG antibodies.

- If serum IgG only is induced in a host, hematogenous spread can be prevented, but viral replication still may occur on the mucosal surface.

IgE antibodies and immediate hypersensitivity: Recent information suggests that viruses that bind to IgE antibodies may trigger immediate hypersensitivity responses through the release of vasoactive mediators. These observations may explain many of the apparent allergic manifestations, such as wheezing and urticaria, that accompany some viral infections.

Complement: Complement enhances the phagocytosis of many viruses.

- This enhanced phagocytosis is due to coating (opsonization) of virions by complement or by complement bound to antibody.
- Complement also can neutralize virus by enhancing either antibody-mediated steric changes on the virus or aggregation of the virus via antibody.
- In addition, complement can directly inactivate antibody-coated, enveloped virions.

Hypogammaglobulinemia: A small minority of patients with impaired B-lymphocyte function (hypogammaglobulinemia limited to impairment of humoral immunity) have a significantly increased frequency of severe poliovirus and enterovirus infections of the nervous system (in addition to more frequent and severe infections with pyogenic bacteria). The risk of central nervous system invasion is related to the duration of viremia, as has been shown in immunosuppressed animals.

The course of most viral infections is typically benign in most of these hypogammaglobulinemic patients, indicating that their weak antibody response and other defence mechanisms may be effective. The development of normal specific resistance to reinfection in hypogammaglobulinemic patients may result, in part, from their ability eventually to produce low levels of serum antibody to virus, as well as from the action of their intact cell-mediated immune system.

CELL-MEDIATED IMMUNITY

Cell-mediated immunity (CMI) was once thought to be mediated solely by T lymphocytes; however, it is now clear that it is mediated by a variety of cell types, cell factors, or both. Virus-infected or virally transformed cells activate strong cell-mediated immune responses. For some viral infections, cell-mediated immune reactions may be more important than antibody in early termination of viral infection and prevention of dissemination within the host. Recent evidence shows that cell mediated immunity functions at the body surfaces, as well as internally. Cell-mediated immune responses to viral infections involve

- T lymphocytes,
- ADCC, (*no Av atkarîgâ ðûnu citotoksicitâte*)
- macrophages,
- natural killer (NK) cells,
- lymphokines, and
- monokines.

T Lymphocytes

Much evidence indicates that T lymphocytes are important in recovery from viral infections. Of the many functional subsets of T cells, those that express specific cytotoxic activity against virus-infected or transformed cells have aroused the most interest.

Cytotoxic T lymphocytes: The generation of virus-specific cytotoxic T lymphocytes (CTLs) is believed to be important in preventing viral multiplication. Presumably, the T lymphocytes prevent virus multiplication by destroying infected cells before mature, infectious virus particles can be assembled. This hypothesis assumes that viral antigens appear on the plasma membrane before the release of virus progeny, a view that is substantiated by studies of many, but not all, infections.

Exposure to a virus-infected cell can cause the antigen-specific T lymphocytes to differentiate into cytotoxic effector T cells, which can lyse virus infected or virally transformed cells. These cytotoxic T cells are specific not only for the viral antigen but also for self major histocompatibility antigens and will lyse virus-infected cells only if these cells also express the correct major histocompatibility complex (MHC) gene products.

Activation of cytotoxic and other T lymphocytes may be one of the earliest manifestations of an immune response.

T-cell effector functions occur as early as 3 to 4 days after initiation of a viral infection. However, T-cell responses often decrease rapidly, within 5 to 10 days of elimination of the virus (although virus-specific memory T cells persist for long periods).

In contrast, antibodies usually become measurable later in the viral infection (after 7 days) and persist at high levels for much longer (often for years). Helper T cells may be as important as cytotoxic T cells in the immune response to a virus infection.

Helper T cells are required for the generation of cytotoxic T cells and for optimal antibody production. In addition, helper T cells, and cytotoxic T cells produce a number of important soluble factors (lymphokines) that can recruit and influence other cellular components of the immune and inflammatory responses. Animal studies indicate that impairing the T-cell defences enhances infections by herpes simplex virus, poxviruses, and Sindbis virus and enhances the development of tumors induced by polyomavirus. Since the host retains some resistance to infections, T lymphocytes probably are not the sole defence against these viruses. Impairment of T lymphocytes also hinders T cell-dependent antibody production. In humans, T-cell impairment is associated mainly with more frequent and severe poxvirus and herpesvirus infections. Nevertheless, these infections still do not develop in most individuals with T-cell deficiencies, even though the prevalence of herpesviruses (and many other viruses) is great.

ANTIBODY-DEPENDENT CELL-MEDIATED CYTOTOXICITY

Effector leukocytes for ADCC have surface receptors that recognize and bind to the Fc portion of IgG molecules.

When IgG binds to virus-specified antigens on the surface of an infected cell, the Fc portion becomes a target for effector cells capable of mediating ADCC. Binding of these effector cells to the Fc portion of IgG bound to the infected-cell surface antigens results in lysis of the infected cell. ADCC is a very efficient way of lysing virus-infected cells because it requires significantly less antibody than does antibody-complement lysis. Lymphocytes, macrophages, and neutrophils are all capable of mediating ADCC against virus infected cells. The lymphocytes with this ability appear to be heterogeneous. Natural killer cells, as well as null lymphocytes with Fc receptors for IgG, appear to be able to mediate ADCC activity.

Macrophages

Macrophages are important in both specific and non-specific responses to viral infections (*e.g.*, herpesvirus infections). Factors that modify macrophage activity can influence the outcome of an infection. Moreover, since macrophages are central to the induction of T and B lymphocyte responses, any effect on macrophages will influence B and T cells.

Macrophages confer protection against viruses through either an intrinsic or an extrinsic process. In the former, virions are disposed of within macrophages acting either as phagocytes or as non-permissive host cells. In the latter case, macrophages retard or ablate virus multiplication in neighbouring cells by destroying virus-infected cells or by producing soluble factors (interferons) that act on these cells.

Phagocytosis of some viruses by macrophages decreases virus levels in body fluids (as during viremia) and thereby impedes virus spread. These effects are produced only if the virus is destroyed or contained by macrophages. If a virus replicates in macrophages, the infected macrophages may aid in transmission of the virus to other body cells.

The permissiveness of macrophages for virus replication may depend

- On the age and genetic constitution of the host and
- On the specific condition of the macrophages.

- Macrophage activation mediated either by products of infection (viral and cellular) or by soluble factors produced by T cells (*e.g.*, gamma interferon) often enhance phagocytosis and the elimination of free virus particles.
- Another important effector mechanism of activated macrophages is their ability to recognize and destroy virus-infected and virus-transformed cells.
- Addition, activated macrophages participate in virus inhibition by producing cytokines (interferon, etc.) and mediating ADCC.

NATURAL KILLER CELLS

Natural killer (NK) cells exhibit cytotoxic activity against a number of tumor cell lines, particularly against virus-infected or virus-transformed cells. Natural killer or natural killer-like cells, which have been found in almost every mammalian species examined and even in some invertebrates, are identified as large granular lymphocytes that possess Fc receptors.

- They can mediate ADCC activity;
- Their non-specific cytotoxic activity is increased by interferon and interleukin-2 (IL-2); and
- They can produce a number of different cytokines including interferon when stimulated with virus or virus-infected cells.

Although natural killer cells display cytotoxic activity against virus-infected or transformed cells, they show little or no cytotoxic activity against normal cells. Unlike that of cytotoxic T lymphocytes, natural killer cell killing

- Is not human leukocyte antigen (HLA) restricted, and
- Natural killer cells do not exhibit conventional immunologic specificity.
- There is evidence that natural killer cells play an important defensive role in virus infections in humans and animals.
- Their importance is believed to be due to their ability to produce cytokines and to kill virus-infected cells.

LYMPHOKINES AND MONOKINES

Soluble factors from T lymphocytes (lymphokines) and macrophages (monokines) regulate the degree and duration of the immune responses generated by T lymphocytes, B lymphocytes, and macrophages.

1. Interleukin-2 and
2. gamma interferon are two such important factors produced by activated T cells.
3. Interleukin-l is a soluble factor produced by macrophages.

All three of these factors are essential for the full differentiation and proliferation of cytotoxic T cells. The two interleukins are also important for antibody production by B lymphocytes.

- Macrophages and T lymphocytes also produce several other important factors that act in both the immune and the inflammatory responses.
- Gamma interferon can activate macrophages to become cytotoxic towards virus-infected cells and can increase the level of phagocytosis and degradation.
- Lymphotoxins produced by T cells also may participate in the destruction of virus-infected cells.
- Virus can stimulate alpha interferon production from macrophages; this enhances natural killer cell function and inhibits virus multiplication in neighbouring cells.

Virus-Induced Immunopathology

A host clearly has numerous mechanisms to recognize and eliminate the viruses that it encounters. However, some viruses persist despite these mechanisms, and then the immune responses may become detrimental to the host and cause immune-mediated disease.

When an antigen (virus) persists, pathologic changes and diseases result from different types of immunologic interactions,

- Including immediate hypersensitivity,
- Antibody-mediated immune complex syndrome,
- And tissue damage caused by cell-mediated effector cells and antibody plus complement.

Of these mechanisms, the immune complex syndrome during viral infections has been studied most intensively. Two major complications of deposition of immune complexes are vascular damage and nephritis. Some viral diseases in which immune complexes have been demonstrated are hepatitis B, infectious mononucleosis, dengue hemorrhagic fever, and subacute sclerosing panencephalitis.

Cytotoxic T cells also mediate immunopathologic injury in murine models of human infections (*i.e.*, infections with lymphocytic choriomeningitis virus and poxviruses). Both cytotoxic T cells and T cells responsible for delayed-type hypersensitivity have also been implicated in the pathology associated with influenza pneumonia and coxsackievirus myocarditis of mice. A delicate balance between the removal of infected cells that are the source of viral progeny and injury to vital cells probably exists for T cells as well as for the other host immune components.

Viruses may sometimes circumvent host defences. An important factor that may impair the function of sensitized T lymphocytes is apparent from the observation that T cells activated by reaction with antigen or mitogen lose their normal resistance to many viruses. Therefore, these activated T lymphocytes develop the capacity to support the replication of viruses, leading to impairment of T lymphocyte function.

ROLES OF IMMUNE FUNCTIONS DURING VIRAL INFECTIONS

A hypothetical model can be constructed that shows how the immune components defend against viruses.

Non-specific Defences

- A primary infection in a non-immune, susceptible host is countered first by the non-specific defence mechanisms.
- The early non-specific responses occur within hours and consist of interferon production, inflammation, fever, phagocytosis, and natural killer cell activity.
- These defences may prevent or abort infection; if they do not, the virus is disseminated by local spread, viremia, or nerve spread. It then may seed to a number of target organs and thereby produce a generalized infection.

Specific Defences Antibody

- The events that lead to a specific immune response begin almost immediately after exposure and result in the production of antiviral antibody and cell-mediated immunity in 3 to 10 days.
- The disseminated antibody response in serum is predominantly IgG (preceded by IgM); the local antibody response in secretions is predominantly secretory IgA (with some IgM).
- The persistence of IgA antibodies in secretions is much shorter (months) than the persistence of IgG antibody in serum (years).
- The role of IgE in secretions is unknown, but it may mediate immediate hypersensitivity and amplify the immune response during infection.
- Antibodies may neutralize virus directly or destroy virus-infected cells via ADCC or complement.
- Clearly, serum antibody confers protection against generalized infections (*e.g.*, measles, polio, and type A hepatitis), in which virus must spread through the antibody-containing bloodstream; inoculation of small quantities of antibody into susceptible individuals prevents viral disease but may not prevent subclinical infection at mucosal surfaces.
- In localized infections of mucosal surfaces, protection does not correlate with the presence of serum antibody, but it does correlate with the presence of local IgA antibody, as has been shown in human studies of viruses restricted to the respiratory tract (*e.g.*, respiratory syncytial virus and influenza virus) or to the gastrointestinal tract (*e.g.*, enteroviruses).
- Under some conditions in which serum antibody is present but local IgA is absent, hypersensitivity instead of protective immunity may occur (*e.g.*, respiratory syncytial virus infection).

- Also, serum antibody may not protect against recurrence of latent infections, such as herpes zoster (shingles) and herpes simplex, both because the virus may be shielded by its intracellular location and because cell-mediated immunity may be the more important defence.
- Antibody may also cause undesirable effects in certain chronic infections. Examples in which small amounts of serum antibody complex with virus and deposit in the kidneys, thereby inducing immune complex disease.

Therefore, serum IgM and IgG antibody seem to be effective in preventing infections of a generalized nature; however, in localized surface infections the presence of secretory IgA antibody appears to correlate much better with protection than the presence of circulating IgG antibody. In persistent infections, serum antibody may be responsible for certain long-term sequelae.

CELL-MEDIATED IMMUNITY

Cell-mediated immunity is essential in recovery from and control of viral infections, especially infections involving oncogenic viruses or viruses that spread directly from cell to contiguous cell.

In these situations antibody cannot reach the virus but virally induced antigens on the surface of the infected cell can be recognized by different effector cells (*e.g.*, cytotoxic T cells).

If the virus reaches target organs, it is more difficult to control. The host defences that may play important roles in target organs are initially inflammation, fever, and interferon and subsequently cell-mediated immunity.

In some situations, cell-mediated immunity may develop before antibody production begins. For example, cytotoxic effector T cells have been found in bronchial washings 3 to 4 days after initiation of intranasal infection in mice; at this time, antibody cannot yet be detected.

Cell-mediated immune responses can cause tissue damage;

- The lung lesions produced in influenza may be examples.
- The lethal effects of lymphocytic choriomeningitis virus in mice are mediated by cytotoxic effector T cells.
- The rash in many exanthems (such as measles) is thought to represent a cell-mediated attack on virus localized within cells of the dermis and its vasculature.

STRESS AND THE IMMUNE SYSTEM

Physical and psychosocial stressors have been shown to compromise immune function. The immune suppressive effects of stress may be more pronounced in individuals that already have limited immune competence, such as infants, individuals with a predisposition to autoimmune disease, and the elderly. An individual's response to a stressor is manifested in physiological, hormonal, behavioural, and immunological changes. These stress-induced responses are initiated by the hypothalamus and translated into action by the hypothalamic-pituitary-adrenal (HPA) axis and the sympathetic nervous system. Products from these two systems (*e.g.*, corticoid hormones and catecholamines) can directly modulate the activity of various immune effector cells.

Stress has a bi-directional effect on the immune system depending on whether it is acute or chronic. Acute stress enhances antigen-specific cell-mediated immunity, alters populations of T-cell subsets and modulates mononuclear cell trafficking.

Acute stressors augment the immune response and result in redistribution of immune cells from the bone marrow into the blood, lymph nodes and skin. Redeployment of immune cells into these compartments will allow for heightened responsiveness in the event of a skin wound, a natural consequence of an encounter with a predator as the acute stressor. Likewise, T cell and natural killer cell function are altered by stressful events. In contrast, chronic stressful life events are thought to suppress the ability of the immune system to respond to challenge and thus increase susceptibility to infectious diseases and cancers.

Although there is convincing evidence linking stress with the onset and progression of certain infectious diseases (*e.g.*, influenza, herpes), relatively little is known about the role of stress in autoimmune diseases (*e.g.*, multiple sclerosis, rheumatoid arthritis, lupus, insulin-dependent diabetes). However, a few studies indicate that stressful life events and poor social support play a role in the onset and exacerbation of autoimmune diseases such as rheumatoid arthritis. Furthermore, intervention studies indicate that cognitive-behavioural stress management decreases the symptomatology of autoimmune disease.

MULTIPLE SCLEROSIS

Multiple sclerosis is the most common demyelinating disease of the CNS occurring at a prevalence of 250,000-350,000 in the US. In 1994, the national annual costs of this disease were estimated to be $6.8 billion. MS usually affects people between the ages of 15-50 and 80 per cent of patients have a relapsing-remitting disease which eventually progresses to a chronic progressive disorder. The MS lesion is characterized by plaques throughout the white matter of the brain and spinal cord.

Demyelination is accompanied by inflammatory cell infiltrates consisting of plasma cells, macrophages/microglia, T and B lymphocytes. In common with other autoimmune diseases, relapsing-remitting MS is more common in women than men, with a ratio of 2:1. Autoimmune responses to myelin components myelin basic protein (MBP) proteolipid protein (PLP) and myelin-oligodendrocyte glycoprotein (MOG) have been detected in MS patients, suggesting an autoimmune etiology for MS.

Stress and Multiple Sclerosis (MS)

Stress was considered to be an important factor in the onset and course of MS in Charcot's original description of the disease. Anecdotal accounts suggest that life stress frequently triggers the development of MS symptoms. Recent studies using standardized assessment of life events have begun to shed light on the idea that psychological stress precedes both the onset and recurrence of MS symptoms in 70-80 per cent of cases. The mechanism involving the role of stress in MS appears to be complex. There is even some evidence of a protective effect of stress under certain conditions. However, in laboratory studies MS patients and controls had similar immune responses following an acute stressor (as measured by NK cell activity, T cell proliferation and changes in cell subsets in the peripheral blood).

More recently, acute life stressors have been shown to be correlated with relapses in MS. Mohr and colleagues conducted a meta-analysis of 14 studies concerning stress and MS and concluded that "there is a consistent association between stressful life events and subsequent exacerbation in multiple sclerosis".

A Viral Etiology for Multiple Sclerosis

The etiology of MS is unknown although epidemiological studies have implicated an infective agent as a probable initiating factor. An epidemiological survey reported the increased risk of developing MS was associated with late infection with mumps, measles and Epstein-Barr virus. In addition, exacerbations of MS are frequently preceded by viral infections. It is also intriguing that the antiviral agent IFN-β, has been reported to have a beneficial effect on relapsing/remitting MS (IFN-β Multiple Sclerosis Study Group, 1993). A number of different viral agents have been isolated from the brains of MS patients, including measles, mumps, parainfluenza type I and human herpes simplex type 6 (HHSV6). In common with other autoimmune diseases, stressful life events may precipitate the onset and clinical relapses in MS patients. One mechanism of stress-induced exacerbation might be via increased glucocorticoid levels resulting in immunosuppression and reactivation of latent viruses such as herpes virus.

Viruses are also known to cause demyelination in animals: measles virus in rats; JHM mouse hepatitis virus, Semliki Forest virus and Theiler's virus in mice; visna in sheep; herpes simplex in rabbits. Therefore, in order to understand the pathogenesis of MS it is most appropriate to study an animal model of virus-induced demyelination such as Theiler's virus infection. Theiler's virus infection in mice represents not only an excellent model for the study of the pathogenesis of MS but also a model system for studying disease susceptibility factors, mechanisms of viral persistence within the CNS and mechanisms of virus-induced autoimmune disease.

Theiler's Virus-induced Demyelination as a Model for MS

Theiler's murine encephalomyelitis virus (TMEV) is a Picornavirus which causes an asymptomatic gastrointestinal infection and occasionally paralysis. There are two main strains of Theiler's virus which are classified according to their neurovirulent characteristics. The virulent GDVII strains of Theiler's virus cause fatal encephalitis following intracranial infection. The persistent TO strains (BeAn, DA, WW, Yale) cause, in susceptible strains of mice, a primary demyelinating disease which is similar to MS. Theiler's virus must establish a persistent infection in the CNS in order to cause later demyelinating disease. Strains of mice that are resistant to developing Theiler's virus-induced demyelination (TVID) are able to clear the early viral infection effectively from the CNS.

Susceptible strains of mice fail to clear the CNS infection, in part due to inadequate natural killer cell (NK) and cytotoxic T cell (CTL) responses. Persistent viral infection of the CNS is a prerequisite for the development of primary inflammatory demyelination.

During the early infection, virus replicates to high levels in the brain and spinal cord. At approximately one month post infection the viral titers are decreased and this coincides with the development of high neutralizing antibody titers. In this phase of the disease, the virus infects neurons and mice may develop polio-like disease *i.e.* flaccid hind limb paralysis. In the late phase of the disease, the virus infects astrocytes, oligodendrocytes and macrophage/microglial cells. Autoimmune reactivity to myelin is detected at both the B and T cell level, during demyelinating disease.

A number of studies have reported that viral persistence and demyelination in susceptible strains of mice are under multigenic control. Genes coding for major histocompatibility complex (MHC) class I and the T cell receptor have been implicated in susceptibility to demyelination. Another gene locus on chromosome 6 not linked to the T cell receptor locus, has also been implicated in demyelination. Two additional loci, one close to Ifng on chromosome 10 and one near Mbp on chromosome 18, have been associated with viral persistence in some strains of mice. Immune recognition of Theiler's virus is clearly an important element in susceptibility to demyelination, as indicated by the genetic association with MHC and the T cell receptor, although other undefined factors are also involved.

Interferon and NK cells in Theiler's Virus Infection

The early events that occur during Theiler's virus infection are crucial in the effective clearance of virus from the CNS. Failure to clear virus results in the establishment of persistent infection of the CNS and subsequent demyelination. The first response to viral infection is the production of Type I interferons which are critical in the early clearance of Theiler's virus from the CNS as demonstrated by experimentation with IFN-α/β receptor knock out mice. These mice die within 10 days of infection with severe encephalomyelitis.

Natural killer (NK) cells are activated early in viral infections and play an important role in natural resistance to certain viruses, tumor surveillance and regulation of hematopoiesis. NK cells are active in the CNS as demonstrated in a rat model of quanethidine-killing induced neuronal destruction where they were shown to be the prime mediators of neuronal killing. In Theiler's virus infection, susceptible SJL mice were found to have a 50 per cent lower NK cell activity when compared to resistant C57BL/6 mice. The low activity of NK cells in the SJL mice is due to a differentiation defect in the thymus that impairs the responsiveness of NK cells to stimulation by IFN-β. When resistant mice were depleted of NK cells by monoclonal antibody to NK 1.1 or anti-asialo-GM1, and then infected with Theiler's virus, they developed severe signs of gray matter disease. Thus NK cells are critical in the early clearance of Theiler's virus from the CNS.

Role of $CD8^+$ and $CD4^+$ T cells in Theiler's Virus Infection

Both $CD8^+$ and $CD4^+$ T cells have been shown to play an important role in early viral clearance, but in later disease these T cell subsets have been implicated in the demyelinating process. In early disease, $CD4^+$ T cells are required for B cells to produce antibodies, one of the most important mediators of Picornavirus clearance. $CD4^+$ T cells also secrete IFN-g which has been shown to inhibit the replication of Theiler's virus *in vitro* and to have a protective role *in vivo*. $CD8^+$ T cells clearly are important in viral clearance as demonstrated by *in vivo* depletion experiments and studies with gene knock-out mice. $CD8^+$ T cell depleted mice fail to clear virus from the CNS and developed more severe demyelinating disease than the immunocompetent controls.

β-2 microglobulin knock-out mice were constructed on a TVID-resistant background and these mice were shown to lack functional cytotoxic T cells. Histological evidence of demyelination developed in the knock-out mice following intracranial infection with Theiler's virus. Introduction of resistant $H\text{-}2D^b$ or $H\text{-}2D^d$ transgene into susceptible strains of mice render these animals resistant to TVID. $CD8^+$ T cells also provide protection against TVID when adoptively transferred to a TVID susceptible BALB/c substrain, BALB/cAnNCr. Taken together, these investigations clearly implicate $CD8^+$ T cells in viral clearance and resistance to demyelination. Indeed cytotoxic T lymphocyte (CTL) activity has been detected in Theiler's virus-infected SJL/J mice and higher CTL activity in TVID-resistant C57BL/6 mice. The CTLs may be important either by recognizing viral determinants or by inhibiting delayed type hypersensitivity (DTH) responses.

Th1/Th2 Responses in TVID

The relative role of Th1/Th2 cells in susceptibility to TVID is complex. A pathogenic role for Th1 cells during the late demyelinating disease is clear. TVID correlates with DTH responses to TMEV. In addition, removal of CD4+ T cells during late disease results in amelioration of clinical signs, although this study did not differentiate Th1 and Th2 T cells. Furthermore, high levels of proinflammatory Th1 cytokines IFN-γ and TNF-α in late disease, correlate with maximal disease activity. In addition, the number of TNF-α producing cells in spinal cord was found to correlate with severity of disease.

In early disease Th1 cytokines are involved in viral clearance. SJL/J mice treated with antibodies to IFN-γ suffered an increase in demyelination. In addition, IFNγg knock-out mice on a TVID-resistant background suffered increased demyelination and mortality when infected with Theiler's virus. These studies suggest the importance of IFN-γ in the resistance to TVID. Administration of the proinflammatory cytokines IL-6 and TNF-α to TVID-susceptible mice resulted in reduced demyelination. However, another proinflammatory cytokine IL-1, induced demyelination in TVID-resistant mice. The differential effects of these cytokines are probably due to their pleotropic effects. For instance IFN-γ is a potent anti-viral agent but also increases inflammation.

Evidence in support of the importance of a Th2 response in protection from TVID comes from Miller and colleagues. They administered ethylene carbonimide-treated splenocytes during early TMEV infection to skew the immune response to TMEV from a predominately Th1 to Th2 response. This procedure proved effective at reducing the later demyelinating disease. In contrast another study by Brahic's group demonstrated that the Th1/Th2 balance did not account for the difference in susceptibility to TVID.

Interestingly, IL-2 secreting tumor cells injected into TVID susceptible mice increased the frequency of virus-specific precursor CTLs and prevented persistent infection. This observation supports the notion that a rapid early CTL response is important in early viral clearance and thus protection from demyelinating disease. TVID-susceptible SJL mice given an immunosuppressive cytokine, TGF-β2 showed a reduction in the number of virus-infected cells and decreased amount of demyelination. The mechanism of action was hypothesized to be TGF-β2 dependent reduction in infiltration or activation of virus-infected macrophages into the CNS. Female SJL/J mice infected with the DA strain of Theiler's virus and then given IL-4 or IL-10 or both cytokines in combination, showed marked decreases in demyelination and inflammation. Thus, immunosuppressive cytokines are beneficial in the treatment of TVID.

A number of studies have been conducted into the expression of cytokines and chemokines during infection with Theiler's virus. Investigators have used different time points, different Theiler's virus isolates and different assay methods for analysis which makes comparisons difficult. Using the DA strain of TMEV, at 40 days p.i. in SJL/J mice, Sato *et al.* using RNA protection assays found that the Th1 cytokines IL-5, IL-1, IL-2 and IL-6 were not detectable in the spinal cord whereas Th2 cytokines, IL-10, and Th1 cytokines TNF-a, IL-12, and IFN-g were elevated compared to controls. In the brains of the same animals, IL-10, IL-12, TNF-α, IL-1, IL-2, IL-6, and IFN-γ were not detected at 40 days p.i. but, IL-4 production was high. In early disease susceptible SJL mice were found to express more IL-12p40 mRNA than TVID-resistant mice. In one study IL-12 was shown to play an important exacerbating role in TVID. However, in another study blocking IL-12 expression did not alter the neuropathogenesis of TVID.

It has also been reported that in DA-infected SJL/J mice at 60 days p.i., mRNA levels for IFN-γ, IL-1, IL-2, IL-6, IL-12, TNF-α, TGF-β1, IL-4, IL-5 and IL-10 were higher compared to controls. These studies were performed using real-time PCR analysis. Interestingly these authors found elevated levels of TGF-β in TVID-susceptible SJL mice which may account for the low CTLs in this strain of mouse.

The Th2 cytokine IL-10 mRNA expression was also observed at particularly high levels in SJL mice, early in disease IL-10 expression may inhibit the CTL response and thus prevent effective viral clearance. Similar results showing increased expression of TNF-α, IL-6 and TGF-β were observed in SJL/J mice infected with DA for 60 days, with an additional result that lymphotoxin-α was also increased.

In summary, Th1 cytokines are generally pathogenic during late demyelinating disease and Th2 cytokines are protective. Th1/Th2 cytokine profiles during early disease are more complicated but clearly the early immunological response to Theiler's virus infection has a profound impact on the later development of demyelinating disease. Strains of mice that are susceptible to TVID, produce elevated levels of TGF-β during early disease which is thought to interfere with the recruitment of effective cytotoxic T cells into the CNS. In addition to defective NK cell response in TVID susceptible mice, the low level of CTLs in the CNS prevents viral clearance and a persistent infection is established which subsequently leads to demyelinating disease. Additional evidence in support of the importance of CTLs in clearing infections comes from studies with mice depleted of their $CD8^+$ T cells. These mice have increased viral titers in the CNS and more severe later demyelinating disease.

Mechanisms of Theiler's Virus-induced Demyelination

Demyelination in the TVID model is partly mediated by:

- Direct viral lysis of oligodendrocytes; immune mechanisms including
- Autoimmunity;

- Bystander demyelination mediated by virus-specific DTH T cells;
- Cytotoxic T cell reactivity. Susceptibility to TVID is correlated with
- Increased MHC class II expression *in vitro* on astrocytes and
- Cerebrovascular endothelial cells following treatment with IFN-γ. Increased MHC class II expression on cells within the CNS may lead to increased antigen presentation and inflammation.

The autoimmune reactivity seen in TVID may result from viral damage to oligodendrocytes and subsequent activation of autoreactive T cells. Futhermore, these autoimmune T cells have been shown to be pathogenic and are able to demyelinate *in vitro* (Dal Canto *et al.*, 2000). The relative contributions of these mechanisms to the demyelinating process, remain to be elucidated.

TVID represents an excellent animal model for MS and therefore we have been investigating the effects of stress in this model in order to gain a better understanding of how stress impacts the human disease, MS.

In our first series of experiments we examined the effect of stress on the early disease induced by Theiler's virus, as a model of MS disease onset. Restraint stress was employed as the stressor because there is a great deal of literature in this area.

STRESS EFFECTS ON THE NEUROPATHOGENESIS OF THEILER'S VIRUS INFECTION

General Restraint Procedures and Experimental Design

Three week old CBA mice (Harlan Labs, Indianapolis, IN) were used in the initial studies since they are of intermediate susceptibility to the BeAn strain of TMEV, with a disease incidence of 70 per cent (Welsh *et al.*, 1987; 1989). Thus, any alterations in disease incidence due to the effects of stress could be readily detected from this baseline. In addition, the neuropathology, rates of viral clearance and immune response to Theiler's virus have been previously characterized in this strain. Additional studies were performed with SJL mice which are highly susceptible to TVID.

Virus

The BeAn strain of Theiler's virus was propagated and amplified in BHK-21 cells. The culture supernatant containing infectious virus was aliquoted and stored at -70^{0}C before use.

Restraint Stress Protocol

Mice were handled for several minutes each day for one week prior to the initiation of restraint stress in order to habituate each mouse to human contact in an attempt to diminish stress due to handling during bleeding, cage changes, and any other contacts which might otherwise have altered stress levels.

Five-week-old mice were randomly assigned to one of three groups, ten mice per group according to a previously reported protocol and treated as follows:

- A control group where mice remained undisturbed in their home cages;
- A group in which food and water (FWD) was withheld for 12 hrs each of five nights per week over a four week period;
- A group in which each mouse was placed in well ventilated restraining tube for 12 hrs each of 5 nights per week.

Half the mice in each of the three groups were either infected intracerebrally with Theiler's virus or similarly inoculated with virus-free BHK cell supernatant. Daily food and water deprivation or restraint began one day prior to infection and five days per week for one month post infection. After the first series of experiments, we did not observe any differences between the food and water deprived mice and the non-restrained mice so in the following experiments the design was simplified to four groups Non-infected/Non restrained; Non-infected/Restrained; Infected/Non-restrained and Infected/Restrained.

THE EFFECTS OF RESTRAINT STRESS ON EARLY THEILER'S VIRUS INFECTION

Restraint stress increased the clinical signs of neurological disease in male CBA mice infected with TMEV. Normally TMEV infection of CBA mice is asymptomatic for the first six weeks of infection. In our first stress study, 80 per cent of the stressed infected mice died during the first three weeks of infection. The restraint protocol caused significant weight loss and induced high levels of glucocorticoids (GCS) in the plasma (450ng/ml after the first 12 hour stress session) (Campbell *et al.*, 2001).

The restrained mice developed thymic and splenic atrophy (Figure 3a&b) and reduced numbers of circulating lymphocytes and increased neutrophils. Stressed mice also developed adrenal enlargement (Welsh *et al.*, 2004). In addition, higher viral titers were observed in the brains and spinal cords of infected/restrained mice when compared to infected/non-restrained mice (Figure 5a&b). Increased levels of GCS have been implicated in the increased mortality of TMEV-infected mice since these effects could be replicated by simply adding corticosterone to the drinking water of mice infected with TMEV (unpublished observations).

The early lesion of TMEV infection is most prominent in the hippocampus and is characterized by neuronal degeneration, astrocytic hypertrophy/hyperplasia, perivascular cuffing and microgliosis. In TMEV-infected mice subjected to restraint stress, the lesions were considerably less pronounced than in the infected non-restrained mice at day 7 p.i. Interestingly, an increase in inflammation was detected at day 24 p.i. in infected/restrained mice. This may be due to the persistence of higher viral titers in the CNS which stimulate increased inflammation in the CNS.

Similar results were found in another study with male and female SJL: that chronic restraint stress (8hrs per night) administered in the first 4 weeks of TMEV infection, decreased body weights, increased clinical symptomatology of infection, and increased plasma GCS levels during the acute viral infection. Although all restraint stressed mice displayed significantly increased GCS levels, female SJL mice showed higher basal and stress-induced increases in GCS.

The results of these studies suggest that restraint stress increased GCS which resulted in immunosuppression, reduced inflammatory cell infiltrate into the CNS and consequently reduced viral clearance. The increased levels of virus replication within the CNS may contribute to the increased mortality observed in the restrained mice.

In more recent studies, the effect of restraint stress on viral dissemination was investigated (Mi *et al.*, 2005a). Stressed mice developed increased levels of virus in the CNS, spleen, lymph nodes, thymus, lungs and the heart when compared to infected/non-restrained mice. Interestingly, inflammatory lesions developed in the hearts of the restrained mice. Furthermore, the virus isolated from the hearts of stressed mice had altered and become more cardiotropic when re-injected into normal mice. These findings suggest that stress-induced immunosuppression allows for increased viral replication and spread to sites that would normally remain uninfected. Viral infection of organs that are not normally considered viral targets may then allow for the development of novel diseases.

Restraint Stress Alters Chemokine/Cytokine mRNAexpression

Experiments were carried out in order to determine the effects of stress on chemokine/cytokine expression in the CNS and spleen (as an example of an immune organ). Groups of male CBA mice were:

- Infected/Restrained for 7 nights,
- Infected/Non-restrained,
- Non-infected/Restrained or
- Non-infected/Non-restrained.

At sacrifice their brains and spleens were removed and RNA isolated and incorporated in RNase Protection Assay to estimate mRNA cytokine and chemokine expression. Infection with TMEV increased the following chemokine expression: lymphotactin (Ltn), interferon-induced protein (IP-10), MIP-1β, monocyte chemoattractant protein-1 (MCP-1) and TCA-3, in the spleen but not the brain at day 2 p.i. The fact that chemokine expression was increased first in the spleen provides evidence that the immune response to TMEV is initiated in the periphery. Ltn, RANTES and IP-10 were elevated in both the spleen and the brain at day 7p.i. and were significantly decreased by restraint in the brain. These chemokines are responsible for the recruitment of $CD4^+$, $CD8^+$ T cells, macrophages and NK cells and thus may account for the diminished inflammatory cell infiltrate in the CNS of stressed mice and subsequently the reduced viral clearance and increased mortality in virus-infected restraint stressed mice (Mi *et al.*, 2004).

In experiments examining cytokine expression, mice were subjected to the restraint paradigm and, at sacrifice, half the brain taken for viral infectivity assays and the other half for RPA analysis of cytokine RNA levels. TMEV infection elevated IFN-γ, LT-β, IL-12p40, IL-6, and IFN-β in the brain at day 2 and 7. Importantly, restraint attenuated the increases in IFN-γ, but elevated IFN-β. RNA levels of IFN-γ, LT-β, and TNF-α were negatively correlated with viral titers in the CNS such that mice with higher cytokine levels had lower virus levels.

Thus, these cytokines may play a role in the clearance of virus from the CNS. TNF-α protein levels, as measured by Western blots, gave similar results to the RPA data for this cytokine.

Interestingly, stress increased the anti-inflammatory cytokine IL-10 in the spleen which may contribute to the decrease in pro-inflammatory cytokine production (Mi *et al.*, 2005b).

The cytokines altered by restraint stress in Theiler's virus infection have pleotropic effects and have vital roles in the neuropathogenesis of this disease. Lymphotoxin-β, a membrane bound form of lymphotoxin, plays a critical role in the resistance to intracellular pathogens including Theiler's virus (Lin *et al.*, 2003). LT-β induces IFN-β and also increases cytotoxic T cell activity which are both important mediators of viral clearance from the CNS. IFN-γ is an important inflammatory mediator produced by NK cells and T cells, which contributes on the one hand to viral clearance and on the other hand to development of demyelination in TVID.

The suppressive effect of stress was first detected at day 2 p.i. and attenuated at day 7 p.i. Stress increased the anti-inflammatory cytokine IL-10 and decreased pro-inflammatory cytokines in the spleen. The increase in IL-10 may have contributed to the decrease in pro-inflammatory cytokines. Interestingly, stress also caused an increase in IFN-β expression in the brain, which may result from the higher levels of virus within the CNS of these mice and this may compensate for the impaired viral clearance caused by decreased production of proinflammatory cytokine during stress.

ELISA assays examined the effects restraint stress on IL-1β and TNF-α levels in serum. No detectable levels of IL-1β were observed in any of the groups of mice but interestingly restraint stress induced high levels of TNF-α in the serum of both infected and un-infected mice (Welsh *et al.*, 2004).

To summarize our findings with regard to the effects of restraint stress on the expression of chemokines and cytokines: stress reduced the expression of chemokines responsible for the recruitment of $CD4^+$, $CD8^+$ T cells, macrophages and NK cells namely: Ltn, RANTES and IP-10. Virus-induced IFN-g expression was also decreased by stress. IFN-γ, TNF-α and LT-β levels were negatively correlated with viral replication in the brain. These cytokines have important roles in the initiation of immune system activation and also have effective anti-viral activities and therefore lower levels of expression may also result in increased viral replication within the CNS

Natural killer (NK) cells are known to be important in the early clearance of TMEV as demonstrated by depletion studies (Paya *et al.*, 1989) and are also exquisitely sensitive to stress. Therefore we examined the effect of restraint stress on NK cell activity in CBA mice infected with TMEV. Twenty-four hours post infection, restraint stress significantly reduced virus-induced NK cell activity in TMEV-infected CBA mice (Welsh *et al.*, 2004) when compared with infected/non-restrained mice. Decreased NK cell activity may also contribute to the reduced ability to clear virus.

In order to characterize the alterations in spleen cell populations that occur over time following TMEV infection and restraint stress, we conducted flow cytometric analysis experiments on splenocytes using combinations of the following directly labeled antibodies:

- CD3-FITC, CD19-PE, CD45-PECy5 (leukocyte marker);
- CD3-FITC, CD8-PE, CD4-PECy7
- F4/80-FITC (macrophage marker), DX5-PE (NK cell marker), CD45-PECy5. Preliminary results indicate that at both day 3 and day 7 p.i. in the spleen, RST stress reduces NK cells, and B cells, while increasing numbers of T cells overall. No significant differences were seen in macrophages or between $CD4^+$ or $CD8^+$ cells (unpublished observations).

Restraint Stress Fails to Render TVID

Experiments were performed in order to examine whether chronic restraint stress applied during the acute phase of Theiler's virus infection, would render the genetically non-susceptible C57BL/6 mice, susceptible to TVID. Despite the fact that chronic restraint stress has been shown to decrease functions of NK, T and B cells, and these immune functions have been shown to be essential for resistance to TVID, chronic restraint stress failed to render resistant C57BL/6 mice susceptible to the demyelination (Steelman *et al.*, 2005). C57Bl/6 mice have a high basal level of NK cell activity and also a robust $CD8^+$ T cell response to TMEV. Although stress may decrease the activity of NK and $CD8^+$ T cells, it may not completely ablate them and the residual cells are then still able to effectively clear virus.

The Effects of Restraint Stress

Life stressors precipitate the onset of MS and we have shown that chronic stress during acute infection with Theiler's virus leads to decreased viral clearance from the CNS. Other studies have shown that increased viral load during acute disease leads to increased demyelinating disease during the late disease (Borrow *et al.*, 1992). Therefore, we hypothesized that stress during the acute viral infection results in higher viral load in the CNS and subsequently increased demyelination in the later disease. Chronic restraint stress, administered during early infection with Theiler's virus, was found to exacerbate the acute CNS viral infection and the subsequent demyelinating phase of disease in SJL male and female mice.

During early infection, stressed mice displayed decreased body weights and locomotor activity, while increased behavioural signs of illness and plasma GCS levels.

During the subsequent demyelinating phase of disease, previously stressed mice had greater behavioural signs of demyelination, worsened rotarod performance, and increased inflammatory demyelinating lesions of the spinal cord, as measured by perivascular cuffing and meningitis (Sieve *et al.*, 2004). Restraint-stressed SJL mice developed higher viral loads in the CNS as compared to non-restrained TMEV-infected mice (unpublished data).

Correlational analysis of all of the dependent variables, found that in the acute phase of disease in SJL mice, plasma corticosterone levels, clinical symptomatology, and loss in body weight were all highly correlated. GCS levels during restraint stress in the acute phase were also highly correlated with: histological indications of meningitis, rotarod performance, and clinical symptomatology in the chronic phase of disease.

Thus plasma GCS levels during stress in the acute phase may be a good predictor of disease course in the chronic phase. Acute phase clinical symptomatology had similar predictive value, with chronic phase clinical symptomatology, rotarod performance and histological indications of meningitis. We have previously reported increased levels of antibody to myelin membranes during the late demyelinating phase of disease (Welsh *et al.*, 1987).

In our more recent study, autoantibodies to myelin basic protein (MBP), proteolipid protein (PLP) or myelin oligodendrocyte glycoprotein (MOG) were detected in virus-infected SJL mice and this represents the first report of antibodies to specific myelin components and demonstrates the value of TMEV-induced demyelination as a model for MS (Sieve *et al.*, 2004). Female SJL mice had higher antibodies to MOG 33-55 than males at day 69 p.i. and previously stressed female mice had decreased antibody titers to MBP when compared to non-restrained infected mice. Antibody titers to the Theiler's virus MBP and PLP were no different between the infected/restrained and infected/non-restrained mice.

In summary, restraint stress during early infection significantly increased both clinical and histological signs of demyelinating disease in SJL mice infected with Theiler's virus. The mice that developed the highest corticosterone levels during the early disease, subsequently developed more severe late demyelinating disease. We propose that stress-induced immunosuppression during early infection with TMEV results in increased levels of virus within the CNS and consequently increased disease severity during the late phase of the disease.

The Effect of Restraint Stress

Stress has been shown to ameliorate experimental allergic encephalomyelitis (EAE), an autoimmune model of MS evoked by injection of spinal cord or myelin components into susceptible strains of mice. The frequency of MBP-specific lymphocytes in the spleen and lymph nodes and both the Th1 and Th2 cytokine responses were suppressed in the stressed mice (Whitacre *et al.*, 1998). Glucocorticoids were implicated as the prime mediators of the disease suppression.

Immunosuppressive therapies such as cyclophosphamide or treatment with rabbit anti thymocyte serum (Lipton and Dal Canto, 1976) or antibody to CD4 T cells (Welsh *et al.*, 1987) have been shown to improve the late demyelinating disease induced by Theiler's virus.

Therefore, since restraint stress induces high levels of immunosuppressive glucocorticoids, if this stressor is applied during the late demyelinating disease we hypothesized that this should result in clinical improvements by reducing inflammatory demyelination. However, experiments with TVID showed that although restraint stress elevated GCS levels, it did not alter the clinical score or histological signs of inflammation. Interestingly, mice infected with Theiler's virus developed high levels of circulating GCS (Welsh *et al.*, 2005). Development of glucocorticoid resistance in restraint stressed mice may factor into these results.

OTHER FACTORS AFFECTING STRESS AND IMMUNITY

There are many interacting factors influencing the immunological response of an animal to stress, these include stressor type (psychological vs. physiological vs. physical), duration of stressor, (chronic vs. acute), genetics, age, and social status. These factors and others may partly explain conflicting conclusions based on the literature. These other factors may include time of sample in relation to time of day (circadian effects), time of sample relative to the onset of stress (1 min vs. 1 h vs. 1 d), blood sample vs. tissue sample, activation of catecholamines or glucocorticoids, pathogen exposure or health status of the animal, and the starting point of the immune system and(or) the balance of Th1 vs. Th2 cells.

Social Status

Social status often times plays a significant role in an animal's response to a stressor than the stressor itself. Pigs identified as dominant had greater NK cytotoxicity than did either intermediate or submissive pigs in response to acute shipping, and heat stress reduced NK cytotoxicity among intermediate pigs compared with other social ranks (McGlone et al., 1993; Hicks et al., 1998). NK cytotoxicity was greater in both dominant and intermediate pigs subjected to acute cold stress, but acute heat reduced NK cytotoxicity in intermediate pigs (Hicks et al., 1998).

While dominant pigs had greater NK, phagocytosis, and leukocyte populations following 14 d of heat and crowding stresses (Sutherland et al., 2006), while NK and percentage of immature macrophages were greater in submissive pigs inoculated with PRRS virus (Sutherland et al., under review). Dominant pigs challenged with Aujeszky disease had greater lymphocyte proliferative response to purified Aujeszky antigen (Hessing et al., 1994). Moreover, it appears that immune responses of mixed dominant pigs are more seriously affected than mixed subordinates (de Groot et al., 2001).

Intermediate pigs had greater lymphocyte proliferation responses than did pigs of other social ranks following acute shipping stress (Hicks et al., 1998), but intermediate pigs exposed to chronic heat stress had reduced responses (Morrow-Tesch et al., 1994). Among pigs subjected to mixing stress, lymphocyte proliferation and total IgG were both greater in dominant pigs than in subordinates (Tuchscherer, et al., 1998). However, social status had no affect on lymphocyte proliferation, chemotaxis or IgG concentration in pigs that were exposed to 14 d of heat and crowding stresses (Sutherland et al., 2006).

Genetics

Genetics affects the immune response of an animal. Early study with cattle showed that Angus cattle had a greater PHA response than did Braham × Angus crosses (Blecha et al., 1984). Others have shown that IgG concentrations were different between Angus and Hereford cattle (Muggli et al., 1987) and immune responses in Angus were greater than in Simmental cattle (Engle et al., 1999). Genetic differences in different breeds of pigs have been reported in the response to antigens or vaccines for sheep red blood cells, E. coli, and others (Meeker et al., 1987). Differences in NK cytotoxicity and lymphocyte proliferation responses have been reported in two commercial lines of pigs (Reed and McGlone, 2000). More recently, studies by Sutherland et al. (2005, 2006) reported several breed effects on various immune components (*i.e.*, neutrophil phagocytosis, NK cytotoxicity).

Genetics has been shown to affect the stress responsiveness of an animal as well. Blecha et al. 1984 showed that Braham × Angus crosses and Angus cattle responded immunologically differently to shipping stress; lymphocyte proliferation was reduced in both breeds. Moreover, Angus calves had greater total IgG and IgM titers against pig red blood cells compared with Simmental and Angus calves had greater lymphocyte proliferation in response to PHA than Simmental. (Engle et al., 1999).

In two commercial lines of pigs the environment in which they were kept influenced their immune status, both genetic lines had similar chemotaxis indoors, but outdoors chemotaxis differed between the two lines (Reed and McGlone, 2000). Large white pigs had greater post stress ACTH levels following exposure to a novel environment than did Meishan, but no immune measures were evaluated (Desautes et al., 1997). Others have investigated the immune competence of two different Australian breeds of pigs to a bacterial challenge; specific cell populations were different between breeds . Recently, studies by Sutherland et al. (2005, 2006) showed numerous breed effects on various immune components (*i.e.*, neutrophil phagocytosis, NK cytotoxicity), but there were no breed × stressor effect on immune status of several breeds of pigs exposed to 14-d of heat and crowding stresses.

STRESS SHIFT TH1/TH2 BALANCE

The stress hormones influence the production of Th1 and Th2 cytokines, thus stress hormones help determine which type of immune response prevails . Cytokines provide the link between the innate and adaptive immune systems and help maintain T-cell homeostasis during infection (Bot et al., 2004). Is it the combination of stress and the disruption in the balance between Th1 and Th2 that causes disease? IL-4 is the hallmark cytokine of Th2 immunity, if IL-4 is over-expressed it negatively interferes with the immune defence mechanisms, thus decreasing the recruitment, expansion, and(or) activity of major effector cells such as the Th1 cells (Bot et al., 2004). During a viral infection, a strong bias towards Th2 responses may interfere with viral clearance. However, if the opposite scenario occurs which consists of elevated Th1 and obliterated Th2 immunity allows normal viral clearance to occur. It is possible that certain stressors may disrupt this balance by interfering either directly or indirectly with the mechanistic process.

A balanced Th1/Th2 response may be favoured in some cases of disease challenge, to achieve a compromise between defence mechanisms and immune homeostasis.

Interluekin-12 or IFN-γ produced by cells of the innate immune systems act on corresponding receptors expressed by differentiating T cells (Hanlon et al., 2002; Trichieri, 2003) that redirect the process from Th2 towards Th1 cells. Thus, if stress disrupts the balance between Th1 and Th2 then disease is the outcome. In several studies conducted in our laboratory, we have theorized based on immune and cortisol responses to these stressors (some cases, cytokine profiles) the impact stress has on Th1 and Th2 balance (Figure 3).

Even though, it is essential to evaluate different subclasses of immunoglobulins along with a more diverse cytokine profile to more definitely speculates we have begun to theorize based on the studies presented here. It seems likely that 4 days of cold stress may shift the Th1/Th2 balance towards a Th1 response; whereas 14 d of heat/crowding may actually result in a balance between Th1 and Th2 response based on enhanced NK and LPS-induced proliferation and reduced total IgG in the stressed animals. At 7 days post PRRS challenge, infected pigs appear to be able to maintain a balanced Th1/Th2 response based on their cytokine and immune profile, thus these animals were able to resolve the infection (Figure 3). Moreover, it is possible that pigs weaned at 28 days of age are skewed towards a Th2 response, whereas pigs weaned at 14 days of age appear to be either shifted towards a Th1 or have a balanced Th1/Th2 based on their cytokine and immune profile (Figure 3). Contrary, pigs that are weaned at 14 d of age and kept on 8 h of light may be shifted towards a Th2 response. Based on these studies, it is theorized that stress does not always suppress the immune system and or disrupt the balance between Th1/Th2. In fact, in some situations stress may enhance some components, while suppressing others in order to shift the balance between Th1 and Th2.

3

Genetics, Immunology and Diseases Resistance of Animals

GENETICS OF SCRAPIE RESISTANCE IN SHEEP

Scrapie is an infectious disease of sheep that affects the central nervous system and is always fatal. Upon necropsy, infected animals will have holes or vacuoles in the tissue of the brain. The disease is classified as a transmissible spongiform encephalopathy (TSE). Some TSE's in other species include bovine spongiform encephalopathy (BSE, Mad Cow Disease), Creutzfeldt-Jakob Disease (CJD) in man, new variant CJD (vCJD) in man thought to result from eating meat from BSE-infected cattle, transmissible mink encephalopathy (TSE), chronic wasting disease (CWD) in some U.S., populations of deer and elk, and feline spongiform ecephalopathy (FSE). Federal and State animal health authorities have considered scrapie a high priority disease for elimination for many years, but the relatively recent evidence that ties vCJD in humans to BSE in cattle has resulted in increased attention on scrapie in sheep.

GENETICS OF SCRAPIE

Scrapie is a 100 per cent fatal, degenerative disease affecting the central nervous system of sheep and goats. The disease has been reported in countries throughout the world with few notable exceptions (Australia and New Zealand). The first case of scrapie was discovered in the United States in 1947. The current incidence is 2/10 of 1 per cent or 1 in 500 U.S., sheep. The incidence of scrapie in the U.S., goat population is not currently known.

While bovine spongiform encephalopathy is believed to be caused by the consumption of contaminated feed (meat and bone meal), scrapie is transmitted during lambing when lambs come into contact with infected placenta and birth fluids from infected ewes. Rams can get scrapie, but are not known to transmit scrapie.

Scrapie is NOT caused by genetics, but the genetic make-up (DNA) of an animal determines whether it will get scrapie if it is exposed to the infective agent. In other words, if a genetically susceptible lamb is exposed to a scrapie-infected placenta, it will develop scrapie. It takes from 2 to 5 years after exposure for an animal to show clinical signs of scrapie. If a genetically resistant lamb is exposed to a scrapie-infected placenta, it will not develop scrapie. No resistant genotypes have been identified in goats.

Incidence

Scrapie was first diagnosed in the U.S., in 1947 in a flock of Suffolk sheep in Michigan that had imported sheep from Canada of U.K., origin for several years. From 1947 through July 2001, scrapie had been diagnosed in over 1,000 flocks, and approximately 1,600 individual cases of natural sheep scrapie and 7 individual cases of natural goat scrapie have been found. Through 1992, the breed distribution was as follows: 87 per cent Suffolk, 6 per cent Hampshire, and 7 per cent other breeds and crosses. While 1,600 appears to be a large number of cases of sheep scrapie, it actually is not since it represents an average of only about 30 cases per year. Relative to most other sheep diseases, the incidence of scrapie is quite low.

Clinical Signs

Early signs of scrapie include subtle changes in behaviour and temperament. These changes may be followed by scratching and rubbing against fixed objects. Other signs are loss of coordination, weight loss despite a good appetite, biting of feet and limbs, and lip smacking. Gait abnormalities such as high-stepping of the forelegs, hopping like a rabbit, and swaying of the back end may be seen. Signs or effects of scrapie usually do not appear until 2 to 5 years after an animal is infected. Sheep may live 1 to 6 months (sometimes longer) after the onset of clinical signs.

Infected animals show no immune response to the infective agent as is the case with viral and bacterial diseases. There is currently no live-animal test to determine if an animal is infected. This is a major area of research, and some promising live-animal tests are in the development and evaluation stages. The scrapie agent is thought to be spread most often from ewe to offspring and to other lambs in contemporary lambing groups through contact of lambs with the placenta and placental fluids of infected ewes. Lateral transmission from infected rams to ewes and lambs, from infected ewes to other ewes, and from an infected environment to adult animals are not thought to be major routes of transmission; although there are documented cases of scrapie where such routes of transmission are thought to have occurred. There is not agreement among scientists on the nature of the infectious agent. However, infected animals have large amounts of an abnormal type of prion protein (denoted as PrP^{Sc}), especially in the central nervous system tissues of the brain and spinal cord. Scrapie-free animals have normal prion protein (PrP^{C}) and no PrP^{Sc}. Some feel that PrP^{Sc}

itself is the infectious agent while others feel that PrP^{Sc} is the result of another infectious agent. However, scientific evidence increasingly supports the theory of PrP^{Sc} itself as the infectious agent.

Prion Protein

Prion protein is a constituent of normal mammalian cells. Sheep prion protein is a protein of 256 amino acids in length. There is some variation among sheep in the particular amino acids that comprise their prion protein. However, the PrP^{Sc} found in a scrapie-infected sheep is of the same amino acid sequence as the normal prion protein (PrP^{C}) found in that sheep. The difference between PrP^{Sc} and PrP^{C} is in its molecular shape. The prion infectious agent theory contends that PrP^{Sc} infects a normal sheep and serves as a template to change the normal shape of PrP^{C} to the infective shape of PrP^{Sc}.

Of the 256 locations for amino acids along the sheep prion protein molecule, amino acid changes in at least three of these locations (amino acids number 136, 154, and 171) have been shown to confer increased or decreased susceptibility to scrapie. Each particular amino acid is specified in the prion protein gene by a group of three nucleotide bases known as a codon. Therefore, these three important locations are referred to as codon 136, codon 154, and codon 171 on the prion protein gene.

The most common amino acids coded for at these three codons are: alanine (A) or valine (V) at codon 136, arginine (R) or histidine (H) at codon 154, and glutamine (Q) or Arginine (R) at codon 171. Since genes occur in pairs, sheep have two prion protein genes. Each gene can be the same in which case the sheep will produce only one type of prion protein. If the genes are different, then two types of prion protein are produced. Just considering these three codons, a population of sheep can contain individuals with one of 27 different prion protein genotypes.

Table. Possible Genotypes for the Sheep Prion Protein at Codons 136, 154, and 171 and a Scrapie Resistance Index for each Genotype

Codons 136	154	171	Scrapie Resistance Index for U.S. Sheep[a]
AA	RR	QQ	3
AA	RR	QR	9
AA	RR	RR	13
AA	RH	QQ	3
AA	RH	QR	9
AA	RH	RR	13
AA	HH	QQ	3
AA	HH	QR	9
AA	HH	RR	13
AV	RR	QQ	1
AV	RR	QR	7
AV	RR	RR	11
AV	RH	QQ	1

AV	RH	QR	7
AV	RH	RR	11
AV	HH	QQ	1
AV	HH	QR	7
AV	HH	RR	11
VV	RR	QQ	0
VV	RR	QR	6
VV	RR	RR	10
VV	RH	QQ	0
VV	RH	QR	6
VV	RH	RR	10
VV	HH	QQ	0
VV	HH	QR	6
VV	HH	RR	10

Note:

[a]Index is sum of numeric value assigned for each individual codon genotype: codon 136: AA=3, AV=1, VV=0; codon 154: RR=RH=HH=0; codon 171: RR=10, RQ=6, QQ=0. Higher values indicate greater expected resistance.

GENETIC VULNERABILITY OR RESISTANCE

Genetic resistance to scrapie depends not only on the prion genotype of the sheep but also on the strain of scrapie present. Genotypes found to be resistant to one strain of scrapie have been shown to be susceptible to another strain. It appears that there are differences between the U.S., and Europe in the strains of scrapie that are present. The fact that the U.S., is free of certain scrapie strains is good justification for the stringent regulations for importation of sheep and goats into the U.S., from countries with scrapie.

Codon 136: Sheep homozygous for alanine (AA) have been shown to be more resistant to scrapie than sheep homozygous for valine (VV) or heterozygous (AV) in European studies. While a lower incidence of scrapie is anticipated in AA sheep in Europe than in the other genotypes, some AA sheep still have been diagnosed with scrapie. AA sheep are not 100 per cent resistant to scrapie. In the U.S., amino acid changes at codon 136 appear to be less important to scrapie susceptibility than in Europe. This may be due to the different strains of scrapie found in the two regions.

Codon 154: Of the three important codons, amino acid changes at 154 appear to have a slightly less dramatic effect on scrapie susceptibility than do the other two, and the susceptible genotypes are not consistent across studies. In some studies, sheep with the arginine (R) allele have a lowered incidence of scrapie, and in other studies, sheep with the histidine (H) allele have a lowered incidence. At the present time, it appears that screening sheep on the basis of codon 154 genotype has little value in increasing resistance to scrapie.

Codon 171: Amino acid changes at codon 171 have a large effect on scrapie susceptibility in sheep in both Europe and the U.S. Virtually no sheep homozygous for arginine (RR) have been identified with scrapie. The one exception is a single RR Suffolk in Japan that was diagnosed with scrapie. The frequency of heterozygous (QR) sheep also is very low among scrapie-infected sheep. However, the frequency of sheep homozygous for glutamine (QQ) is very high among scrapie-infected sheep.

A scrapie resistance index for each genotype in U.S., sheep. The higher the number, the greater the expected resistance to scrapie. The index is weighted heavily in favour of RR and QR genotypes at codon 171, less heavily in favour of the AA genotype at codon 136, and neutral with respect to the genotypes at codon 154.

SUSCEPTIBILITY VERSUS SCRAPIE-INFECTED

It must be remembered that a susceptible genotype like QQ at codon 171 does not imply that the animal is scrapie-infected. Scrapie is not a genetic disease. Scrapie is not caused by a particular genotype. An infectious agent causes scrapie. In order to have scrapie, both an infectious agent and a susceptible genotype need to be present. For example, Australia and New Zealand are scrapie-free, but Suffolk, Cheviot, Merino, and Poll Dorset sheep of susceptible genotypes are found in these countries. There is no scrapie in these countries because the scrapie agent is not present.

Likewise, susceptible genotypes are found in many breeds of sheep in the U.S., but almost 90 per cent of the scrapie cases are in the Suffolk breed. This may be due to the major mode of transmission of the disease from an infected ewe to her newborn lambs. Scrapie was brought into the U.S., in Suffolk sheep. A possible scenario that followed was that infected Suffolk ewes infected their lambs, and infected females from infected ewes continued to pass the disease to their lambs.

However, infected Suffolk rams would not tend to infect the ewes they were mated to or their lambs, so infected Suffolk rams mated to ewes of a different breed, as is common in crossbreeding systems in the U.S., would not tend to pass scrapie onto that breed.

While scrapie is primarily a disease of Suffolk sheep in the U.S., the disease is found in the Suffolk, Cheviot, Swaledale, Bleu du Maine, Herdwick, Poll Dorset, Shetland, and Soay breeds in the U.K., Texel breed in The Netherlands, Suffolk and Corriedale breeds in Japan, Romanov and Lacaune breeds in France, Rygja breed in Norway, and Icelandic breed in Iceland. This is not an exhaustive list of sheep breeds or countries with scrapie, but a sample to indicate that scrapie is found in several breeds. A discussion of theories on how scrapie initially becomes established in a breed of sheep would be interesting.

Breeding for Scrapie Resistance in the U.S.

Selection for resistant prion protein genotypes need only be conducted in breeds where scrapie is found, *i.e.* Suffolks and, perhaps, other blackfaced breeds that have been "improved" by illicit crossing with the Suffolk. With the current strain(s) of scrapie present in the U.S., selection for the arginine (R) allele at codon 171 appears to be sufficient.

A flock where every ewe is of the susceptible genotype QQ can be converted to a flock of QR and RR resistant ewes fairly quickly by simply purchasing and using only RR rams. With a normal ewe replacement rate of 20 per cent per year, over 2/3 of the ewe flock will be of the QR or RR genotypes after five years of RR ram use; even with no selection of ewes or ewe lambs on prion protein genotype. Conversion of the flock to QR and RR ewes will be even faster if, in addition to using RR rams, replacement ewe lambs are preferentially selected from QR or RR dams and if QQ ewes are preferentially culled.

GENOMICS, IMMUNOLOGY AND DISEASES IN NON- SALMONID FISH

Considering that 70 per cent of the international fishing grounds are overexploited and that the current volume of captures by fishing efforts has practically reached a maximum level, the increased consumption of fishery related products must be sustained by aquaculture. Indeed, it has recently been estimated that approximately 30 per cent of the fisheries products that are consumed in the world are provided by aquaculture and this aquatic production will increase in the near future.

However, mortalities due to disease can occasionally be high in fish farms. Although there are several commercial vaccines that help in the prevention of numerous diseases, further studies are needed for the improvement of existing vaccines and for the development of new vaccines and vaccination strategies. Aquaculture can greatly benefit from the use of molecular and biotechnological tools to identify and characterize genes and regulatory genetic networks of potential use.

In this sense, molecular biology can be applied in aquaculture in the diagnosis of diseases, in the design of new vaccines, in the control of growth and reproduction, and in increasing disease resistance of cultivated species. Moreover the availability of genetic maps of the appropriate density is of high interest for the identification of genomic regions with characters of interest in production by means of assisted marker selection programmes.

This knowledge acquired in fish can be used not only to improve aquaculture production but can also be applied in other industries. In fact, for a long time now, fish have had an impact in Genomics development. Approximately 30 years ago, a popular tropical fish named *Danio rerio* (zebrafish) was chosen as a great candidate for the genetic analysis due to numerous interesting features such as its short life cycle (3 months to reach sexual maturity), relatively high egg clutches throughout all the year, easy culture and external development with transparent embryos.

All this combined with large scale mutagenesis experiments conducted at the beginning of the 90s allowed zebrafish studies to fill a gap in the vertebrate development biology because of the ability to help in the study of genes through mutant phenotypes, as in *Drosophila melanogaster* o *Caenorrhabditis elegans*.

Since then great advances on the knowledge and understanding of vertebrate development and human disease have been accrued using this model fish. Fish became an important actor in genomic studies (DNA sequencing and data mining) in 1993, when Sydney Brenner suggested the "pufferfish", *Takifugu rubripes* (fugu) as a genome model. On top of its attraction to gourmets in Japan and China fugu has one of the smallest vertebrate genomes. This characteristic already known from its freshwater relative *Tetraodon nigroviridis* in 1968, constitutes a great advantage to access a gene catalogue for a modest cost compared to higher vertebrates. It is important to point out that in recent years available fish genomic resources have increased dramatically, especially for salmonids.

CLONING OF IMMUNE RELATED GENES

A hypothesis that is becoming quite popular among comparative immunologists is that innate immunity of lower vertebrates constitutes an important protection against pathogens for this group of animals. The reason is the relative inefficiency of their acquired immune response due to the evolutionary status and their poikilothermic nature. In fact, innate parameters are considered as relatively independent of temperature and more active at the lower range temperatures at which fish live.

However, acquired immunity parameters such as antibody production and lymphocytic activity are more effective at higher temperatures. This translates into a limited antibody repertoire and lower memory and a very slow lymphocyte proliferation in contrast with the almost instantaneous innate response.

Despite of all this, a few non- specific immune genes have been cloned in fish, although this group has grown significantly in the last years. What follows is a review of the "innate and specific" genes characterized up to now in fish (model and commercial species). Most of these studies are based on the cloning and characterization of individual genes, complete sequencing, phylogeny, expression analysis, etc., and recently also the profile expression analysis.

Salmonid Fish

Salmonids, especially rainbow trout (*Oncorhynchus mykiss*), are the group in which the molecular basis of the immune response has been more extensively studied. Among other genes, there have been sequencing and expression studies on interleukins (IL): IL-1β, IL-6, IL-11 and IL-18 and Tumor Necrosis Factor-alpha (TNF-α). Interferon (IFN) and related genes such as Mx have been also studied because of the importance of viral aetiology in diseases and the lack of treatments. In rainbow trout the following genes have been characterized: two Toll Like Receptors (TLRs); IFN regulatory factors (IRFs); Mx proteins; a macrophage activating factor (MAF) similar to IFN-g, expression and gene structure of Inducible Nitric Oxide Synthase (iNOS). Both in rainbow trout and Atlantic salmon (*Salmo salar*) the guanylate binding protein (GBP) induced by IFN-g in mammals has been characterized.

Several antimicrobial peptides (AMPs) have been sequenced and their expression characterized, the same was done with complement factors such as C4 and molecules type C1, anaphylatoxins C3a, C3a receptor and several chemokines.

Transforming Growth Factor-beta (TGF-β) has also been characterized and an Immunoglobulin T (IgT) has been described as well. Concerning IFN-γ inducible chemokines a CXC, CXCL8 type and another with homology with the subgroup CXCL9, CXCL10, CXCL11, apparently with two forms and inducible by viral infections have been identified.

Two chemokines, CK1 and CK2 have been characterized. β1,3-glucan receptors in macrophages have been found in Atlantic salmon. A type C lectin receptor has been sequenced and its expression characterized and a lectin associated to pathogens recognition has been detected in serum. A protein associated to IL-1 receptor has been cloned. Two IgM isotypes and an IgD isotype have been cloned. IFN type I genes and some of the inducible proteins have been cloned and their expression studied, some IFN-g have been identified. A lectin has been partially characterized in Chinook salmon (*Oncorhynchus tshawytscha*) embryos.

Non- Salmonid European Fish

In comparison with those reported in salmonids there are not many characterized genes in non- salmonid fish species. The non- salmonid cloned genes up to date. In sea bream (*Sparus aurata*) several genes induced by interferon (α or γ) such as Mx or IRF-1 have been characterized. Viral infections are able to induce the expression of these factors suggesting an anti-viral function. Sunyer *et al.* have underlined the diversity of functional forms of complement factor 3, as already described in trout.

A type F lectin has been characterized. Several factors involved in the immune and inflammatory response have been studied such as TNF, IL-1 or its receptors or TGF. All of these factors are expressed constitutively. In contrary to what is expected with the mammalian perspective, TNF does not increase its expression level after a lipopolysaccharide (LPS) treatment, whilst IL-1 does.

However, TNF shows pro-inflammatory and proliferatory functions when administered *in vivo*, suggesting a similar role as in mammals. There is also evidence of other roles not directly immune such as the regulation of fat tissue in this species. TLR-9 has high expression levels in the immune organs (spleen, head kidney) and in the mucosal and epithelial barriers.

However, its expression did not change in the spleen when fish were infected with bacteria. A second form was found, generated by alternative splicing, although its biological meaning has to be further studied. Recently Major Histocompatibility Complex (MHC) class II alpha chain has been characterized and is constitutively expressed in several tissues and the expression was increased in kidney cells when incubated with bacteria and yeast cells. In addition the CD8a co-receptor has recently been cloned and characterized in sea bream. As in sea bream several genes modulated by interferon α, β and γ have been characterized in turbot (*Psetta maxima*) such as Mx and IRF-1.

Recently, class II α and β MHC and TNF have been cloned. The expression profile in the life cycle has also been studied for hepcidin and T cell receptors. In sole (*Solea senegalensis*), only the Mx gene has been characterized so far. In sea bass (*Dicentrarchus labrax*) there has been a growing effort in the characterization of immune genes. Caspase genes such as caspase 3 and 9, cyclooxygenase-2 (COX-2), T cell receptor-β, MHC class II, CD8α, hepcidin and interleukins such as IL-1, IL-10 and IL-12 have all been characterized recently. The light chain of IgM has also been cloned. It is interesting to point out the study on the biological function of IL-1 that has been proposed as an immunostimulant or adjuvant to be used in aquaculture.

Non- Salmonid Fish Out of Europe

β1,3-glucan receptors have been characterized in catfish (*Ictalurus punctatus*) neutrophils. Also in this species an IgD, Mx and IFN-γ similar sequences have been recently described. In the carp (*Cyprinus carpio*) the α1-anti-protease has been purified and characterized. Two Mannose Binding Protein (MBP) homologues and an MBP associated serine protease have been characterized. Among the different characterized molecules we can quote the following: a chimerical immunoglobulin IgM-IgZ; the protein Nitric Oxide Synthase-2 NOS2; a factor similar to TGF-β-2; a chemokine CXC similar to subgroup CXCL9, CXCL10, CXCL11, a chemokine CC similar to C4-CC, a chemokine receptor CXC and two IL-11 paralogues.

In the herbivorous carp (*Ctenopharyngodon idellus*) the α2-macroglobulin has been purified and characterized. In the Japanese flounder (*Paralichthys olivaceous*) the following immune genes have been cloned: an IgD cDNA; IFN receptor factors; Mx and the chemokines CXC type CXCL8 and two CC chemokines, C6-CC and C4-CC, with a high homology with mammalian CCL11. Three isoforms with homology with mammalian TGF-b-1/4/5, β-2 and β-3 have been described in plaice (*Pleuronectes platessa*). In halibut (*Hippoglossus hippoglossus*) the Mx proteins have also been characterized. In cod (*Gadus *morhua*) a soluble and membrane associated IgM form with an unusual alternative splicing and an IgD have been described. In the stripped sea bass (*Morone saxatilis*)a type F lectin has been characterized.

In the cobia (*Rachycentron canadum*), the most important cultured fish in Taiwan, a mannose specific lectin has been cloned and characterized that exhibited a bactericidal and mitogenic activity. The primary structure of a Japanese eel (*Anguilla japonica*) lectin from the epithelial mucus has been characterized. The gene and promoter of viperine (an antiviral protein) from Chinese perch (*Siniperca chuatsi*) have been cloned.

Model Species of Primitive Fish

The lamprey (*Lampetra fluviatilis*), belonging to the most primitive fish, the agnathans, have been used as a model to study the evolutionary relations with other model fish: fugu, *Tetraodon*, zebrafish, goldfish (*Carassius auratus*) and other species. Although the studies of the immune system are not very abundant, the first fish chemokine is a lamprey CXC that codes a mammal type CXCL8 peptide. A MBP has also been cloned and characterized. Although structurally similar sequences can be found between groups this does not necessarily indicates a functional similarity but rather how conserved the defence related mechanisms can be throughout evolution.

An immunoglobulin isotype has been identified in fugu (*Takifugu rubripes*, fugu), whose structure and expression analysis suggest differences from the IgH locus isotypes previously described; IFN-γ, TLRs, IRFs phagocytic oxidase subunits (oxidase NADPH) and Macrophage Colony-Stimulating Factor (M-CSF) receptor sequences have been also identified. In *Tetraodon nigroviridis*, freshwater fugu, comparative genomics shows an independent expansion in vertebrates of type I IFN receptors and their ligands. Janus kinases (JAKs)-Signal Transducers and Activators of Transcription (STATs) pathway (JAK-STAT pathway) genes have also been characterized.

Several IgZ isotypes have been recently described in zebrafish. A molecular and functional analysis of the following genes have been conducted in zebrafish: IFN, TLRs, several JAK-STAT genes and Mx proteins and their promoters. Sequences of the M-CSF and two chemokines, a CXC similar to mammalian CXCL14 and CXCL12 type have been identified. In goldfish studies have been mostly focused in interferon and associated proteins. TLRs, whose expression increases in activated macrophages, IFN regulatory factors, JAK-STAT genes and antiviral proteins such as Mx, Interferon Stimulated Gene (ISG) and dsRNA Protein Kinase (PKR) have been characterized.

EXPRESSED SEQUENCE TAGS (ESTS)

Immune response understanding is crucial for minimising losses in aquaculture. The use of immunostimulants, vaccines and genetic selection programmes has helped to attain this goal. The use of genomic tools such as ESTs libraries, subtractive hybridizations (SSH) and microarrays have given essential information to identify homologous genes, new genetic functions, expression profiles, routes, candidate genes. EST production, directly from organs related with the function under study or by SSH, has generated multiple databases with hundreds or thousand of genes, which constitute the platform needed for microarray construction.

The developing and application of bioinformatics tools in parallel has permitted an accurate management of a large number of sequences for expression profiles and gene annotation. The developing of microarrays for the simultaneous analysis of the expression of hundreds to thousands of genes is a basic tool for the identification of signatures and candidate genes. The main advantage of the modern techniques in genomics is the large quantity of results produced but this also implies two different risks: the massive production of data in few individuals leads to the choice of models with too high parameters (overparameterization) and obtaining of false positives.

Obtaining consistent results by this strategy demands an appropriate experimental design, a correct application of statistics in data analysis, and recently, the convenience of results modelling using genetic nets has been demonstrated in order to correctly interpret gene expression patterns.

The increase of EST databases has been dramatic in recent years. Salmonids are the group in which this is more apparent. More than 175 cDNA libraries have been constructed from a wide variety of tissues and different developmental stages and more than 300.000 salmonid cDNA sequence reads have been combined from a consortium comprising groups from Canada (Ben Koop and Willie Davidson and the Genomics Research on Atlantic Salmon Project, GRASP; Susan Douglas *et al.* and the Institute for Marine Biosciences, IMB-NRC); France (Yann Guiguen *et al.* and INRA-SCRIBE); Norway (Bjorn Hoyheim *et al.* and the Norwegian School of Veterinary Science, NSVS) and the U.S.A. (Caird Rexroad III and the USDA/ARS National Center for Cool and Cold Water Aquaculture).

These sequences have been assembled into over 40.000 unique contigs. A preliminary microarray of 3.557 cDNAs has been constructed and assessed for its ability to provide new data in the study of cellular and tissue responses to pollutants, diseases and stress, as well as for reproduction and development. On the basis of these results, a larger array of 16.006 genes has been constructed and initial results have shown sensitivity of gene expression patterns to disease challenge, and to small environmental and physiological changes.

BASSMAP, an EU funded project, is focused on sea bass genomics. A Bacterial Artificial Chromosome (BAC) library was constructed with an insert mean of 164 kb and a final cover equivalent to 7 times of total genome. The BAC clones are being used to generate ESTs in order to detect genetic markers such as Single Nucleotide Polymorphisms (SNPs) and microsatellites. BRIDGEMAP is another EU funded project focused on sea bream genomics, where 1.500 ESTs have been generated with the aim of improving the knowledge of several aspects of the biology of this species. EU has funded and is supporting several research projects that have the common goal of increasing the knowledge of genomics in aspects such as health (AVINSI, AQUAFIRST, IMAQUANIM), welfare (WEALTH, STRESSGENE), reproduction (PROBASS, CRYOCITE, PUBERTIMING), growth and nutrition (FISHCAL, fPPARS). Moreover the network "Marine Genomics Europe" (MGE) has a major goal for the development, use and dissemination of genomic approaches to the study of marine organism biology and marine ecosystems.

One of the goals of the fish and shellfish node has been the production of genomic tools, including cDNA libraries, molecular markers (macro and microsatellites, SNPs), microarrays, etc., integrated in a bioinformatics platform. These tools will dramatically improve the available genomic resources that will help solving numerous scientific questions. Despite of all these efforts there is a long way in front of us. As an objective data, while the GeneBank number of sequences for rainbow trout is 244.984 and 236.009 for Atlantic salmon, there are only 200 for turbot, 2.448 for sea bream and 24.452 for sea bass. As a comparison there are 833.880 zebrafish ESTs.

IMMUNE RESPONSE AND DISEASE RESISTANCE

Another approach that is being used to characterize genes related with immune response and disease resistance if the study of differential expression of genes using Suppression Subtractive Hybridization (SSH). SSH is a powerful technique that allows the comparison of two mRNA populations, cloning genes that express in one but not in the other. Two pioneer SSH examples are the identification of T cell receptors and the identification of activated genes in *Xenopus laevis* gastrulation. Since then several modifications of the technique have been described.

Alonso and Leong used SSH Chinook salmon and staghorn sculpin (*Hemilepdotus spinosus*) to determine differentially expressed genes against Poly I:C, a potent IFN inducer, finding that the overexpressed genes were quite similar to those described as IFN inducible in mammals. Bayne *et al.* identified rainbow trout immune genes constructing a subtracted library with livers from fish injected with *Vibrio* bacterine. The resulting library consisted in 300-600 bp fragments with 25 genes related with the immune system, of which 15 had not been previously described in salmonid fish and 12 not in any fish at all. The library included acute phase genes such as amyloid A protein, transferrine and precerebeline type protein, complement proteins and lectins, a putative antimicrobial peptide, several membrane receptors, such as TLRs and IL-1 receptor.

O'Farrell *et al.* also used SSH to identify changes in host cells against viral infections (rainbow trout/Viral Hemorrhagic Septicemia, VHS). 24 genes were identified as induced by the virus, most of them were IFN inducible. Zhang *et al.* used SSH to study the model grass carp/Grass Carp Hemorrhagic Virus (GCHV) to conclude that IFN and IFN induced genes are the main tool against virus. Also, with a viral infection model using Chinese perch and Infectious Spleen and Kidney Necrosis Virus (ISKNV), He *et al.* found genes related with the immune response and apoptosis and with the proteasome degradation pathway of ubiquinated protein that was found also in the SSH library generated by O'Farrell *et al.* and also by Dios *et al*.

Another approach was cDNA libraries generation from primed organs and randomly sequencing of a group of clones. These were successful approaches but with high cost and low efficacy. The same approach was used by Fernandez-Gonzalez *et al.* to detect immune genes in carp experimentally infected with *Icthyophthirius multifilis* sampled at 3 and 72 hours post-infection. In a total of 3.500 ESTs, 82 ortologues with immune relevance, previously described in other organisms, were found. 61 of them have not been previously described in carp. Among them the complete Prostaglandin D2 Synthetase (PGDS), the chemokine SCYA103 and a second βm2 macroglobulin gene were found.

The expression modulation by this parasite was determined by RealTime-PCR (RT-PCR). Tsoi *et al.* used SSH to determine the differential expression of Atlantic salmon genes against the furunculosis etiological agent *Aeromonas salmonicida*.

Subtracted cDNA libraries were prepared from three immune organs at two times after infection. A forward and a reverse library were constructed and 200 clones of each library were sequenced, giving a total of 1.778 ESTs that were annotated according functional categories and deposited in GenBank. Numerous genes involved in signalling, innate immunity and other processes were identified.

They include genes that are involved in acute phase and other more novel genes such as tachylectin, hepcidin, genes similar to precerebeline or methyltransferase, a putative protein that binds saxitoxine, etc. A subgroup of genes was studied with more detail by virtual Northern or RT-PCR to verify the differential expression as a result of the infection. Matejusova *et al.* used SSH to determine *Gyrodactylus salaris* infected Atlantic salmon gene expression profiles. Dios *et al.* used this technique to determine gene profile expression in sea bream brain after nodavirus infection that has the CNS as target. Forward and reverse libraries were generated one day post-infection and the ESTs expressed in infected tissues were catalogued as belonging to stress an immune response. In the reverse library (ESTs expressed in controls when compared with infected tissues) the most expressed genes were ribosomal and mitochondrial.

PHYSICAL PLATFORMS OF MICROARRAYS

Microarrays are physical platforms or chips (usually glass slides) with genes or gene sequences printed, which allow for the simultaneous analysis of the expression of hundred or thousands of genes. The study of these expression profiles in tissues or cell pools constitute the basis for functional genomics. Microarrays can be prepared by printing ESTs, generated from cDNA libraries (subtracted or not) or by short oligos (25-70 bp), designed from the ESTs specific regions such as 3' Untranslated Regions (3'UTRs) or code regions, if alternative splicing studies are the goal.

Sometimes cDNA microarrays are prone to the ambiguous EST identification, as they can produce cross-hybridizations among homologous genes and they are not able to distinguish different products of the same gene resulting from differential splicing. In contrast, oligo microarrays avoid some of these problems, but are more expensive. Thus, its application in projects of species involving an important research using arrays could be justified.

Comparative studies between different platforms do not permit a definitive conclusion in this matter. In fact, controversial results between oligo and cDNA platforms have been described. The use of microarrays allows the detection of gene expression profile changes under different experimental conditions such as pathogens, probiotics, developmental stages, contaminants, etc..

The use of microarrays in fish diseases studies was based on human cDNA microarrays. Commercially available human cDNA microarrays were used to compare differential expression in the livers of Atlantic salmon infected with *A. salmonicida* compared to healthy fish. cDNA probes were prepared from total RNA isolated from livers of control salmon and infected salmon by reverse transcription in the presence of 33P-dCTP and independently hybridized to human GENEFILTERS GF211 microarrays. Of the 4.131 known genes on the microarray, 241 spots gave clearly detectable signals using labelled RNA from the control salmon liver.

Of these, 4 spots were consistently found to have a greater than 2-fold increase in infected salmon compared with controls when using the same pair of filters to generate hybridization data from triplicates. These up-regulated genes were ADP/ATP Translocase (AAT2), Na+/K+ ATPase, Acyloxyacyl Hydrolase (AOAH), and Platelet-Derived Growth Factor (PDGF-A). A BlastN search revealed an AAT2 homolog from Atlantic salmon, and a reverse transcriptase polymerase chain reaction assay using primers based on this sequence confirmed its up-regulation (approx. 1.8-fold) during early infection. This work demonstrates the feasibility of using human microarrays to facilitate the discovery of differentially expressed genes in Atlantic salmon.

This was corroborated by Renn *et al.*, which used a microarray prepared with 4.500 genes from a specific cichlid *Astalotilapia burtoni* brain cDNA library. This microarray was used with different fish species and the degree of concordance in expression profiles (number of genes and changes in the levels of expression) was consistent. Rise *et al.* used microarrays constructed with ESTs previously described to study macrophage and haematopoietic kidney gene expression modulated by *Piscirickettsia salmonis* infection. Results were validated by RT-PCR. In infected salmon macrophages, 71 different transcripts were up-regulated and 31 different transcripts were down-regulated. In infected haematopoietic kidney, 30 different transcripts were up-regulated and 39 different transcripts were down-regulated.

Ten antioxidant genes, including glutathione *S*-transferase, glutathione reductase, glutathione peroxidase, and cytochrome b558 and subunits, were up-regulated in infected macrophages but not in infected haematopoietic kidney. Changes in redox status of infected macrophages may allow these cells to tolerate *P. salmonis* infection raising the possibility that the treatment with antioxidants may reduce haematopoietic tissue damage caused by this rickettsial infection. The down-regulation of transcripts involved in adaptive immune responses (*e.g.*, T cell receptor chain and C-C chemokine receptor 7) in infected haematopoietic kidney but not in infected macrophages may contribute to infection-induced kidney tissue damage.

Molecular biomarkers of *P. salmonis* infection, characterized by immune-relevant functional annotations and high fold differences in expression between infected and non- infected samples, may aid in the development of anti-piscirickettsial vaccines and therapeutics. Purcell *et al.* also used this microarray to study Atlantic salmon gene profile against a DNA vector or an Infectious Haematopoietic Necrosis Virus (IHNV) DNA vaccine. Eighty different genes were significantly modulated in the DNA vector group while 910 genes were modulated in the IHNV DNA vaccinated group relative to control group. RT-PCR was used to examine expression of selected immune genes at the Intra Muscular (I.M.) site and in other secondary tissues.

In the localized response (I.M. site), the magnitude of gene expression changes was much greater in the vaccinate group relative to the DNA vector group for the majority of genes analyzed. At secondary systemic sites (*e.g.* gill, kidney and spleen), type I IFN-related genes were up-regulated in only the IHNV DNA vaccinated group. The results presented here suggest that the IHNV DNA vaccine induces up-regulation of the type I IFN system across multiple tissues, which is the functional basis of early anti-viral immunity.

In a similar way Martin *et al.* used this microarray to study the response of Atlantic salmon against an *A. salmonicida* vaccine and found that the greatest increase in expression identified in the array analysis was a liver antibacterial peptide, hepcidin, which was increased 11-fold following the challenge. Roberge *et al.* also used this microarray to determine the levels for gene expression in *Saprolegnia* infected salmon, confirming the importance of non- specific immune response in the resistance against this disease.

MacKenzie *et al.* used another microarray developed by Krasnov *et al.* including 1.380 genes printed in six replicates. They studied the ability of cortisol to directly modulate the transcriptional response of rainbow trout macrophages to the cellular activator LPS. The results indicate that cortisol significantly inhibits the well-described LPS-dependent induction of the expression of TNF-alpha2, a pro-inflammatory cytokine through a complex network of interactions. Gerwick *et al.* used an oligo microarray to study gene profile in the inflammatory process of de *Listonella* (*Vibrio*) *anguillarum* bacterine injected to rainbow trout livers with Freund adjuvant. Microarray analysis determined that individual variability was high probably due to variable resistance to the disease. Li and Waldbieser have also reported the construction and use of a microarray for catfish aimed to the study of innate immune response.

The high density microarray was prepared from oligos based on catfish ESTs. This platform was used to study the gene profile in catfish spleens 2, 4, 8 and 24 hours post-LPS injection. 38 genes were modulated by LPS treatment. The expression of 9 genes determined by RT-PCR was positively correlated with microarray data. Byon *et al.* determined the antiviral response in Japanese flounder using a microarray. Non-specific immune response genes such as Macrophage Inflammatory Protein 1-a (MIP 1-a) receptor of Natural Killer (NK) and Kupffer cells and Mx1 protein gene were observed to be up-regulated by the VHSV G-protein DNA vaccine at 1 and 3 days post-immunization.

Also, specific immune-related genes including the CD20 receptor, CD8 alpha chain, CD40 and B lymphocyte cell adhesion molecule were also up-regulated during that time. In a later work Byon *et al.* determined that humoral defence-related genes such as complement component C3, complement regulatory plasma proteins, IgM, IgD, MHC class II-associated invariant chain and CD20 receptor were observed to be up-regulated by the VHSg recombinant protein vaccine at 1 or 21 days post-vaccination.

On the other hand, cellular defence-related genes such as CD8 alpha chain, T-cell immune regulator, MIP 1-a and apoptosis-associated protein were not detected. With a second version of this microarray Matsuyama *et al.* determined the immune response of Japanese flounder against *Edwardsiella tarda*. Among the 1.187 analyzed genes, 42 genes were up-regulated during the course of infection either in vaccinated or non-vaccinated fish.

These genes included immune-related genes, such as Matrix Metalloproteinases (MMP) MMP-9, MMP-13, CXC chemokine, CD20 receptor and hepcidin. Some immune-related genes were down-regulated after the *E. tarda* challenge, *i.e.* interferon inducible Mx protein, MHC class II-associated invariant chain, MHC class II alpha and MHC class II beta encoding genes, immunoglobulin light chain precursor, immunoglobulin light chain and IgM. Kurobe *et al.* using cDNA microarray containing 871 unique cDNAs including 91 putative immune-related genes studied the gene expression of *in vitro* grown kidney cells stimulated with mitogens such as Concanavalin A (ConA), Phorbol Myristate Acetate (PMA), LPS or infected with hirame rhabdovirus (HRV). The number of genes whose expression was increased or decreased by these factors was: 17 by Con A, 139 by PMA, 76 by LPS and 182 by HRV infection. The treatment of ConA for 1 and 6 h affected the expression of only a few of the immune-related genes. PMA down-regulated much more genes from the ones it up-regulated.

Apoptosis-related factors such as c-fos, NGF induced protein IB and NR13 genes were among the genes whose expression was induced by PMA. LPS induced the expression of inflammation-related genes, such as IL-1β, monocyte chemotactic protein 1 and collagenase. The expression of many genes was induced after 3 h HRV infection but some of them were decreased to the basal level after 6 h HRV infection. The expression of some genes of unknown function was induced or reduced by Con A, PMA or LPS or by HRV infection in different time periods. Dios *et al.* studied gene profile expression of nodavirus infected sea bream. cDNA SSH libraries were generated 1 day post-infection.

Some of the genes were included in functional categories of stress and immune system. To check the modulation of expression profiles, samples were taken 1, 3 and 7 days post-infection and hybridized with a macroarray with 765 genes constructed from PCR products with more than 300 bp from the SSH forward (385 genes) and reverse (380) libraries. Significant changes of antiviral genes were detected.

CLONED AND GENETICALLY MODIFIED ANIMALS

Several animal species have already been genetically modified, and at least eleven have been cloned, though some scientists doubt the health of those clones that survived to birth. Some of these efforts are commercial, either for agribusiness or for sale directly to consumers as pets. Others are scientific experiments, usually defended as advancing, directly or indirectly, the cause of medicine for humans.

The cloning or genetic modification of pets serves no justifiable purpose. These efforts serve only to play upon one set of emotions-our affection for our companion pets-in order to desensitize another set of emotions-our repugnance at the idea of treating them as artifacts that can be "designed" and manufactured.

The modification of livestock and the possibility of cloned meat entering the food chain are very controversial. So is the possible use of genetically modified animals to "grow" either pharmaceutical products or organs for transplant into humans.

CLONING

There have been published reports of the following species being cloned: carp, sheep, mice, cattle, goats, pigs, cats, rabbits, mules, horses, rats, and a deer. Some closely related species have also been cloned (a banteng, a wild cow, and a mouflon, a kind of sheep). A gaur, a wild ox, was cloned but died within two days. Attempts have also been made, without success, to clone monkeys, dogs, pandas, chickens, and at least two extinct species: the Tasmanian tiger and the woolly mammoth. The mammoth experiment used an elephant surrogate and tissue found in permafrost. Three major British institutions announced in July 2004 that they were setting up a tissue bank to preserve the DNA of endangered species, even after their extinction. Future cloning is seen as a possibility.

The Roslin Institute, where the first mammal was cloned, maintains records of all published mammalian cloning experiments up to July 2002 - 50 papers detailing 68 experiments, with 386 surviving clones. They conclude that the "overall efficiency of cloning is typically between 0 and 3 per cent (number of live offspring as a percentage of the number of nuclear transfer embryos), irrespective of the species, the donor cell type or technique." There is no evidence that efficiency has significantly improved since.

Cloning for Livestock

About 300 bulls have been cloned, with the aim of improving the quality of breeding stock. Cloning is too expensive, at around $20,000 per bull, to clone directly for meat, but breeding bulls are worth much more than that. The meat and milk of cloned cattle is presently kept off the market pending FDA approval. Nevertheless, BIO is actively promoting the use of cloned and transgenic animals for human food, as well as for pharmaceuticals.

The FDA is investigating the possibility of selling meat from cloned pigs as well as cattle, and in 2003 released a draft executive summary well in advance of the report it was supposed to summarize. "The FDA wants to gauge public reaction to the prospect of food from cloned farm animals before it decides whether to require government approval of the products before they are sold. That decision is expected to take another year."

Pet Cloning

In 1998 Arizona billionaire John Sperling gave $3.7 million to Texas A&M University to clone his pet dog, Missy (the "Missyplicity Project"). Sperling is controversial. He became wealthy as founder of the University of Phoenix, a distance learning university that has been accused by many of being a "diploma mill." He has since used his assets to support a number of idiosyncratic endeavors.

The dog-cloning effort failed, and the team, reportedly against Sperling's wishes, began parallel efforts to clone a cat. The birth of the first cloned domestic cat was announced by the Texas A&M research team in February 2002. Born on December 22, 2001, "CopyCat" or "CC" was produced by fusing an ovarian tissue cell from an adult cat with a cat egg, and implanting the clonal embryo into an adult cat. This cloning "success" occurred after 188 failed attempts. Sperling retained Lou Hawthorne, a publicist from Marin County, California, to handle public relations for his dog-cloning effort. Hawthorne subsequently established "Genetic Savings and Clone" as a profit-making venture to provide pet cloning services.

The company is offering to clone cats for $50,000. They also offer "gene banking" services for up to $1395, plus up to $150/year, all of which can be credited against the future cost of cloning. They announced in April 2004 that five customers had paid the fee, work had already begun on three other cats for staff members and one more slot was available, to make "nine lives." They hope to increase production to several thousand a year, and to reduce the cost substantially.

GENETIC MODIFICATION

Science, Mice and Patents

The most commonly genetically modified animal is almost certainly the mouse. It is small, short-lived and sufficiently similar to humans to be an almost ideal laboratory animal. As a result, mice have not only been cloned and modified, they have led to an actual industry in the production of "knockout mice," that is, mice with a particular gene or set of genes inactivated for research purposes. Trans Genic Inc asserts, "Currently, we are able to produce almost 1,000 strains of Knockout mouse in a year." "Pharming". Cattle, sheep, goats, chickens, rabbits and pigs have been genetically modified with the aim of producing human proteins that are useful, generally as medicines. The gene transfer process is typically very inefficient, and cloning is seen as another way of propagating the GM animal. A 1999 USDA report cited estimates that there was a $24 billion market for human proteins, and theoretically 600 transgenic cows could supply the worldwide demands for some drugs. In practice, however, several companies that have pursued this line have gone bust, and the profit potential seems less than it once did.

Genetic modification of animals in order to improve the prospects of organ transplants is also being investigated.

Genetically Modified Fish as Pets

A tropical fish genetically modified to glow in the dark went on sale in Taiwan in 2003 for about $17 each. A different variety of zebrafish, called "GloFish," which were created in Singapore, reached the United States market in January 2004.

The distributor says that GloFish were originally developed to fluoresce only in the presence of pollutants, but that is not the form in which they are being sold. They cost about $5 each, and are intended to live in aquariums, but can breed and, in the right conditions, live in the wild.

The Food and Drug Administration (FDA) approved the sale without ceremony. A coalition led by the Center for Food Safety filed suit against the decision, but sales went ahead. In California, the Fish and Game Commission initially banned the fish but later agreed to hold hearings at the request of the distributor.

Allergy-free Cats

A company called Transgenic Pets, in Syracuse, NY, was widely reported in 2001 to be working with scientists at the University of Connecticut to "remove the allergen gene" from cats. The company hoped to raise $2 million and sell the modified animals for $1,000 each. Funding problems ended the project.

Genetic Modification for Aquaculture

Most discussion of bioengineered food focuses on plants, but work on animals and fish is well under way. Genetically modified salmon have already been created, though FDA approval is not expected before at least 2006 and the target date has repeatedly been delayed. The Biotechnology Industry Organization (BIO) and the developers, Aqua Bounty Farms, claim that the GE salmon grow faster but not larger than ordinary salmon, but this is strongly disputed. Opponents also cite studies showing dramatic population crashes and unpredictable environmental impacts.

Salmon are not the only fish species being modified. Acting FDA Commissioner Lester M. Crawford summarized the position in a speech given in March 2004: "Less well known is that catfish and tilapia have been also genetically modified to grow faster and more efficiently than their non-transgenic counterparts. Rainbow trout has been engineered to increase its contents of omega 3 fatty acids, and shellfish is being modified to reduce its allergenicity and make it grow faster."

The matter-of-fact, if not approving, tone of these comments is disturbing, as it comes from the head of the agency that is supposed to be regulating these technologies. Other countries, including Canada, have moved much faster than the United States to ban or at least place a moratorium on the genetic modification of fish. Malcolm Grant, Chair of the UK Agriculture and Environment Biotechnology Commission, points out that

"Once the fish has escaped, there's virtually nothing that can be done to recall it... Genetic biotechnology has opened a new chapter in the relationship between man and animals. We must therefore prepare now for developments that may be many years away." He also argues that pet cloning is "trivial, distasteful and could be sold to gullible owners."

Genetically Modified Farm Animals

Acting Commissioner Crawford continued: "Cows can be bioengineered to produce several varieties of milk: milk with a lower level of a protein that's allergenic to some infants; milk that is more easily digested by people who are lactose intolerant; milk that has more naturally occurring antimicrobial enzyme, and therefore has longer shelf life; and milk that makes better cheese because it has altered distribution of caseins or less fat."

Genetic Modification for Livestock

Research is also underway to use genetic modification to improve the health of cows and pigs. Advocates hope to produce cattle that would be resistant to Mad Cow disease, for example. There have also been reports of cows being genetically modified to "produce milk with higher than normal levels of protein, which would speed the process of making cheese."

CHIMERAS

Some researchers have created embryos with genetic material from both a human and an animal, also known as chimeras. Most claim this is for research purposes only, and such embryos would never be implanted or brought to term. But some bioethicists are unwilling to draw a line that would prevent it.

For example, Jason Scott Robert and Francoise Baylis assert that they take "no stance at all" on whether "interspecies hybrids or chimeras from human materials should be forbidden or embraced." But much of their article is devoted to their contention that "the arguments against... creating novel part-human beings... are largely unsatisfactory."

The prospect of such human-animal chimeras being born raises a number of troubling questions. Does such an organism have human rights? What if it were 99.9 per cent human and 0.1 per cent chimpanzee? What of the reverse situation? The mixing of species can occur at three different levels. First, some DNA from one organism can be inserted into another organism's genome. Most often, however, these are described as transgenic animals rather than chimeras. For example, scientists have produced transgenic mice which contain some human genes.

Another type of chimera involves a blastocyst containing components from multiple species. James Grifo has used this technique for fertility research. After the US federal government informed him he could no longer continue his experiments, his team moved to China. There, they removed the nucleus from a fertilized rabbit egg and inserted a nucleus from a human somatic cell. The resulting embryos, which still contained rabbit mitochondrial DNA, were allowed to grow for 14 days before destruction.

Finally, scientists have placed cells from one species, typically human stem cells, into a multicellular embryo of another species. In 2004, researchers were surprised to discover that injecting human stem cells into a pig embryo resulted in a fetus whose cellular components were intermingled down to the genetic level. Many cells contained chromosomal DNA of both pig and human origin.

Opposition

Several environmental and animal rights organizations have expressed opposition to pet cloning, including Friends of the Earth and the Humane Society of the United States, the largest animal welfare organization in the country. Jeremy Rifkin from the Foundation on Economic Trends and Stuart Newman of the New York Medical College and the Council for Responsible Genetics have pursued a novel path of opposition. They filed a patent application with the US Patent and Trademark Office for chimeric embryos and animals containing human cells. They did not intent to create a "humouse." Instead, they tried to force the PTO to take a position and, if the patent is granted, to prevent chimeras from being developed.

CLONING AND GENETICALLY ALTERED ANIMALS

At Eurogroup for Animals, we believe that humans have a duty to safeguard animals' welfare and health and we oppose all human activity that causes distress or suffering. In particular in the area of animal breeding, we are of the opinion that animals genetic constitution should not be changed if doing so causes suffering to themselves or to future generations.

Genetic selection must always seek to maximise the wellbeing of the resultant animal. Animal breeding should support a diverse gene pool in order that the genetic resources to maximise wellbeing are sustained for future generations. Techniques and technologies used in animal reproduction must not be used if they cause distress or suffering.

For these reasons Eurogroup is opposed to the cloning of animals and would urge the EU to introduce an immediate ban on the cloning of animals for food production, and on the sale of imported food products from cloned animals and their offspring.

Eurogroup is concerned that delaying a decision will mean that food from cloned animals will enter the supply chain uncontrolled and without consideration of the opposition of EU citizens and consumers. Under Article 13 of the Lisbon Treaty, in the EU it is a legal obligation to pay full regard to the welfare requirements of animals when formulating and implementing the Union's agriculture, fisheries, transport, internal market, research and technological development and space policies.

Our concerns are based on the fact that some of the developments and applications of animal cloning and other genetic alteration techniques:

- Involve procedures that may cause animals pain, suffering or distress;
- Use a very large number of animals;

- Encourage a wider variety of applications leading to increased animal use;
- Increase the perception of animals as commodities for human use and/or gain, such as research tools or units of production;
- Are progressing at a rate that is outstripping public understanding and ethical and public debate.

CONCERNS RELATING TO HUMAN AND ANIMAL HEALTH

The main applications of cloned and other genetically altered (GA) animals (and their offspring) that are of concern at the present time are:

- The creation of genetically manipulated (GA) and cloned animals;
- The subsequent use of these GA animals (and their offspring):
    - As livestock on farms (used to standardize/maximise quantity and reduce the costs of processing/producing animal derived food products *e.g.* milk, meat, eggs);
    - As disease models;
    - In fundamental research *e.g.* to understand gene function;
    - In toxicity testing;
    - As bioreactors to produce biologically active compounds for experimental and/or medical purposes;
    - As sources of cells, tissues and organs for xenotransplantation;
    - In the creation of cloned pets, sports animals and 'living art'.

However, any new biotechnology, or new application of existing technologies, that is developed and/or tested in animal models, or that causes the animals pain, suffering, distress or lasting harm is of serious concern to Eurogroup. Examples include tissue engineering and the development of nanotechnology generally. Production of cloned and other GA animals

GENERAL ETHICAL AND ANIMAL WELFARE CONCERNS

Numbers of Animals Used

Use of animals in experiments is a matter of serious public concern and pressure to reduce numbers has contributed to a downward trend in some countries. Creation and use of GA animals is reversing this trend and there has been an exponential rise in the number of GA animals used in scientific procedures each year in some EU member states.

For example, in the UK, the number of GA animals has risen from around 50,000 in 1990 to 900,000 in 2004. In Germany, Ireland, Finland, Sweden and the Netherlands, there is also increasing creation and use of GA animals. GA animals can be produced by a number of different techniques, all of which are inherently wasteful with respect to the number of embryos that are manipulated relative to the number of GA offspring subsequently produced. Current estimates suggest only a 3-5 per cent success rate when generating new GA animals. The remaining offspring are surplus to requirements and are killed. A large number of animals are therefore used to provide sufficient eggs or embryos for genetic manipulation, and to act as recipients and foster mothers for the manipulated embryos.

These animals will usually be killed, either before harvesting the eggs or embryos, or, in the case of recipients, once their young are weaned. Thus GA technology is wasteful of animal life and the ethical implications of such wastage are important and need to be acknowledged.

Potential for Pain, Suffering or Distress During Creation of GA or Cloned Animals

The procedures used to produce GA and/or nuclear transfer cloned animals involve hormonal and surgical interventions that can cause pain, suffering and distress. These include; superovulation, vasectomy, semen and embryo collection and embryo transfer. Many of the manipulated embryos die during gestation. This may also cause suffering, although this depends on the stage of development at which death occurs and the species involved.

Adverse Effects as a Consequence of Genetic Modification and Cloning

Where GA animals are created as models of specific diseases, they can experience a range of adverse effects associated with the condition in question, which can have profound effects on their health and welfare. However, being genetically altered does not necessarily compromise the welfare of individual animals, and indeed some GA animals are indistinguishable from their non-GA siblings.

It also needs to be acknowledged that adverse effects may only become apparent when animals are subsequently maintained in a less well defined or controlled, environment than that of the laboratory or experimental farm. Nevertheless, in many cases, genetic alteration can have a deleterious effect on animal welfare and the harms caused depend on a number of factors.

Studies have shown that some *in vitro* culture procedures carried out during genetic manipulation or cloning protocols can lead to unpredictable complications in the animals subsequently produced. An example of this is Large Offspring Syndrome (LOS), which affects sheep, mice and cows following nuclear transfer.

As well as causing complications for the mother during birth, LOS encompasses a range of debilitating pathologies for the offspring including malformations in the liver, brain and urogenital tract, immune dysfunction, placental abnormalities, stillbirth, fetal overgrowth, respiratory failure and circulatory problems. A further concern is that there is currently no mechanism to ensure consistency in the training of personnel in specific GA technologies and procedures, or to ensure that experimental and other refinements are disseminated throughout the biotechnology community. This can have a profound influence on the levels of pain, suffering and distress experienced by animals undergoing these procedures. It can also have a negative impact on the success rates achieved and levels of animal wastage.

Concerns Regarding Mutagenesis Programmes

Mutagenesis (using chemicals such as ENU, or physical mutagens such as radiation, to increase the natural mutation rate of DNA) is the quickest method for producing large numbers of GA mice. This technique is being widely applied both in Europe and beyond, with mutagenesis programmes aiming to explore the function of every gene in the mouse genome.

This project presents a number of animal welfare concerns:

- The number of animals involved in mutagenesis programmes is vast; *e.g.* around 35-36,000 for a 3 year project, or around 50 animals per mutant line established;
- The process of mutagenising animals has significant animal welfare implications for the animals involved, for example males require 12-14 weeks to recover their fertility following treatment with a mutagen. Furthermore, only around 50 per cent of mutagenised males are able to go on to sire offspring with the remainder being culled;
- The mutations induced are by their very nature unpredictable and the scientific usefulness of mutagenised animals cannot therefore be predicted, nor can the effect of any mutation on the health and welfare of the animals. This makes the justification for producing GA mice in this way highly questionable.

CONCERNS REGARDING KNOCK-IN AND KNOCK-OUT TECHNOLOGY

A more targeted approach to the production of GA animals uses DNA constructs inserted into the animals genome to either completely remove a gene of interest (knock-out), or to replace a given gene with an altered version (knock-in). This is done either in the whole animal, or within specific tissues of an animal (conditional).

The animal welfare concerns include:

- At the current level of efficiency, the numbers of animals used is high - at least 200 animals will be used in the production of a single GA animal;
- The site of insertion into the host genome and the number of copies of the DNA construct inserted cannot always be controlled unless ES cell manipulation is used. This can be a problem because the incorporation of the construct DNA at an incorrect location can result

in the random inactivation of other genes or alterations in the expression of surrounding genes, both of which can impact on the health and welfare of the animals produced;

- When a knockout animal is generated the level, or pattern of expression observed for other genes can be altered to compensate for the lost gene. Thus any effects observed in the GA animal may not only reflect the loss of the gene of interest, which means that investigation of the effects is not always straightforward. The use of knock-out as an alternative to knock-in or conditional technology, therefore needs careful consideration and justification.

Special Concerns for Non-human Primates

This submission relates to all animals used in biotechnologies, but Eurogroup has particular concerns about the application of such technologies to non-human primates. Macaques have already been produced by nuclear transfer cloning in the USA and recent technical advances show that the production of GA primates is currently increasing. Eurogroup firmly believes that the genetic modification of non-human primates should not be allowed for any purpose, given the ethical issues raised by such developments, the large number of animals required to produce each GA animal, and the associated potential for harms.

ANIMAL MODELS OF DISEASE

A common justification for the creation of GA animals is that they will provide, or contribute to, 'improved', more predictive models of disease. This is an oversimplification because a) this is not necessarily always true, and b) even where a new GA model is more appropriate, it may be used alongside other, older models by different researchers. There is no mechanism for ensuring only the most relevant are used and that newer models are available to all researchers. In such cases the GA animal is not the new *definitive* model but just an *additional* one. The motivation for the research may merely be an interest in the model for its own sake, but a medical application may be used to justify the work since this is likely to be more acceptable publicly and politically. Basic, fundamental research carried out within academic research establishments is not regulated under Directive 86/609, so it may not undergo an ethical review with appropriate assessment and weighing of harms and benefits. This directive is under review and is expected to be adopted end 2010. The revised directive may incorporate basic, fundamental research with proper review, however only if implemented and enforced properly.

There is also currently no requirement for GA animals to be cryopreserved and stored within central archive facilities or depositories. Such methods can reduce repetition and duplication of work by providing a central resource for use by the wider scientific community and protect against adverse events such as environmental disasters or genetic drift. They also reduce the need for live transportation of GA animals, with associated welfare problems, because frozen gametes or embryos could be sent instead.

GA ANIMALS IN TOXICITY TESTING

GA mice and rats are increasingly used in genotoxicity and carcinogenicity testing, within studies that are done to fulfil regulatory requirements for the marketing of chemicals and pharmaceuticals. Such animals are likely to suffer equivalent (or even more severe) levels of pain and distress to those experienced by animals in traditional tests, but it has been claimed that fewer animals will be needed.

Eurogroup believes that reducing the numbers of animals used in research and testing is an important goal, provided that this can be done without increasing the level of suffering experienced by individual animals. However, relatively severe adverse effects have been reported in some GA strains used in toxicity testing. For example, mortality rates are higher in *c-neu* and *c-myc* mice used in carcinogenicity testing than in conventional mice used in the same type of test. Many GA mice used in carcinogenicity tests are more susceptible to developing cancer and so will develop tumours more rapidly, which could make it more difficult to implement humane endpoints. Reducing numbers is thus not automatically a positive outcome for animals - the impact on individuals must be taken into account and it may be justifiable to use more animals who will suffer less.

In any case, the contribution that biotechnologies can make to reducing animal numbers in carcinogenicity and genotoxicity is not consistent, largely due to actual or potential regulatory requirements. In carcinogenicity testing, GA mice were introduced to try to reduce animal numbers and the time taken to obtain test results. However, there are proposals to add additional control groups (a positive control and treated and untreated controls using non-GA mice) that would decrease the magnitude of the reduction if they are adopted. It is also uncertain whether testing on one GA strain will be regarded as sufficient by regulators, in which case the reductions will be further diminished by requirements for results obtained using other strains.

For genotoxicity testing, GA models have distinct scientific advantages over existing *in vivo* assays when used as second tier tests for *in vitro* genotoxins. The reduction in numbers of animals used would be fairly substantial, perhaps from 50 to 20 per substance tested, but again it is not certain that a test on one GA model would be regarded as sufficient. There are potentially much greater savings in animals if GA tests can be used in place of very large tests of heritable mutation which are currently used, albeit rarely, for chemicals of high concern.

Conversely, using GA animal models in toxicity testing could increase the use of animals by making some tests more practical, or by increasing the amount of information they produce. For example, the use of GA animals could make investigations feasible that would otherwise require very large and impractical numbers of non-GA animals.

Regulators might be inclined to ask for the GA test in cases where the conventional test would not have been requested (and could therefore presumably have been done without) because it was regarded as too cumbersome and possibly uninformative. Eurogroup believes that, in toxicity testing as in the other research fields discussed in this document, the focus should be on developing *in vitro* alternatives to replace animals and not on developing different animal models.

Animals as 'Bioreactors'

This category of GA animal use includes:

- "Pharmed" animals who produce therapeutic substances *e.g.* pigs who express the blood protein Factor IX in milk, and goats that express the anti-clotting agent Atryn in their milk;
- Animals producing specialist materials *e.g.* goats who produce spiders' silk proteins in their milk for use to make 'biosteel'. This has both medical and non-medical applications (*e.g.* in sutures and bullet-proof vests respectively) (Nexia Biotechnologies, Quebec);

The substance produced may have an adverse effect on the animal, either at the point of expression, or if it can enter the animal's bloodstream. For example, a strain of rabbits genetically engineered to express human erythropoietin (EPO) in the mammary glands also expresses the protein at low levels in other organs, resulting in greatly elevated numbers of red blood cells, infertility and premature death. Using animals in this way, and referring to them as 'bioreactors', reinforces the perception of animals as units of production and/or biological tools, rather than as sentient beings with the ability to experience pain, suffering and distress.

Xenotransplantation

The use of GA animals to supply organs, tissues or cells for transplantation into humans is a highly controversial issue which has been the subject of a great deal of debate. There are many legal, scientific, human health, animal welfare and ethical concerns, which have been described in a number of documents. Only the ethical and welfare issues relating to animals are addressed here.

These include:

- The ethics of genetically modifying animals of any species as a source of cells, tissues and organs for human transplantation;

- The harms associated with the initial creation of GA animals as source animals;
- The suffering and/or distress associated with production and maintenance systems for high health status source herds. This includes hysterotomy-derivation, early weaning practices, and barren husbandry environments, which have a serious negative impact on animal welfare because they prevent animals from satisfying their physical, social and behavioural needs.

Furthermore, development of xeno technology to a point where it can be used still requires a great deal of pre-clinical research. To date, such research has included studies of efficacy, physiology, immunology, and infection risks in a range of species including primates, goats and dogs.

This research, by its very nature, causes considerable suffering. Experiments involving organ transplantation require major surgery, which in itself causes suffering that is exacerbated by tissue rejection and immunosuppressive treatment.

Xenotransplantation is also an example of a biotechnology where over-optimistic claims are made to justify the approach, the funding and the use of animals. For example, in September 1995, the UK company Imutran *"envisaged the first xenotransplants of transgenic pig hearts into human patients taking place in 1996"*. Yet despite some progress, particularly with cell transplants, the transplant of whole organs is no closer and xenografts still rarely survive for more than a few months.

Cloning Companion Animals

Eurogroup believes that, without doubt, some applications of modern biotechnology are trivial, scientifically unnecessary and ethically unjustifiable.

Examples include;

- The cloning of champion racing and show jumping horses for sport;
- The generation of a green fluorescent rabbit 'GFP Bunny' as transgenic "art";
- The cloning of companion animals for example cats, purely to satisfy humans' emotional requirements.

CONCERNS RELATING TO AGRICULTURAL PRODUCTION

Gene mapping was/is the most widely used technique in agriculture to enhance selective breeding schemes, however as more and more 'super' animals exist this is being overtaken by the import/export of embryos and/or sperm from cloned 'super' animals.

Examples of agricultural applications of gene mapping and other genetic altering techniques that have given rise to ethical and animal welfare concerns include:

Increasing Productivity or Changing Body Composition

• Gene mapping has been used primarily to select individuals for breeding with the aim of increasing productivity *i.e.* growth rates, litter sizes and production traits such as egg laying, milk volume and meat quantity and quality (including the proportion of lean meat to fat). Whilst still being practiced to create 'super' individuals for subsequent breeding, gene mapping is being/has been replaced by the import/export of embryos and/or sperm from cloned 'super' livestock (primarily from the US).

Farmed species have also been genetically manipulated to alter the composition of meat and milk. For example, pigs and cows respectively have been genetically altered to have higher levels of Omega 3 in their muscle, and to express higher levels of casein in their milk.

Increasing Disease Resistance

Animals are genetically manipulated to be resistant to disease, for example, cattle have been engineered to express the antibiotic lysostaphin in their milk, which results in increased resistance to mastitis.

Animals (including pigs, sheep, mice and rabbits) have also been modified to express antibodies providing immunity to specific diseases, for example mice have been generated with protection against prion disease.

Making Animals More 'environmentally Friendly'

An example of this application is the 'Enviropig', which has been engineered to contain the enzyme phytase in the pigs' saliva so that they can digest sources of dietary phosphorus. This results in faeces with a lower phosphorus content, which in turn reduces the pollution of surface and ground water with phosphorus.

ETHICAL AND ANIMAL WELFARE CONCERNS

The selective breeding of farm animals has been conducted for thousands of years, and has given rise to a number of welfare concerns. However, Eurogroup believes that the use of cloning or other GA technologies to speed this process, or to introduce genes that could never be incorporated into the genomes of farm animals by any natural process, is a serious ethical and welfare issue. Directly altering an animal's genome is viewed by many as an unacceptable assault on the integrity of the animal that is incompatible with the concept of respecting farmed animals, and minimising the harms that are caused to them for human benefit. These views are important and should be respected as a legitimate part of the debate on biotechnology and farmed animal welfare.

Eurogroup also questions the necessity of further increasing production in farm animals. In many cases, productivity is already pushing animals to their physical and metabolic limits, so with any further increase there is an enhanced likelihood of animal welfare problems. Enhancing selective breeding, by gene mapping or genetic modification, can also cause suffering if the trait that is selected for has a negative impact on the rest of the animals' physiology. For example, hens who produce high numbers of eggs suffer from osteoporosis because the majority of the calcium they ingest is used in eggshell production.

There can also be less direct effects on welfare, in that some GA animals may receive lower standards of husbandry than conventional animals. For example, clinical mastitis is a major welfare problem in dairy systems with sub-optimal standards of hygiene, and early detection is reliant on routine inspections by parlour staff at milking. The creation of cattle resistant to mastitis may encourage the perception that mastitis is no longer a problem. This could not only compromise standards of parlour hygiene, but may reduce the level of attention paid to each animal at milking. This would increase the potential for other clinical or welfare problems to go undetected.

"High productivity" animals may also be at risk if their husbandry is not appropriate. It may be possible for them to be properly managed and cared for in the controlled environment of a breeding company or experimental farm, but there are serious concerns regarding the welfare of such animals once they are released into commercial agriculture.

Concluding Remarks

Modern biotechnologies have had, and will continue to have, a serious adverse impact on animals, particularly with regard to their use in scientific research and agriculture. This adverse impact relates to the numbers of animals used and the nature of the harms caused to them. In addition, directly altering an animal's genome, as occurs in many applications of biotechnology, is viewed by many as altering the integrity of the animal in a way that is incompatible with the concept of respecting animals, and minimising the harms that are caused to them for human benefit. Lastly, the technology is progressing at a rate that is outstripping public understanding and ethical and public debate.

The development and application of novel biotechnologies therefore poses new challenges for existing regulatory regimes in a number of fields of science, medicine, agriculture and the environment. Eurogroup believes that the broader issues surrounding the ethical and social acceptability of such uses of animals, as set out in this submission, cannot be effectively addressed within the current regulatory systems. The following principles are fundamental to ensuring that the lives and welfare of animals involved in all modern and future biotechnologies are awarded due priority.

- It is critically important that all relevant regulatory systems are updated to take into account the animal welfare, ethical and social implications and societal concerns of the development and intended use of all modern biotechnologies.

- Biotechnology is applied in many different fields so there needs to be effective liaison, co-ordination and definition of responsibilities within and between all the relevant legislative and regulatory bodies concerned with a particular issue. This includes, for example, the different bodies regulating use of animals in experiments and those setting requirements for product regulation.
- The regulatory framework for each technology must encompass a process which enables a critical scrutiny of the potential harms to animals and the intended benefits, and a careful and fair weighing of these. This applies to broad research directions as well as individual projects and the further application of new technologies that result from these. Critical assessment of justification needs to be done prior to the development and/or application of a technology and must then be reviewed regularly to check whether the harms and benefits are as expected so that appropriate action can be taken if necessary.
- A mechanism should be set in place to ensure that the justification and clinical relevance of all research involving the production and use of GA animals is critically scrutinised, such that animals are not used simply because the technology is available. This also needs to ensure that animal models of disease are regularly reviewed, so that redundant models are no longer routinely used for research purposes.
- There needs to be greater transparency with regard to the use of animals in biotechnology throughout Europe. Clearer information on the numbers of animals, and nature and level of any suffering that they experience, is essential in order to be able to identify issues of concern and assess trends. It is also vital that the public is well informed and therefore able to engage in constructive debate on the associated ethical issues.
- Restrictions should be placed on the species of animal that it is permissible to genetically modify. Non-human primates should not be genetically modified or cloned for any purpose, nor used as source animals for cells, tissues or organs.
- The production of GA livestock where the intention is to modify traits such as increased lean to fat ratio, growth rate, or litter size should not be allowed, as levels of productivity are already causing serious welfare problems.
- There should be far greater effort devoted to developing and validating alternatives to animal use in all fields. There should be greater commitment to, and endorsement of, the principles of the Three Rs of reduction, refinement and replacement in animal experiments.
  Examples especially relevant to modern biotechnology are:
  - The development of GA germ cells for *in vitro* testing;

- The production of drugs, proteins, or material by bacteria rather than 'bioreactor' animals;
- Generating cells, tissues and organs for treatment or transplantation using a patients own cells, eg human bladders.

CURRENT CONTEXT OF GENETICALLY ENGINEERED ANIMALS

Genetic engineering technology has numerous applications involving companion, wild, and farm animals, and animal models used in scientific research. The majority of genetically engineered animals are still in the research phase, rather than actually in use for their intended applications, or commercially available.

COMPANION ANIMALS

By inserting genes from sea anemone and jellyfish, zebrafish have been genetically engineered to express fluorescent proteins — hence the commonly termed "GloFish." GloFish began to be marketed in the United States in 2003 as ornamental pet fish; however, their sale sparked controversial ethical debates in California — the only US state to prohibit the sale of GloFish as pets. In addition to the insertion of foreign genes, gene knock-out techniques are also being used to create designer companion animals.

For example, in the creation of hypoallergenic cats some companies use genetic engineering techniques to remove the gene that codes for the major cat allergen.

Companion species have also been derived by cloning. The first cloned cat, "CC," was created in 2002. At the time, the ability to clone mammals was a coveted prize, and after just a few years scientists created the first cloned dog, "Snuppy". With the exception of a couple of isolated cases, the genetically engineered pet industry is yet to move forward. However, it remains feasible that genetically engineered pets could become part of day-to-day life for practicing veterinarians, and there is evidence that clients have started to enquire about genetic engineering services, in particular the cloning of deceased pets.

Wild Animals

The primary application of genetic engineering to wild species involves cloning. This technology could be applied to either extinct or endangered species; for example, there have been plans to clone the extinct thylacine and the woolly mammoth. Holt et al point out that, "As many conservationists are still suspicious of reproductive technologies, it is unlikely that cloning techniques would be easily accepted. Individuals involved in field conservation often harbour suspicions that hi-tech approaches, backed by high profile publicity would divert funding away from their own efforts." However, cloning may prove to be an important tool to be used alongside other forms of assisted reproduction to help retain genetic diversity in small populations of endangered species.

Farm Animals

As reviewed by Laible, there is "an assorted range of agricultural livestock applications [for genetic engineering] aimed at improving animal productivity; food quality and disease resistance; and environmental sustainability." Productivity of farm animal species can be increased using genetic engineering. Examples include transgenic pigs and sheep that have been genetically altered to express higher levels of growth hormone.

Genetically engineered farm animals can be created to enhance food quality. For example, pigs have been genetically engineered to express the Ä12 fatty acid desaturase gene (from spinach) for higher levels of omega-3, and goats have been genetically engineered to express human lysozyme in their milk. Such advances may add to the nutritional value of animal-based products.

Farm species may be genetically engineered to create disease-resistant animals. Specific examples include conferring immunity to offspring via antibody expression in the milk of the mother; disruption of the virus entry mechanism (which is applicable to diseases such as pseudorabies); resistance to prion diseases; parasite control (especially in sheep); and mastitis resistance (particularly in cattle).

Genetic engineering has also been applied with the aim of reducing agricultural pollution. The best-known example is the Enviropig; a pig that is genetically engineered to produce an enzyme that breaks down dietary phosphorus (phytase), thus limiting the amount of phosphorus released in its manure. Despite resistance to the commercialization of genetically engineered animals for food production, primarily due to lack of support from the public, a recent debate over genetically engineered AquAdvantage Atlantic salmon may result in these animals being introduced into commercial production.

Effort has also been made to generate genetically engineered farm species such as cows, goats, and sheep that express medically important proteins in their milk. According to Dyck et al, "transgenic animal bioreactors represent a powerful tool to address the growing need for therapeutic recombinant proteins." In 2006, ATryn® became the first therapeutic protein produced by genetically engineered animals to be approved by the Food and Drug Administration (FDA) of the United States. This product is used as a prophylactic treatment for patients that have hereditary antithrombin deficiency and are undergoing surgical procedures.

Research Animals

Biomedical applications of genetically engineered animals are numerous, and include understanding of gene function, modeling of human disease to either understand disease mechanisms or to aid drug development, and xenotransplantation.

Through the addition, removal, or alteration of genes, scientists can pinpoint what a gene does by observing the biological systems that are affected. While some genetic alterations have no obvious effect, others may produce different phenotypes that can be used by researchers to understand the function of the affected genes. Genetic engineering has enabled the creation of human disease models that were previously unavailable. Animal models of human disease are valuable resources for understanding how and why a particular disease develops, and what can be done to halt or reverse the process. As a result, efforts have focused on developing new genetically engineered animal models of conditions such as Alzheimer's disease, amyotrophic lateral sclerosis (ALS), Parkinson's disease, and cancer. However, as Wells (13) points out: "these [genetically engineered animal] models do not always accurately reflect the human condition, and care must be taken to understand the limitation of such models."

The use of genetically engineered animals has also become routine within the pharmaceutical industry, for drug discovery, drug development, and risk assessment.

As discussed by Rudmann and Durham: "Transgenic and knock out mouse models are extremely useful in drug discovery, especially when defining potential therapeutic targets for modifying immune and inflammatory responses...Specific areas for which [genetically engineered animal models] may be useful are in screening for drug induced immunotoxicity, genotoxicity, and carcinogenicity, and in understanding toxicity related drug metabolizing enzyme systems."

Perhaps the most controversial use of genetically engineered animals in science is to develop the basic research on xenotrans-plantation — that is, the transplant of cells, tissues, or whole organs from animal donors into human recipients.

In relation to organ transplants, scientists have developed a genetically engineered pig with the aim of reducing rejection of pig organs by human recipients. This particular application of genetic engineering is currently at the basic research stage, but it shows great promise in alleviating the long waiting lists for organ transplants, as the number of people needing transplants currently far outweighs the number of donated organs.

However, as a direct result of public consultation, a moratorium is currently in place preventing pig organ transplantation from entering a clinical trial phase until the public is assured that the potential disease transfer from pigs to humans can be satisfactorily managed. According to Health Canada, "xenotransplantation is currently not prohibited in Canada. However, the live cells and organs from animal sources are considered to be therapeutic products (drugs or medical devices)...No clinical trial involving xenotransplantation has yet been approved by Health Canada".

ETHICAL ISSUES OF GENETIC ENGINEERING

Ethical issues, including concerns for animal welfare, can arise at all stages in the generation and life span of an individual genetically engineered animal. The following sections detail some of the issues that have arisen during the peer-driven guidelines development process and associated impact analysis consultations carried out by the CCAC. The CCAC works to an accepted ethic of animal use in science, which includes the principles of the Three Rs (Reduction of animal numbers, Refinement of practices and husbandry to minimize pain and distress, and Replacement of animals with non-animal alternatives wherever possible).

Together the Three Rs aim to minimize any pain and distress experienced by the animals used, and as such, they are considered the principles of humane experimental technique. However, despite the steps taken to minimize pain and distress, there is evidence of public concerns that go beyond the Three Rs and animal welfare regarding the creation and use of genetically engineered animals.

4

Cell Physiology

HUMAN BODY STRUCTURE

Human beings are debatably the most complex organisms on this planet. Imagine billions of microscopic parts, each with its own identity, working together in an organized manner for the benefit of the total being. The human body is a single structure but it is made up of billions of smaller structures of four major kinds:

CELLS

Cells contain long be recognized as the simplest units of living matter that can maintain life and reproduce themselves. The human body, which is made up of numerous cells, begins as a single, newly fertilized cell.

Organs

Organs are more compound units than tissues. An organ is an organization of several different kinds of tissues so arranged that together they can perform a special function. For example, the stomach is an organization of muscle, connective, epithelial, and nervous tissues. Muscle and connective tissues form its wall, epithelial and connective tissues form its lining, and nervous tissue extends throughout both its wall and its lining.

Tissues

Tissues are somewhat extra complex units than cells. By definition, a tissue is an organization of a great many similar cells with varying amounts and kinds of neo-living, intercellular substance between them.

Systems

Systems are the most complex of the component units of the human body. A system is an organization of varying numbers and kinds of organs so arranged that together they can perform complex functions for the body. Ten major systems compose the human body:

- Skeletal
- Muscular
- Nervous
- Endocrine
- Cardiovascular
- Lymphatic
- Respiratory
- Digestive
- Urinary
- Reproductive.

ANATOMICAL TERMINOLOGY

Before we get keen on the following learning units, it is necessary to learn some useful terms for describing body structure. Knowing these terms will make it much easier for us to understand the content of the following learning units.

Three groups of terms are introduced here: directional terms, terms describing planes of the body, and terms describing body cavities.

Directional Terms: Directional terms describe the positions of structures relative to other structures or locations in the body.

Superior or Cranial: Towards the head end of the body; upper (example, the hand is part of the superior extremity).

Inferior or Caudal: Away from the head; lower (example, the foot is part of the inferior extremity).

Anterior or Ventral: Front (example, the kneecap is located on the anterior side of the leg).

Posterior or Dorsal: Back (example, the shoulder blades are located on the posterior side of the body).

Medial: Towards the midline of the body (example, the middle toe is located at the medial side of the foot).

Lateral: Away from the midline of the body (example, the little toe is located at the lateral side of the foot).

Proximal: Towards or nearest the trunk or the point of origin of a part (example, the proximal end of the femur joins with the pelvic bone).

Distal: Away from or farthest from the trunk or the point or origin of a part (example, the hand is located at the distal end of the forearm).

PLANES OF THE BODY

Medical professionals often pass on to sections of the body in terms of anatomical planes (flat surfaces). These planes are imaginary lines-vertical or horizontal-drawn through an upright body. The terms are used to describe a specific body part.

Coronal Plane (Frontal Plane): A verticle plane running from side to side; divides the body or any of its parts into anterior and posterior portions.

Sagittal Plane (Lateral Plane): A verticle plane running from front to back; divides the body or any of its parts into right and left sides.

Axial Plane (Transverse Plane): A horizontal plane; divides the body or any of its parts into upper and lower parts.

Median Plane: Sagittal plane through the midline of the body; divides the body or any of its parts into right and left halves.

BODY CAVITIES

The cavities, or spaces, of the body contain the internal organs, or viscera. The two main cavities are called the ventral and dorsal cavities. The ventral is the larger cavity and is subdivided into two parts (thoracic and abdominopelvic cavities) by the diaphragm, a dome-shaped respiratory muscle.

Thoracic cavity: The upper ventral, thoracic, or chest hollow contains the heart, lungs, trachea, esophagus, large blood vessels, and nerves. The thoracic cavity is bound laterally by the ribs (covered by costal pleura) and the diaphragm caudally (covered by diaphragmatic pleura).

Abdominal and Pelvic Cavity: The lower part of the ventral (abdominopelvic) cavity can be further divided into two portions: abdominal portion and pelvic portion.

The abdominal cavity contains most of the gastrointestinal tract as well as the kidneys and adrenal glands. The abdominal cavity is bound cranially by the diaphragm, laterally by the body wall, and caudally by the pelvic cavity. The pelvic cavity contains most of the urogenital system as well as the rectum. The pelvic cavity is bounded cranially by the abdominal cavity, dorsally by the sacrum, and laterally by the pelvis.

Dorsal Cavity: The smaller of the two main cavities is called the dorsal cavity. As its name implies, it contains organs lying more posterior in the body. The dorsal cavity, again, can be divided into two portions. The upper portion, or the cranial cavity, houses the brain, and the lower portion, or vertebral canal houses the spinal cord.

BODY FUNCTIONS AND LIFE PROCESS

BODY FUNCTIONS

Body functions are the physiological or psychological functions of body systems. The body's functions are eventually its cells' functions. Survival is the body's most important business. Survival depends on the body's maintaining or restoring homeostasis, a state of relative constancy, of its internal environment. More than a century ago, French physiologist, Claude Bernard (1813-1878), made a remarkable observation. He noted that body cells survived in a healthy condition only when the temperature, pressure, and chemical composition of their environment remained relatively constant. Later, an American physiologist, Walter B. Cannon (1871-1945), suggested the name homeostasis for the relatively constant states maintained by the body. Homeostasis is a key word in modern physiology.

It comes from two Greek words-"homeo," meaning the same, and "stasis," meaning standing. "Standing or staying the same" then is the literal meaning of homeostasis.

However, as Cannon emphasized, homeostasis does not mean something set and immobile that stays exactly the same all the time. In his words, homeostasis "means a condition that may vary, but which is relatively constant." Homeostasis depends on the body's ceaselessly carrying on many activities. Its major activities or functions are responding to changes in the body's environment, exchanging materials between the environment and cells, metabolizing foods, and integrating all of the body's diverse activities.

The body's ability to perform many of its functions changes gradually over the years. In general, the body performs its functions least well at both ends of life-in infancy and in old age. During childhood, body functions gradually become more and more efficient and effective. During late maturity and old age the opposite is true. They gradually become less and less efficient and effective. During young adulthood, they normally operate with maximum efficiency and effectiveness.

Life Process

All living organisms have certain characteristics that distinguish them from non-living forms. The basic processes of life include organization, metabolism, responsiveness, movements, and reproduction. In humans, who represent the most complex from of life, there are additional requirements such as growth, differentiation, respiration, digestion, and excretion. All of these processes are interrelated.

No part of the body, from the smallest cell to a complete body system, works in isolation. All function together, in fine-tuned balance, for the well being of the individual and to maintain life. Disease such as cancer and death represent a disruption of the balance in these processes.

The subsequent is a brief description of the life process:

Organization: At all levels of the organizational scheme, there is a division of labour. Each component has its own job to perform in cooperation with others. Even a single cell, if it loses its integrity or organization, will die.

Metabolism: Metabolism is a broad term that includes all the chemical reactions that occur in the body. One phase of metabolism is catabolism in which complex substances are broken down into simpler building blocks and energy is released.

Responsiveness: Responsiveness or irritability is concerned with detecting changes in the internal or external environments and reacting to that change. It is the act of sensing a stimulus and responding to it.

Movement: There are many types of movement within the body. On the cellular level, molecules move from one place to another. Blood moves from one part of the body to another. The diaphragm moves with every breath. The ability of muscle fibres to shorten and thus to produce movement is called contractility.

Reproduction: For most people, reproduction refers to the formation of a new person, the birth of a baby. In this way, life is transmitted from one generation to the next through reproduction of the organism. In a broader sense, reproduction also refers to the formation of new cells for the replacement and repair of old cells as well as for growth. This is cellular reproduction. Both are essential to the survival of the human race.

Growth: Growth refers to an increase in size either through an increase in the number of cells or through an increase in the size of each individual cell. In order for growth to occur, anabolic processes must occur at a faster rate than catabolic processes.

Differentiation: Differentiation is a developmental process by which unspecialized cells change into specialized cells with distinctive structural and functional characteristics. Through differentiation, cells develop into tissues and organs.

Respiration: Respiration refers to all the processes involved in the exchange of oxygen and carbon dioxide between the cells and the external environment. It includes ventilation, the diffusion of oxygen and carbon dioxide, and the transport of the gases in the blood. Cellular respiration deals with the cell's utilization of oxygen and release of carbon dioxide in its metabolism.

Digestion: Digestion is the process of breaking down complex ingested foods into simple molecules that can be absorbed into the blood and utilized by the body.

Excretion: Excretion is the process that removes the waste products of digestion and metabolism from the body. It gets rid of by-products that the body is unable to use, many of which are toxic and incompatible with life. The ten life processes described above are not enough to ensure the survival of the individual. In addition to these processes, life depends on certain physical factors from the environment. These include water, oxygen, nutrients, heat, and pressure.

LEVELS OF STRUCTURAL ORGANIZATION

The human body contains multiple levels of structural organization:

- Chemical,
- Cellular,

- Tissue,
- Organ,
- Organ system
- Organism levels.

The simplest stage of structural organization of living organisms is the chemical level. Atoms of various elements combine to form larger, more complex structures termed molecules. Organic molecules aggregate to form cellular organelles responsible for specific cell functions such as cell membranes that regulate the movement of chemical substances into and out of the cell, mitochondria, convert energy of organic nutrients into atp, and ribosomes, are involved in the production of protein molecules.

Cells are the structural and functional units of life. Each organism begins life as a single cell formed when a sperm injects the male genetic material (paternal chromosomes) into the ovum, forming a zygote, or fertilized ovum. Growth and development of a zygote through the stages of embryo, fetus, new born, child and adult requires two fundamental processes: mitosis and cellular differentiation.

Mitosis is a cell replication process-a type of cell xeroxing that result in an increase in the number of somatic cells in an organism. During mitosis, all the chromosomes and other cellular components in the parent cell are replicated so that each daughter cell receives a full set of 46 chromosomes and all essential cell components. Each somatic cell is formed from an existing cell by the process of mitosis. The process of cellular differentiation allows cells, by selective expression of genes, to become anatomically distinct and functionally specialized. Although all cells contain 46 chromosomes and hence the complete human genome, cells generally only express about 15 per cent of the genes they contain.

Cells of parallel structure and function congregate to form tissues. There are 4 principle types of tissues in the human organism: epithelial tissue, connective tissue, muscular tissue and neural tissue. Two or more types of tissues are combined within the same structure to form an organ such as the heart, liver, kidney or brain. Most organs contain all 4 of the principle types of tissues. Individual organs that function cooperatively to accomplish a common purpose are grouped together into ORGAN SYSTEMS.

Examples include the cardiovascular system that functions to circulate the blood, the gastrointestinal system functions to digest and absorb nutrients and the urinary system that removes metabolic wastes, excess minerals and water from the blood. There are eleven organ systems in the human body that are combined to form the complete human organism.

In humans, portions of the body which are closer to the head end are "superior" (Latin "upper"); those which are farther away are "inferior" ("lower") — "superior" corresponds to cranial ('at the skull'), or cephalic (head), and "inferior" corresponds to caudal ('at the tail'). Objects near the front are "anterior"; those near the rear are "posterior" — these correspond to the terms "ventral", forward surface, and "dorsal" rear surface.

The terms "anterior" and "posterior" are confusing when referring to most animals, however, and are particularly unsuitable for quadrupeds. In this case, "rostral/cranial" and "caudal" are more appropriate. However the word posterior is commonly used (in common slang usage) as a substantive meaning the buttocks or an adjective referring to them.

In humans, anatomical terms of motion refer to changes away from the standard anatomical position, such as the position of the forearm with the palm directed anteriorly (or upwards when seated) is known as the supine position. Where the palm faces posteriorly (or downwards when seated), this is the prone position.

Turning the hand from prone to supine is called supination; turning the hand from supine to prone is pronation. Pronation results in crossing of the radius (bone) with respect to the ulna. To avoid confusion with "medial" and "lateral", different terms are used when describing the sides of the forearm.

RELATION DIRECTIONS

Structures near the midline are called medial and those near the sides of animals are called lateral. Therefore, medial structures are closer to the midsagittal plane, lateral structures are further from the midsagittal plane. Structures in the midline of the body are median, or medial. For example, your cheeks are lateral to your nose and the tip of the nose is in the median line. Ipsilateral means on the same side, contralateral means on the other side and bilateral means on both sides.

Specialized terms are second-hand to describe location on appendages, parts that have a point of attachment to the main trunk of the body. Structures that are close to the point of attachment of the body are proximal or central, while ones more distant from the attachment point are distal or peripheral. For example, the hands are at the distal end of the arms, while the shoulders are at the proximal ends.

These terms can also be used relatively to organs, for example the proximal end of the urethra is attached to the bladder. Structures on or closer to the body's surface are superficial (or external) and those further inside are profound or deep (or internal).

When speaking of inner organs, visceral means attached to or associated with an organ, while parietal refers to a structure associated with or attached to the body wall (the chest wall or the abdominal wall). For example, whilst the pleura is a single structure, for convenience the term "visceral pleura" is used to refer to that part attached to the outer surface of the lung, and "parietal pleura" to refer to that part attached to the inside of the chest wall.

RELATION DIRECTIONS IN THE LIMBS

Anatomists and medical personnel use specific DIRECTIONAL TERMS to describe where body parts are located.

- *Superior*: towards the head or the upper part of the body or structure; "above". Example: the nose is superior to the chin.
- *Inferior*: towards the lower part of the body or structure; "below". Example: the mouth is inferior to the nose.
- *Anterior (ventral)*: towards or at the front of the body; "in front of". Example: the breastbone is anterior to the spine.
- *Posterior (dorsal)*: towards or at the back of the body; "behind". Example: the heart is posterior to the breastbone.
- *Medial*: towards or at the midline of the body or structure. (The midline is an imaginary vertical line that divides the body into equal right and left sides.) Example: the heart is medial to the lungs.
- *Lateral*: away from the midline of the body or structure. Example: the eyes are lateral to the bridge of the nose.
- *Ipsilateral*: on the same side of the body. Example: the left arm and left leg are ipsilateral.
- *Contralateral*: on the opposite side of the body. Example: the left arm and right leg are contralateral.
- *Proximal*: closer to the point of attachment of a limb to the body trunk. Example: the elbow is proximal to the hand.
- *Distal*: farther from the point of attachment of a limb to the body trunk. Example: the knee is distal to the thigh.
- *Superficial*: towards or at the body surface. Example: the skin is superficial to the skeleton.
- *Deep*: away from the body surface; more internal. Example: the lungs are deep to the ribs.

In the limbs of most animals, the terms cranial and caudal are used in the regions proximal to the carpus (the wrist, in the forelimb) and the tarsus (the ankle in the hindlimb). Objects and surfaces closer to or facing towards the head are cranial; those facing away or further from the head are caudal. Nearer the carpal joint, the term dorsal replaces cranial and palmar replaces caudal. Similarly, nearer the tarsal joint the term dorsal replaces cranial and plantar replaces caudal.

For example, the top of a dog's paw is its dorsal surface; the underside, either the palmar (on the forelimb) or the plantar (on the hindlimb) surface. The sides of the forearm are named after its bones: Structures closer to the radius are radial, structures closer to the ulna are ulnar, and structures relating to both bones are referred to as radioulnar. Similarly, in the lower leg, structures near the tibia (shinbone) are tibial and structures near the fibula are fibular (or peroneal).

Volar (sometimes used as a synonym for "palmar") refers to the underside, for both the palm and the sole (plantar), as in volar pads on the underside of hands, fingers, feet and toes.

The terms valgus and varus are used to refer to angulation of the distal part of a limb at a joint. For example, at the elbow joint, in the anatomical position, the forearm and the upper arm do not lie in a straight line, but the forearm is angulated laterally with respect to the upper arm by about 5-10°. The forearm is said to be "in valgus". Angulation at a joint may be normal (as in the elbow) or abnormal.

PLANES IN THE HUMAN BODY

The study of anatomy often involves dissection, in which the body or its organs are sectioned (cut) along an imaginary flat surface called a plane. A section is the exposed flat surface that results from the cut made through the body or organ.

The most frequently used planes are the sagittal, frontal and transverse planes. These planes lie at right angles to each other.

- A sagittal plane is a vertical plane that divides the body or organ into right and left portions, a cut along a sagittal plane produces a sagittal section.
  (a) A midsagittal plane is exactly at the midline of the body or organ, and divides the body or organ into equal right and left sides.
  (b) A vertical plane that divides the body or organ into unequal right and left sides is a parasagittal plane.
- A vertical plane that divides the body or organ into anterior and posterior portions is a frontal (coronal) plane. a cut made along a frontal plane produces a frontal section.
- A transverse (horizontal) plane runs parallel to the ground and divides the body into superior and inferior portions. A cut made along a horizontal plane produces a transverse (horizontal) section. The transverse section is also sometimes called a cross-section.
- The mid-clavicular line, a line running vertically down the surface of the body passing through the midpoint of the clavicle.
- The mid-pupillary line, a line running vertically down the face through the midpoint of the pupil when looking directly forwards.
- The mid-inguinal point, which is the point midway between the anterior superior iliac spine and the pubic tubercle.
- Tuffier's line, which is a transverse line passing across the lumbar spine between the posterior iliac crests.

Additionally, reference may be made to structures at specific levels of the spine (*e.g.* the 4th cervical vertebra, abbreviated "C4"), or the rib cage (*e.g.* the 5th intercostal space, abbreviated "5ICS").

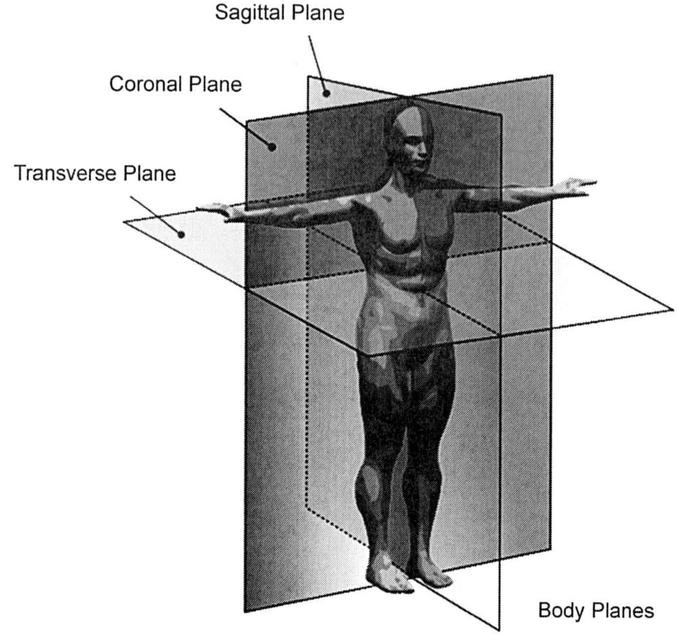

Fig. Surface and other Landmarks in Humans

STANDARD ANATOMICAL POSITION

Anatomical terms are applied to the subject (human or animal) in the standard anatomical position. This is typically a (standing) posture similar to that seen during life, rather than lying on a table. For humans, the body is standing erect, feet together and toes pointed forward, arms at the sides and palms facing forward (forearms supine).

In other species, *e.g.* quadrupeds, the standard anatomical position is described as standing erect with the head facing forwards in a neutral position. In humans, the anatomical position of the skull has been agreed by international convention to be the Frankfurt plane, a position where the lower margins of the orbits and the upper margins of the ear canals all lie in the same horizontal plane. This is a good approximation to the position where the subject is standing upright and facing forwards.

BODY CAVITIES

Spaces within the body that contain internal organs are called BODY CAVITIES. The two principal body cavities are the DORSAL and VENTRAL body cavities.

- The dorsal body cavity is located near the posterior surface of the body. It is further subdivided into a cranial cavity and a vertebral canal.

(a) The cranial cavity is a bony cavity formed by the skull. It contains the brain.

(b) The vertebral canal is also called the spinal canal. It is a bony cavity formed by the vertebrae of the backbone. It contains the spinal cord. Since the spinal cord emerges from the brain, the cranial and vertebral cavities are continuous with one another.

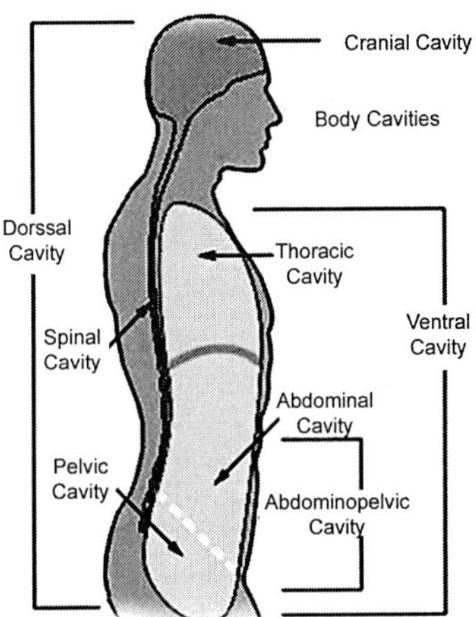

- The ventral body cavity is located in the anterior part of the body. The ventral body cavity walls are made of skin, connective tissue, bone, and muscles. The organs inside the ventral body cavity are called the viscera. The ventral body cavity is further subdivided into the thoracic and abdominopelvic cavities by the diaphragm, a large, dome-shaped muscle used in breathing.

(a) The thoracic cavity is surrounded by the ribs and muscles of the chest. It is further subdivided into the two pleural cavities and the mediastinum. Each pleural cavity contains one lung. The mediastinum is medial to the pleural cavities. The mediastinum is not a cavity. It is defined as a region or mass of tissue that extends from the breastbone (sternum) to the vertebral column. The mediastinum contains the pericardial cavity, which encloses the heart. The mediastinum also contains other thoracic organs and structures (for example: the thymus, aorta and esophagus).

(b) The abdominopelvic cavity is inferior to the thoracic cavity and the diaphragm. The abdominopelvic cavity is subdivided into two portions, which are not separated by any physical partition. The superior portion is the abdominal cavity, which contains the stomach, small intestine, part of the large intestine, spleen, liver, gall bladder, and pancreas. The inferior part is the pelvic cavity, which contains the urinary bladder, the internal male and female reproductive organs, and the lower part of the large intestine.

(c) Abdominopelvic cavity regions:

i. The umbilical region is deep to and surrounding the navel.
ii. The epigastric region is superior to the umbilical region.
iii. The hypogastric (pubic) region is inferior to the umbilical region.
iv. The right and left hypochondriac regions are lateral to the epigastric region.
v. The right and left lumbar regions are lateral to the umbilical region.
vi. The right and left iliac (inguinal) regions are lateral to the hypogastric region.

CELL STRUCTURE AND FUNCTION

CELLS

Often thought of as the smallest unit of a living organism, a cell is made up of many even smaller parts, each with its own function. Human cells vary in size, but all are quite small. Even the largest, a fertilized egg, is too small to be seen with the naked eye.

Human cells have a membrane that holds the contents together. However, this membrane is not just a sac. It has receptors that identify the cell to other cells. The receptors also react to substances produced in the body and to drugs taken into the body, selectively allowing these substances or drugs to enter and leave the cell. Reactions that take place at the receptors often alter or control a cell's functions. An example of this is when insulin binds to receptors on the cell membrane to maintain appropriate blood sugar levels and to allow glucose to enter cells.

Within the cell membrane are two major compartments, the cytoplasm and the nucleus. The cytoplasm contains structures that consume and transform energy and perform the cell's functions. The nucleus contains the cell's genetic material and the structures that control cell division and reproduction. Inside every cell are mitochondria. Mitochondria are tiny structures that provide the cell with energy.

Inside a Cell

Although there are different types of cells, most cells have the same components. A cell consists of a nucleus and cytoplasm and is contained within the cell membrane, which regulates what passes in and out. The nucleus contains chromosomes, which are the cell's genetic material, and a nucleolus, which produces ribosomes.

Ribosomes produce proteins, which are packaged by the Golgi apparatus so that they can leave the cell.

The cytoplasm consists of a fluid material and organelles, which could be considered the cell's organs. The endoplasmic reticulum transports materials within the cell. Mitochondria generate energy for the cell's activities. Lysosomes contain enzymes that can break down particles entering the cell. Centrioles participate in cell division.

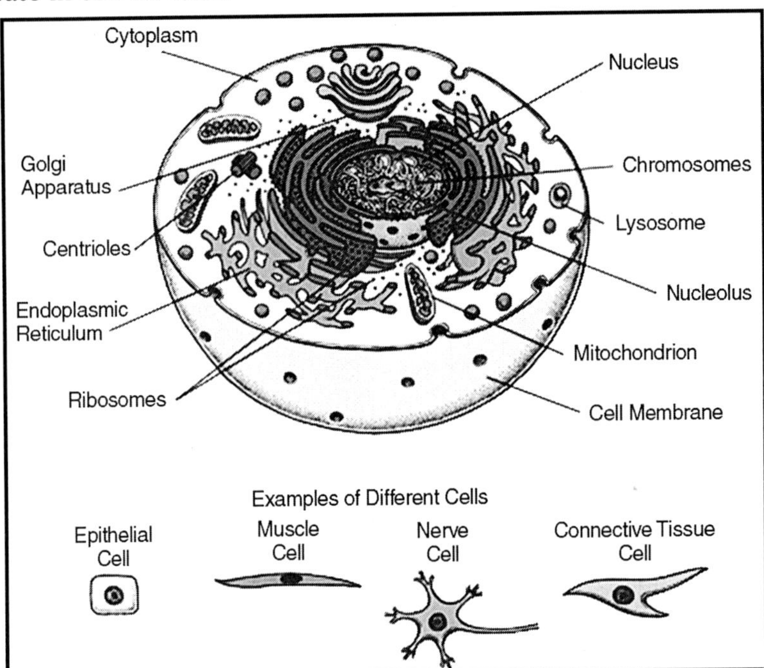

The body is composed of many different types of cells, each with its own structure and function. Some, such as white blood cells, move freely, unattached to other cells. Others, such as muscle cells, are firmly attached one to another. Some cells, such as skin cells, divide and reproduce quickly. Others, such as nerve cells, do not divide or reproduce except under usual circumstances. Some cells, especially glandular cells, have as their primary function the production of complex substances, such as a hormone or an enzyme.

For example, some cells in the breast produce milk, some in the pancreas produce insulin, some in the lining of the lungs produce mucus, and some in the mouth produce saliva. Other cells have primary functions that are not related to the production of substances—for example, muscle cells contract, allowing movement. Nerve cells generate and conduct electrical impulses, allowing communication between the central nervous system (brain and spinal cord) and the rest of the body.

CELL STRUCTURE

The interior of the cell is divided into the nucleus and the cytoplasm. The nucleus is a spherical or oval shaped structure at the center of the cell. The cytoplasm is the region outside the nucleus that contains cell organelles and cytosol, or cytoplasmic solution. Intracellular fluid is collectively the cytosol and the fluid inside the organelles and nucleus.

Membranes

Membranes are the gateways to the cell. The plasma membrane, is the selective barrier surrounding the cell. It provides a barrier to the movement of molecules between the intra and extracellular fluids. Recall that extracellular means outside the cell. The plasma membrane also serves to anchor adjacent cells together and to the extracellular matrix. Various signals and inputs can alter the sensitivity and permeability of membranes.

The Fluid Mosaic Model: Membrane Structure

Membranes are made of a double layer of lipids, mainly phospholipids, containing embedded proteins. The embedded proteins are important as facilitators in moving molecule through the membrane. The membrane itself is organized into a bimolecular layer, meaning that the non-polar region is organized in the middle (away from water as it is hydrophobic) and the polar regions are oriented towards the outside: the extracellular fluid and the cytosol. Another way to think of it is two rows of pins with their heads to the outside and the needle part to the inside.

Heads, needles, needles, heads. Like a sandwich. As the phospholipid molecules are not chemically bound to each other and thus each molecule is free to move independently, the overall bi-layer structure has a flexible fluidity. Cholesterol molecules are also embedded in the plasma membrane and serve to deliver substances to cell organelles by forming vesicles.

The proteins embedded in membrane are categorized into two classes:

1. Peripheral membrane proteins are proteins on the membrane surface, mainly the cystolic side where they interact with cytoskeletal elements in order to influence cell shape and motility. These proteins are not amphipathic and are bound to polar regions of the integral proteins.
2. Integral membrane proteins span the entire width of the membrane, thus crossing through both the polar and non-polar regions of the structure. These proteins cannot be removed from the membrane without disrupting the lipid bi-layer.

It is important to realize that membrane functions are dependent on the chemical composition and any asymmetries in composition between the two surfaces of the membrane and the specific proteins that are attached to or associated with the membrane. The plasma membrane also has an extracellular surface layer of monosaccharides that are linked to the membrane lipids and proteins. This layer is called the glycocalyx and is important in the intercellular recognition process.

Membrane Junctions

Integrins are transmembrane proteins that bind to specific proteins in the extracellular matrix and to membrane proteins on adjacent cells. Integrins help to organize cells into tissues. They are also responsible for transmitting signals from the extracellular matrix to the cell interior.

If two cells are adjacent, but separated, they may be junctured by desmosomes. Desmosomes are dense accumulations of protein at the cytoplasmic surface of the plasma membranes of both separate cells. They are infiltrated with protein fibres that extended into either cell. The purpose and function of desmosomes is to hold adjacent cells firmly in place in areas that are subject to stretching, such as skin.

Another type of membrane junction is the tight junction. These junctions are formed by the actual physical joining of the extracellular surfaces of two adjacent plasma membranes. Tight junctions are important in areas where more control over tissue processes is needed, such as the epithelial cells in the intestine that are involved in absorption.

Finally, gap junctions are actual protein channels that link the cytosols of adjacent cells. The drawback to this 'direct link' is that it only permits smaller molecules to pass through.

Cell Organelles

Cell organelles are the little workhouses within the cell. All the functions of life take place in each individual cell. Organelles can be released by breaking the plasma membrane, through homogenization and ultracentrifuging the mixture. The organelles are of different size and density and will settle out at specific rates.

Overview of organelles:

- The nucleus is in the center of most cells. Some cells contain multiple nuclei, such as skeletal muscle, while some do not have any, such as red blood cells. The nucleus is the largest membrane-bound organelle. Specifically, it is responsible for storing and transmitting genetic information. The nucleus is surrounded by a selective nuclear envelope. The nuclear envelope is composed of two membranes joined at regular intervals to form circular openings called nuclear pores. The pores allow RNA molecules and proteins modulating DNA expression to move through the pores and into the cytosol. The selection process is controlled by an energy-dependent process that alters the diameter of the pores in response to signals. Inside the nucleus, DNA and proteins associate to form a network of threads called chromatin. The chromatin becomes vital at the time of cell division as it becomes tightly condensed thus forming the rodlike chromosomes with the enmeshed DNA. Inside the nucleus is a filamentous region called the nucleolus. This serves as a site where the RNA and protein components of ribosomes are assembled. The nucleolus is not membrane bound, but rather just a region.

- Ribosomes are the sites where protein molecules are synthesized from amino acids. They are composed of proteins and RNA. Some ribosomes are found bound to granular endoplasmic reticulum, while others are free in the cytoplasm. The proteins synthesized on ribosomes bound to granular endoplasmic reticulum are transferred from the lumen (open space inside endoplasmic reticulum) to the golgi apparatus for secretion outside the cell or distribution to other organelles. The proteins that are synthesized of free ribosomes are released into the cytosol.
- The endoplasmic reticulum (ER) is collectively a network of membranes enclosing a singular continuous space. As mentioned earlier, granular endoplasmic reticulum is associated with ribosomes (giving the exterior surface a rough, or granular appearance). Sometimes granular endoplasmic reticulum is referred to as rough ER. The granular ER is involved in packaging proteins for the golgi apparatus. The agranular, or smooth, ER lacks ribosomes and is the site of lipid synthesis. In addition, the agranular ER stores and releases calcium ions Ca^{2+}.
- The golgi apparatus is a membranous sac that serves to modify and sort proteins into secretory/transport vesicles. The vesicles are then delivered to other cell organelles and the plasma membrane. Most cells have at least one golgi apparatus, although some may have multiple. The apparatus is usually located near the nucleus.
- Endosomes are membrane-bound tubular and vesicular structures located between the plasma membrane and the golgi apparatus. They serve to sort and direct vesicular traffic by pinching off vesicles or fusing with them.
- Mitochondria are some of the most important structures in the human body. They are they site of various chemical processes involved in the synthesis of energy packets called ATP (adenosine triphosphate). Each mitochondrion is surrounded by two membranes. The outer membrane is smooth, while the inner one is folded into tubule structures called cristae. Mitochondria are unique in that they contain small amounts of DNA containing the genes for the synthesis of some mitochondrial proteins. The DNA is inherited solely from the mother. Cells with greater activity have more mitochondria, while those that are less active have less need for energy producing mitochondria.
- Lysosomes are bound by a single membrane and contain highly acidic fluid. The fluid acts as digesting enzymes for breaking down bacteria

and cell debris. They play an important from in the cells of the immune system.

- Peroxisomes are also bound by a single membrane. They consume oxygen and work to drive reactions that remove hydrogen from various molecules in the form of hydrogen peroxide. They are important in maintaining the chemical balances within the cell.
- The cytoskeleton is a filamentous network of proteins that are associated with the processes that maintain and change cell shape and produce cell movements. The cytoskeleton also forms tracks along which cell organelles move propelled by contractile proteins attached to their various surfaces. Like a little highway infrastructure inside the cell.

Three types of filaments make up the cytoskeleton:

1. Microfilaments are the thinnest and most abundant of the cytoskeleton proteins. They are composed of actin, a contractile protein, and can be assembled and disassembled quickly according to the needs of the cell or organelle structure.
2. Intermediate filaments are slightly larger in diameter and are found most extensively in regions of cells that are going to be subjected to stress. Desmosomes in the skin will contain filaments. Once these filaments are assembled they are not capable of rapid disassembly.
3. Microtubules are hollow tubes composed of a protein called tubulin. They are the thickest and most rigid of the filaments. Microtubules are present in the axons and long dendrite projections of nerve cells. They are capable of rapid assembly and disassembly according to need. Microtubules are structured around a cell region called the centrosome, which surrounds two centrioles composed of 9 sets of fused microtubules. These are important in cell division when the centrosome generates the microtubluar spindle fibres necessary for chromosome separation.

Finally, cilia are hair-like motile extensions on the surface of some epithelial cells. They have a central core of 9 sets of fused microtubules. In association with a contractile protein, these microtubules produce movement in cilia. Ciliar movements propel the luminal contents of hollow organs lined with ciliated epithelium.

CELL STRUCTURE AND FUNCTION

Physiology - science that describes how organisms FUNCTION and survive in continually changing environments

Levels of Organization

Chemical Level - includes all chemical substances necessary for life; together form the next higher level

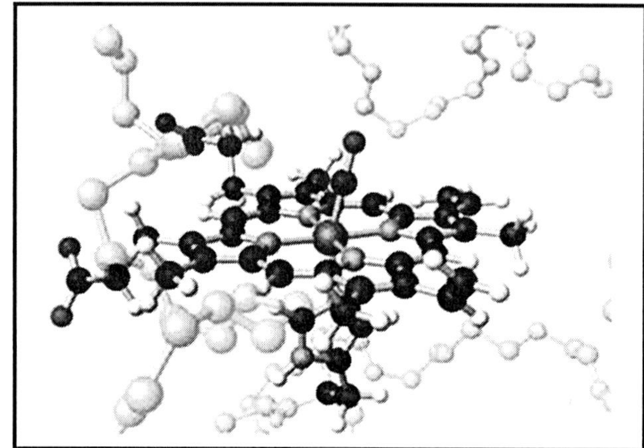

Cellular Level - cells are the basic structural and functional units of the human body and there are many different types of cells (*e.g.*, muscle, nerve, blood, and so on)

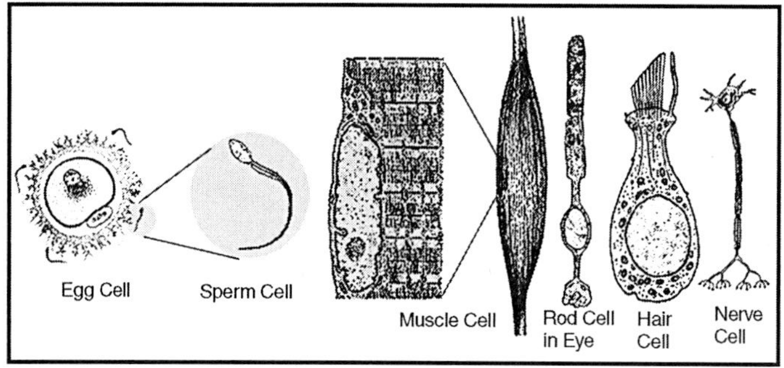

Tissue Level - a tissue is a group of cells that perform a specific function and the basic types of tissues in the human body include epithelial, muscle, nervous, and connective tissues.

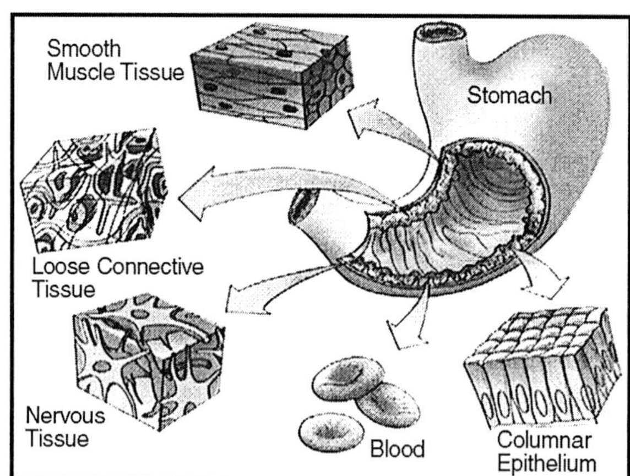

Organ Level - an organ consists of 2 or more tissues that perform a particular function (*e.g.*, heart, liver, stomach, and so on)

System Level - an association of organs that have a common function; the major systems in the human body include digestive, nervous, endocrine, circulatory, respiratory, urinary, and reproductive.

There are two types of cells that make up all living things on earth: prokaryotic and eukaryotic.

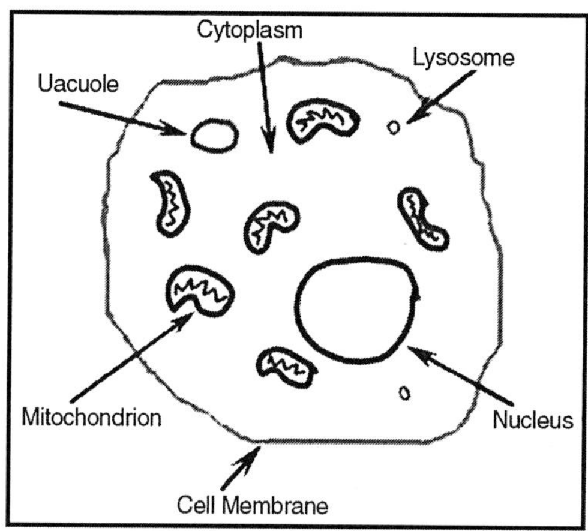

Fig. Parts of the Cell.

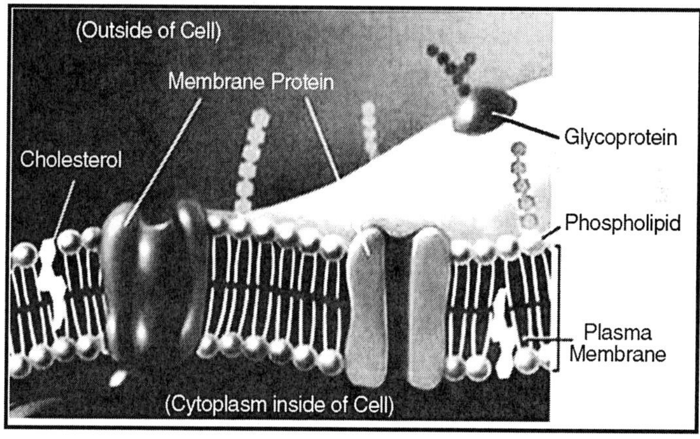

Fig. Cell, or Plasma, Membrane - encloses Every Human Cell.

Prokaryotic cells, like bacteria, have no 'nucleus', while eukaryotic cells, like those of the hum an body, do. So, a human cell is enclosed by a cell, or plasma, membrane.

Enclosed by that membrane is the cytoplasm (with associated organelles) plus a nucleus.

- Structure - 2 primary building blocks include protein (about 60 per cent of the membrane) and lipid, or fat (about 40 per cent of the membrane). The primary lipid is called phospholipid, and molecules of phospholipid form a 'phospholipid bilayer' (two layers of phospholipid molecules). This bilayer forms because the two 'ends' of phospholipid molecules have very different characteristics: one end is polar (or hydrophilic) and one (the hydrocarbon tails below) is non-polar (or hydrophobic):

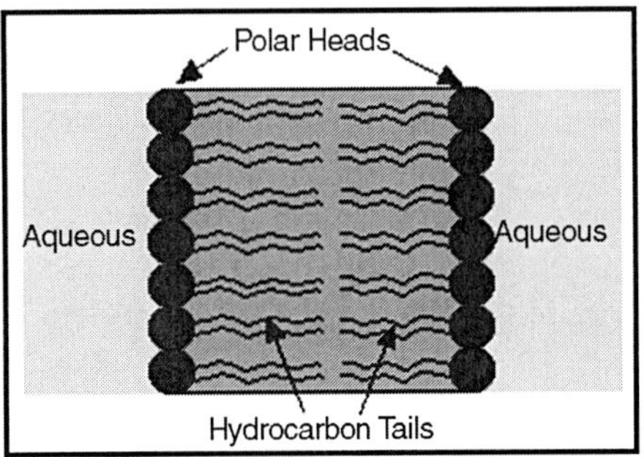

- Functions include:
  - Supporting and retaining the cytoplasm
  - Being a selective barrier
    i. The cell is separated from its environment and needs to get nutrients in and waste products out. Some molecules can cross the membrane without assistance, most cannot. Water, non-polar molecules and some small polar molecules can cross. Non-polar molecules penetrate by actually dissolving into the lipid bilayer. Most polar compounds such as amino acids, organic acids and inorganic salts are not allowed entry, but instead must be specifically transported across the membrane by proteins.
  - Transport
    i. Many of the proteins in the membrane function to help carry out selective transport. These proteins typically span the whole membrane, making contact with the outside environment and the cytoplasm. They often require the expenditure of energy to help compounds move across the membrane
  - Communication (via receptors)

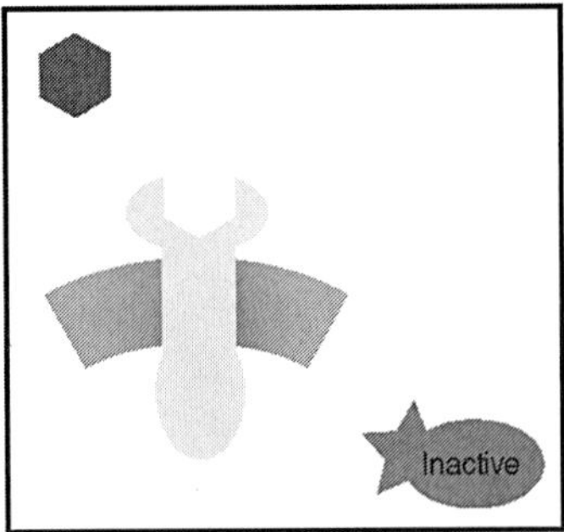

  - Recognition

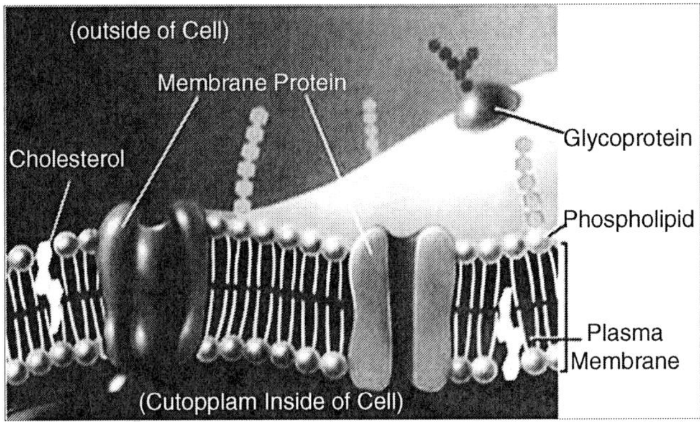

Cytoplasm and Organelles

- Cytoplasm consists of a gelatinous solution and contains microtubules (which serve as a cell's cytoskeleton) and organelles (literally 'little organs')

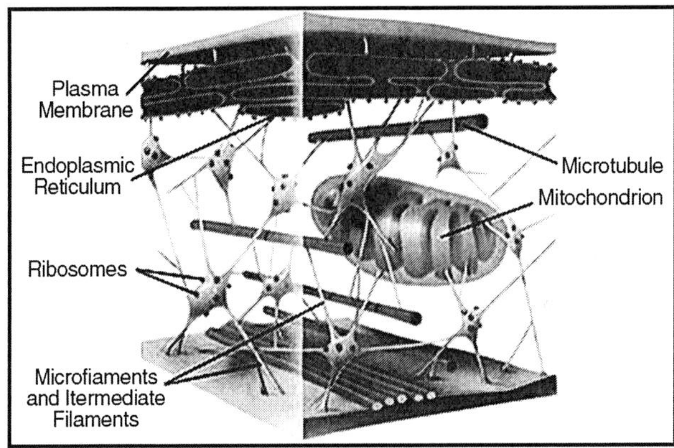

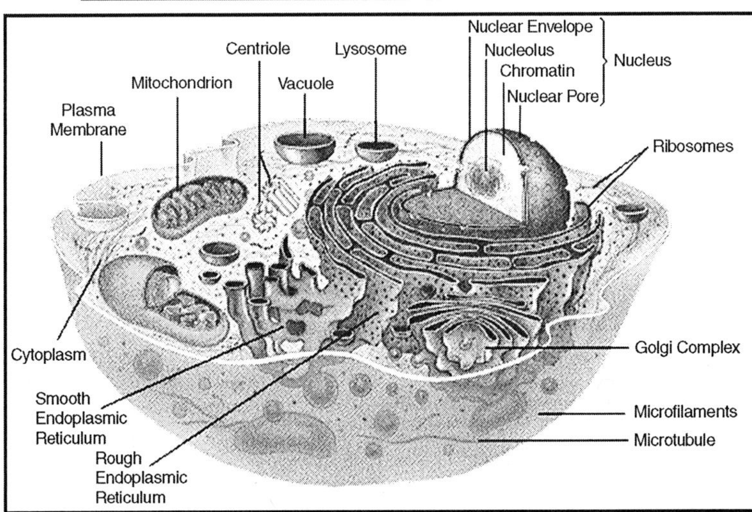

- Cells also contain a nucleus within which is found DNA (deoxyribonucleic acid) in the form of chromosomes plus nucleoli (within which ribosomes are formed)

Eukaryotic organelles include

- Endoplasmic reticulum -
  - Comes in 2 forms: smooth and rough; the surface of rough ER is coated with ribosomes; the surface of smooth ER is not
  - Functions include: mechanical support, synthesis (especially proteins by rough ER), and transport
- Golgi complex -
  - Consists of a series of flattened sacs
  - Functions include: synthesis (of substances likes phospholipids), packaging of materials for transport (in vesicles), and production of lysosomes
- Lysosomes -
  - Membrane-enclosed spheres that contain powerful digestive enzymes
  - Functions include destruction of damaged cells (which is why they are sometimes called 'suicide bags') and digestion of materials absorbed by phagocytosis (such as bacteria)
- Mitochondria -
  - Have a double-membrane: outer membrane and highly convoluted inner membrane

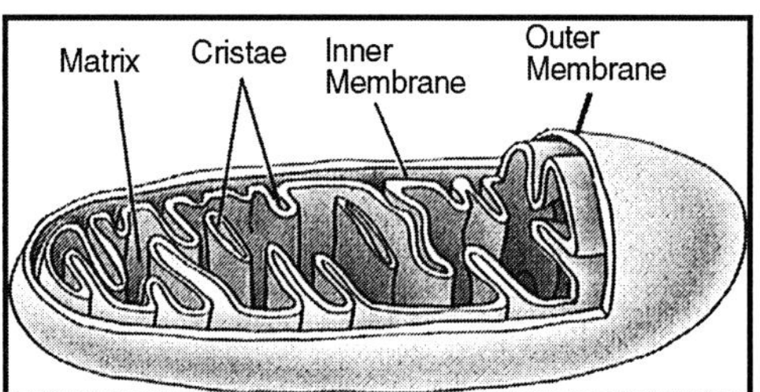

  - Inner membrane has folds or shelf-like structures called cristae that contain elementary particles; these particles contain enzymes important in ATP production
  - Primary function is production of adenosine triphosphate (ATP)
- Ribosomes-
  - Composed of rRNA (ribosomal RNA) and protein
  - May be dispersed randomly throughout the cytoplasm or attached to surface of rough endoplasmic reticulum
  - Often linked together in chains called polyribosomes or polysomes
  - Primary function is to produce proteins
- Centrioles -

  - Paired cylindrical structures located near the nucleas
  - Play an important role in cell division
- Flagella and cilia - hair-like projections from some human cells
  - Cilia are relatively short and numerous (*e.g.*, those lining trachea)
  - A flagellum is relatively long and there's typically just one (*e.g.*, sperm)

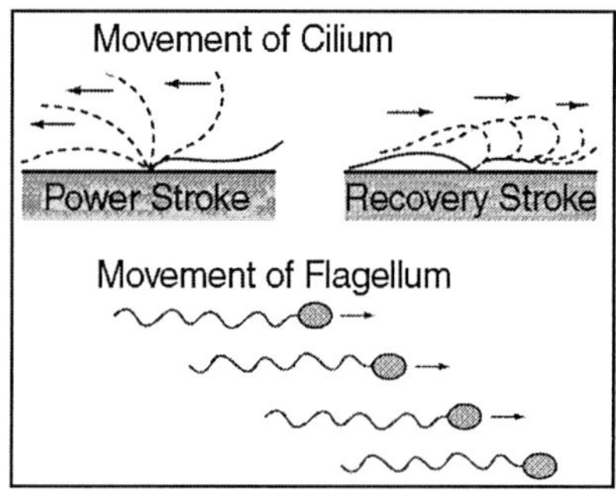

- Villi - projections of cell membrane that serve to increase surface area of a cell (which is important, for example, for cells that line the intestine)

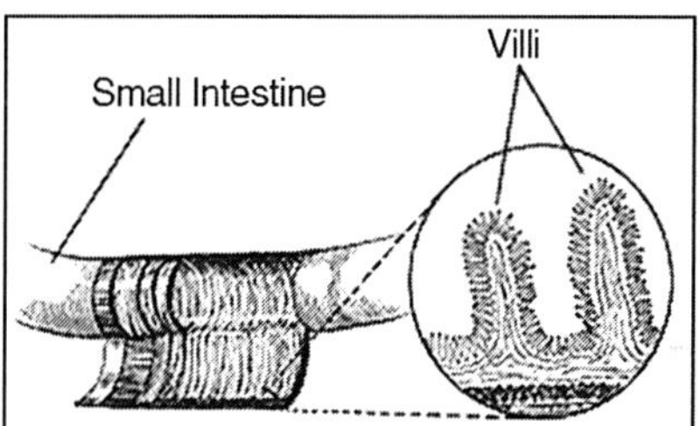

Movement Across Membranes

1 - Passive processes - require no expenditure of energy by a cell:

- Simple diffusion = net movement of a substance from an area of high concentration to an area of low concentration.

The rate of diffusion is influenced by:

   i. Concentration gradient
   ii. Cross-sectional area through which diffusion occurs
   iii. Temperature
   iv. Molecular weight of a substance
   v. Distance through which diffusion occurs

- Osmosis = diffusion of water across a semipermeable membrane (like a cell membrane) from an area of low solute concentration to an area of high solute concentration
- Facilitated diffusion = movement of a substance across a cell membrane from an area of high concentration to an area of low concentration.

- This process requires the use of 'carriers' (membrane proteins). In the example below, a ligand molecule (*e.g.*, acetylcholine) binds to the membrane protein.
- This causes a conformational change or, in other words, an 'opening' in the protein through which a substance (*e.g.*, sodium ions) can pass.

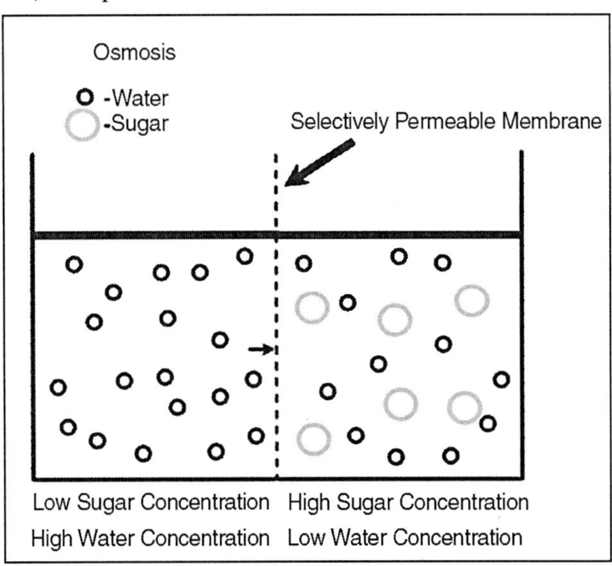

2 - Active processes -

Require the expenditure of energy by cells:

i Active transport = movement of a substance across a cell membrane from an area of low concentration to an area of high concentration using a carrier molecule

ii Endo- and exocytosis - moving material into (endo-) or out of (exo-) cell in bulk form

– Phagocytosis (Endocytosis)

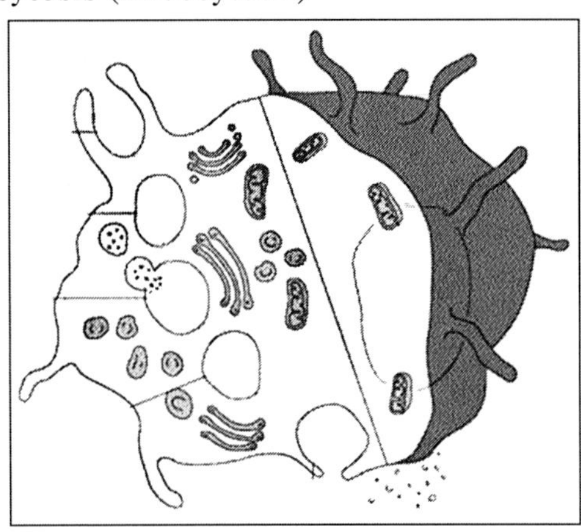

Exocytosis

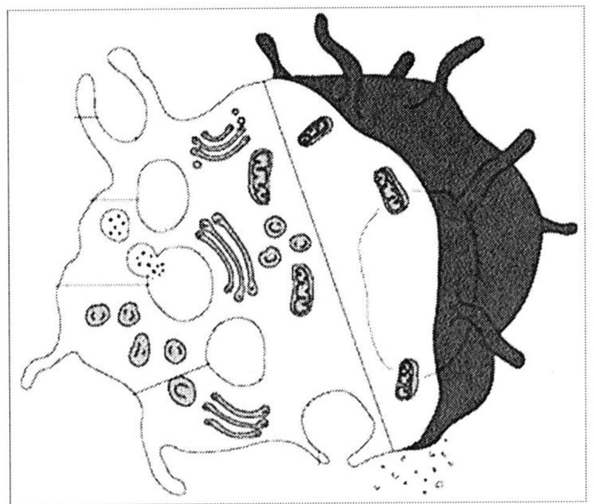

Characteristics of Facilitated Diffusion and Active Transport - both require the use of carriers that are specific to particular substances (that is, each type of carrier can 'carry' one type of substance) and both can exhibit saturation (movement across a membrane is limited by number of carriers and the speed with which they move materials).

BODY TISSUES

WHAT ARE THE FOUR TYPES OF TISSUE FOUND IN THE HUMAN BODY?

Tissues are groups of similar cells that perform a common function. There are four categories of tissues in the human body: epithelial, connective, nervous, and muscle. Epithelial tissue protects your body from moisture loss, bacteria, and internal injury. There are two kinds of epithelial tissues:

- Covering and lining epithelium covers or lines almost all of your internal and external body surfaces; for example, the outermost layer of your skin and other organs, and the internal surface lining of your lymph vessels and digestive tract.
- Glandular epithelium secretes hormones or other products such as stomach acid, sweat, saliva, and milk.

Connective tissue generally provides structure and support to the body. *There are two types of connective tissue:*

- Loose connective tissue holds structures together. For example, loose connective tissue holds the outer layer of skin to the underlying muscle tissue. This tissue is also found in your fat layers, lymph nodes, and red bone marrow.
- Fibrous connective tissue also holds body parts together, but its structure is a bit more rigid than loose connective tissue. Fibrous connective tissue is found in ligaments, tendons, cartilage, and bone.

Nervous tissue forms the nervous system, which is responsible for coordinating the activities and movements of your body through its network of nerves. Parts of the nervous system include the brain, spinal cord, and nerves that branch off of those two key parts.

Nervous tissue consists of two kinds of nerve cells:

- Neurons are the basic structural unit of the nervous system. Each cell consists of the cell body, dendrites, and axon.
- Neuroglia, or glial cells, provide support functions for the neurons, such as insulation or anchoring neurons to blood vessels.

Muscle tissue differs from other tissue types in that it contracts. Muscle tissue comes in three types: cardiac, smooth, and skeletal. Those muscle tissues are made up of muscle fibres.

The muscle fibres contain many myofibrils, which are the parts of the fibre that actually contract.

There are three kinds of muscle tissues:

- Skeletal muscle is attached to bones and causes movements of the body.
- Cardiac muscle is found in the heart.
- Smooth muscle lines the walls of blood vessels and certain organs such as the digestive and urogenital tracts.

TISSUES AND ORGANS

Related cells joined together are collectively referred to as a tissue. The cells in a tissue are not identical, but they work together to accomplish specific functions. A sample of tissue removed for examination under a microscope (biopsy) contains many types of cells, even though a doctor may be interested in only one specific type.

Connective tissue is the tough, often fibrous tissue that binds the body's structures together and provides support. It is present in almost every organ, forming a large part of skin, tendons, and muscles. The characteristics of connective tissue and the types of cells it contains vary, depending on where it is found in the body.

Inside the Torso

The body's functions are conducted by organs. Each organ is a recognizable structure—for example, the heart, lungs, liver, eyes, and stomach—that performs specific functions.

An organ is made of several types of tissue and therefore several types of cells. For example, the heart contains muscle tissue that contracts to pump blood, fibrous tissue that makes up the heart valves, and special cells that maintain the rate and rhythm of heartbeats. The eye contains muscle cells that open and close the pupil, clear cells that make up the lens and cornea, cells that produce the fluid within the eye, cells that sense light, and nerve cells that conduct impulses to the brain.

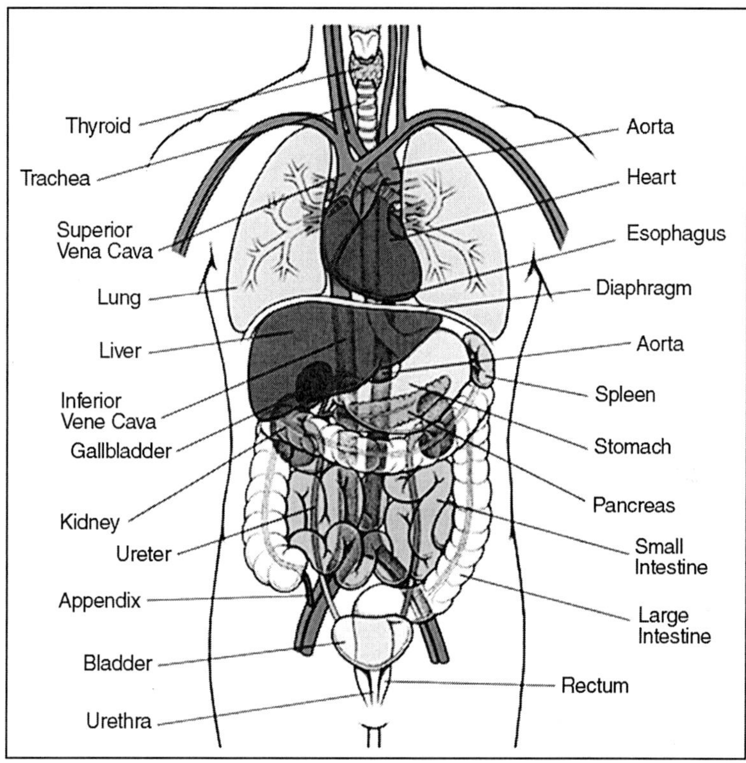

Even an organ as apparently simple as the gallbladder contains different types of cells, such as those that form a lining resistant to the irritative effects of bile, muscle cells that contract to expel bile, and cells that form the fibrous outer wall holding the sac together.

MEMBRANES

MOVEMENT OF MOLECULES ACROSS CELL MEMBRANES

Diffusion

Diffusion is essentially the movement of molecules from a region of higher concentration to a region of lower concentration as a result of thermal motion. Diffusion is an important process in human physiology. Specifically, diffusion is the mechanism of movement of oxygen, nutrients and other molecules across the capillary walls and the movement of other molecules across membranes. The amount of material crossing a surface per unit of time is called flux and depends upon the difference in concentrations between two compartments where movement is potentially going to occur.

When diffusion between two compartments is equal, meaning no net movement, the system has reached diffusion equilibrium. Net flux is zero and there are no further changes in concentration. Difference in concentration, temperature, and surface area of diffusion are all positively correlated with direction and magnitude of net flux.

While the mass of molecules in solution are negatively correlated with direction and magnitude of net flux. The time that it takes for diffusion to occur increases in proportion to the square of the distance over which molecules diffuse. Diffusion, therefore, is only useful for moving molecules over small distances.

Diffusion through Membranes

The magnitude of net flux can be measured as:

$F = k_p A(C_0 - C_i)$ where,

k_p = permeability constant for a particular molecule at a particular temperature

A = surface area of membrane

C_0 = extracellular concentration of the substance

C_i = intracellular concentration of the substance

Remember that membranes slow down diffusion and molecules will move slowly than through a water layer of equal thickness. for structural reasons a water layer is easier than a membrane to diffuse through.

Role of Electric Forces on Ion Movement

Membrane potential is the separation of electric charges across a membrane. The separation of charges influences the movement of ions across the membrane. This can act independently of or in conjunction with, or in opposition to, the force generated by concentration differences. Electrochemical gradient refers to these two forces collectively: the force due to charges and the force due to concentration differences.

Diffusion through the Lipid Bi-layer

Non-polar molecules can dissolve in the non-polar fatty acid chains of the membrane phospholipids and therefore non-polar molecules have larger permeability constants than polar molecules.

Diffusion of Ions through Protein Channels

Protein channels formed by integral proteins allow ions to diffuse across the membrane. Different cells have different permeabilities to these ions. The diameter of the channel and the polar groups on the protein subunits forming channel walls determine the permeability of the channels by various ions and molecules.

Regulation of Diffusion through Ion Channels

Channel gating is the opening and closing of ion channels which changes the permeability of a membrane. It is controlled by three modulators:

1. Modulation of allosteric or covalent channel-proteins in ligand-sensitive channels
2. Modulation of channel proteins due to changes due to changes in membrane potential in voltage-gated channels.
3. Modulation of channel proteins due to stretching in mechanosensitive channels.

Several factors and influence a single channel and any one ion can pass through several different channels.

Mediated Transport Systems

There are integral membrane proteins called transporters that mediate movement of molecules that are too polar or too large to move across a membrane by diffusion.

In order to accomplish this, a solute (molecule to be transported) binds to a specific site on a transporter on one surface of the membrane. The transporter then changes shape in order to expose the bound solute to the opposite side of the membrane.

The solute then dissociates from the transporter and finds itself on the other side of where it started. Depending on the membrane, and the needs of the cellular environment, there may be many types of transporters present with specific binding sites for particular types of substances.

Solute flux magnitude through a mediated transport system is positively correlated with the number of transporters, the rate of conformational change in the transporter protein, and the overall saturation of transporter binding sites which is dependent on the solute concentration and affinity of the transporter. These are important factors to consider in getting large materials through a membrane.

Facilitated Diffusion

Facilitated diffusion moves solutes from a region of higher concentration to a region of lower concentration until the concentrations become equalized on both sides of the membrane.

Active Transport

This form of molecule movement requires energy in order to move solute against its electrochemical gradient. Energy is required to either:

1. Alter the affinity of the binding site on different sides of the membrane
2. Alter the rates at which the binding site on the transporters is shifted from one side of the membrane to the other.

Furthermore, there are two ways in which a flow of energy can be coupled to transporters.

1. Primary active transport requires energy is provided by ATPase.

Sodium, potassium—ATPase (Na, K—ATPase) is present in plasma membranes which works by moving 3 Na^+ ions out of a cell and 2 K^+ ions in, resulting in a net transfer of positive charge outside the membrane.

Calcium—ATPase in plasma membranes moves Ca^{2+} ions from the cytosol to the extracellular fluid, while Ca—ATPase in membranes of organelles moves Ca^{2+} from cytosol into the organelle lumen (space). Hydrogen—ATPase in plasma membranes moves hydrogen ions (H^+ or protons) out of cells.

Secondary active transport provides energy from the flow of ions from an area of higher concentration to one of lower concentration. Allosteric modulation modifies the affinity of the binding site. There are technically two types of secondary active transport.

1. Cotransport occurs if a molecule moves in the same direction as the ion providing the energy. An example is the movement of amino acids using sodium ions.
2. Countertransport occurs when the molecule moves in the opposite direction as the ion providing the energy. An example is the movement of calcium ions using sodium ions.

In sum, with ions the movement is from high to low concentration, and molecules from low to high.

Osmosis

Osmosis is the net diffusion of water across a membrane. Aquaporins are proteins that form channels in the lipid bi-layer for the polar water molecules to diffuse through. There will be a net diffusion of both compartments leading to diffusion equilibrium with no change in volume in either compartment if the compartments are separated by a membrane that is permeable to both a solute and water.

However, if the membrane is only permeable to water (*i.e.* not to the solute) then diffusion equilibrium will be reached with a net increase in volume of the compartment that had a higher osmolarity to begin with. Osmolarity is the total solute concentration of a solution and is measured in units called osmols. Therefore, water concentration in a solution is negatively correlated with the number of solute particles. Osmotic pressure is the pressure that must be applied to prevent the net flow of water into a solution separated by a membrane. The osmotic pressure increases with increases in osmolarity. Water will then move from regions of lower osmotic pressure to regions of higher osmotic pressure.

When a system reaches equilibrium, the osmolarities of intra- and extracellular fluids are the same. An isotonic solution is a solution which cells will neither swell nor shrink, this is assuming that the cells are placed into a solution of non-penetrating solutes with the same osmolarity as the extracellular fluid. The key thing is that there is no net movement in an isotonic solution. In an hypotonic solution, the solution contains less non-penetrating solutes, and the cells therefore absorb water and the cells swell. Finally, a hypertonic solution is one in which the solution contains more non-penetrating solutes and water moves out of the cells and they shrink. It is important to understand that penetrating solutes do not contribute to the tonicity of the solution.

Endocytosis

Endocytosis is a transportation process that requires energy. The main mechanism is that regions of the plasma membrane fold into the cell which forms small pockets on the inside of the cell. These pockets pinch off into membrane-bound vesicles inside the cell.

Fluid endocytosis refers to when the vesicles formed enclose a small volume of extracellular fluid. However, if certain molecules in the extracellular fluid happen to bind to specific proteins on the plasma membrane and are then carried into the cells with extracellular fluid, the process is then called adsorptive endocytosis. Collectively, these two processes are also called pinocytosis and are demonstrated by most cells.

Some cells will engulf large foreign particles via a process called phagocytosis. This only happens in specialized cells that are relatively few in number and occurrence. The type of particles engulfed include bacteria and cell debris. Endosomes are usually fused with endocytic vesicles at some point in the process, and the contents of the packets are then passed into organelles such as Lysosomes.

Both pinocytosis and phagocytosis are examples of endocytic processes. The big thing to remember is that the movement of particles is from the outside of the plasma membrane to the inside.

Exocytosis

In order to move things from the inside of the cell to the outside, membrane-bound vesicles in the cytoplasm will fuse with the plasma membrane and release their contents outside the cell. The bound vesicle material then assimilates into the plasma membrane. In this fashion, portions of the plasma membrane lost during endocytosis can be replaced. Additionally, the process provides a route by which membrane impermeable molecules, such as protein hormones, that are synthesized by cells can be released into the extracellular fluid. Finally, the process of exocytosis is triggered by stimuli that leads to an increase in cystolic calcium concentration which in turn activates proteins required for the vesicle membrane to fuse with the plasma membrane and thus repairing any 'holes' from prior processes.

Epithelial Transport

The luminal (or apical or mucosal) membrane is the plasma membrane surface of an epithelial cell that faces a hollow or fluid filled chamber. The basolateral (or serosal) membrane is the surface of plasma membrane on the opposite side usually adjacent to a network of blood vessels.

Substances can cross a layer of epithelial cells via two pathways:

1. The paracellular pathway refers to diffusion between adjacent cells in the epithelium. This pathway is limited to small ions and water because of the presence of tight junctions.
2. The transcellular pathway refers to the movement into an epithelial cell from one side, then diffusion through the cytosol and exit through the opposing membrane.

The transport and permeability characteristics of the luminal and basolateral membranes are not the same due to the presence of different ion channels and transporters. Substances, therefore, are able to move from a region of lower concentration on one side to a higher concentration on the other.

Glands

Gland cells secrete organic molecules synthesized by their own cellular processes and they also secrete salts and water, moving them from one extracellular compartment to another.

The rate of secretion is controlled by chemical or neural signals and work by:

1. Altering the rate of synthesis
2. Altering the rate of exocytosis via calcium channels. Altering the pumping rate of transporters and opening rate of ion channels

Two types of glands:

1. Endocrine glands will release their secretions directly into the interstitial fluid surrounding the gland cells. Endocrine glands secrete hormones. Exocrine glands utilize ductworks in order to connect to epithelial surfaces. The secretions flow through the ductworks or onto the surface of the epithelium. Sweat and salivary glands are examples of exocrine function.

ORGAN SYSTEMS, BODY CAVITIES, AND BODY MEMRANES

ORGAN SYSTEMS

Integumentary System

The major organ of the integumentary system is the skin. It also includes nails, hairs, muscles that move hairs, the oil and sweat glands, blood vessels, and nerves leading to sensory receptors.

Cardiovascular System

In the *cardiovascular system*, the heart pumps blood and sends it out under pressure into the blood vessels. In humans, blood is always contained in blood vessels, never leaving these vessels unless the body suffers an injury.

While blood is moving throughout the body, it distributes heat produced by the muscles. Blood transports nutrients and oxygen to the cells and removes their waste molecules, including carbon dioxide. Despite the movement of molecules into and out of the blood, it has a fairly constant volume and pH. This is particularly due to exchanges in the lungs, the digestive tract, and the kidneys. The red blood cells in blood transport oxygen, and the white blood cells fight infections. Platelets are involved in blood clotting.

Lymphatic and Immune Systems

The *lymphatic system* consists of lymphatic vessels, lymph nodes, the spleen, and other lymphatic organs. This system collects excess tissue fluid and plays a role in absorbing fats and transporting lymph to cardiovascular veins. It also purifies lymph and stores lymphocytes, the white blood cells that produce antibodies. The *immune system* consists of all the cells in the body that protect us from disease. The lymphocytes, in particular, belong to this system.

Digestive System

The *digestive system* consists of the mouth, esophagus, stomach, small intestine, and large intestine (colon). It also includes these associated organs: teeth, tongue, salivary glands, liver, gallbladder, and pancreas. This system receives food and digests it into nutrient molecules, which can enter the cells of the body. The neo-digested remains are eventually eliminated.

Respiratory System

The *respiratory system* consists of the lungs and the tubes that take air to and from them. The respiratory system brings oxygen into the body and removes carbon dioxide from the body at the lungs. The removal of carbon dioxide helps adjust the acid–base balance of the blood.

Urinary System

The *urinary system* contains the kidneys, the urinary bladder, and the tubes that carry urine. The kidneys rid the body of metabolic wastes, particularly nitrogenous wastes. They also help regulate the salt–water balance and acid–base balance of the blood.

Skeletal System

The bones of the *skeletal system* protect body parts. For example, the skull forms a protective encasement for the brain, as does the rib cage for the heart and lungs. The skeleton helps move the body because it serves as a place of attachment for the skeletal muscles. The skeletal system also stores minerals, notably calcium, and produces blood cells within red bone marrow.

Muscular System

In the *muscular system*, skeletal muscle contraction maintains posture and accounts for the movement of the body and its parts. Cardiac muscle contraction results in the heartbeat. The walls of internal organs, such as the bladder, contract due to the presence of smooth muscle. Muscle contraction releases heat, which helps warm the body.

Nervous System

The *nervous system* consists of the brain, spinal cord, and associated nerves. The nerves conduct nerve impulses from sensory receptors to the brain and spinal cord, where integration occurs. Nerves also conduct nerve impulses from the brain and spinal cord to the muscles and glands, allowing us to respond to both external and internal stimuli.

Endocrine System

The *endocrine system* consists of the hormonal glands, which secrete chemical messengers called *hormones* into the bloodstream. Hormones have a wide range of effects, including regulation of cellular metabolism, regulation of fluid and pH balance, and helping us respond to stress. Both the nervous and endocrine systems coordinate and regulate the functioning of the body's other systems. The endocrine system also helps maintain the functioning of the male and female reproductive organs.

Reproductive System

The *reproductive system* has different organs in the male and female. The male reproductive system consists of the testes, other glands (such as the prostrate), and various ducts that conduct semen to and through the penis. The testes produce sex cells called *sperm.* The female reproductive system consists of the ovaries, oviducts, uterus, vagina, and external genitals. The ovaries produce sex cells called *eggs.* When a sperm fertilizes an egg, an offspring begins development.

BODY CAVITIES

The human body is divided into two main cavities: the ventral cavity and the dorsal cavity. Called the *coelom* in early development, the*ventral cavity* later becomes the thoracic, abdominal, and pelvic cavities. The thoracic cavity contains the lungs and the heart. The thoracic cavity is separated from the abdominal cavity by a horizontal muscle called the*diaphragm*. The stomach, liver, spleen, pancreas, gallbladder, and most of the small and large intestines are in the abdominal cavity. The pelvic cavity contains the rectum, the urinary bladder, the internal reproductive organs, and the rest of the small and large intestine. Males have an external extension of the abdominal wall called the *scrotum,* which contains the testes.

The *dorsal cavity* has two parts:

(1) The cranial cavity within the skull contains the brain.

(2) The vertebral canal, formed by the vertebrae, contains the spinal cord.

BODY MEMBRANES

Body membranes line cavities and the internal spaces of organs and tubes that open to the outside. The body membranes are of four types: mucous, serous, and synovial membranes and the meninges.

Mucous membranes line the tubes of the digestive, respiratory, urinary, and reproductive systems. They are composed of an epithelium overlying a loose fibrous connective tissue layer. The epithelium contains specialized cells that secrete mucus. This mucus ordinarily protects the body from invasion by bacteria and viruses. Hence, more mucus is secreted and expelled when a person has a cold and has to blow her/his nose. In addition, mucus usually protects the walls of the stomach and small intestine from digestive juices. This protection breaks down when a person develops an ulcer.

Serous membranes line and support the lungs, the heart, and the abdominal cavity and its internal organs. They secrete a watery fluid that keeps the membranes lubricated. Serous membranes support the internal organs and compartmentalize the large thoracic and abdominal cavities.

Serous membranes have specific names according to their location. The pleurae (sing., *pleura*) line the thoracic cavity and cover the lungs. The pericardium forms the pericardial sac and covers the heart. The peritoneum lines the abdominal cavity and covers its organs. A double layer of peritoneum, called mesentery, supports the abdominal organs and attaches them to the abdominal wall. *Peritonitis* is a life-threatening infection of the peritoneum.

Synovial membranes composed only of loose connective tissue line the cavities of freely movable joints. They secrete synovial fluid into the joint cavity. This fluid lubricates the ends of the bones so that they can move freely. In rheumatoid arthritis, the synovial membrane becomes inflamed and grows thicker, restricting movement.

The *meninges* (sing., meninx) are membranes found within the dorsal cavity. They are composed only of connective tissue and serve as a protective covering for the brain and spinal cord. Meningitis is a life-threatening infection of the meninges.

PHYSIOLOGY OF THE HEART

The work of the heart is to pump blood to the lungs through pulmonary circulation and to the rest of the body through systemic circulation. This is accomplished by systematic contraction and relaxation of the cardiac muscle in the myocardium.

Conduction System

An effective cycle for productive pumping of blood requires that the heart be synchronized accurately. Both atria need to contract simultaneously, followed by contraction of both ventricles. Specialized cardiac muscle cells that make up the conduction system of the heart coordinate contraction of the chambers.

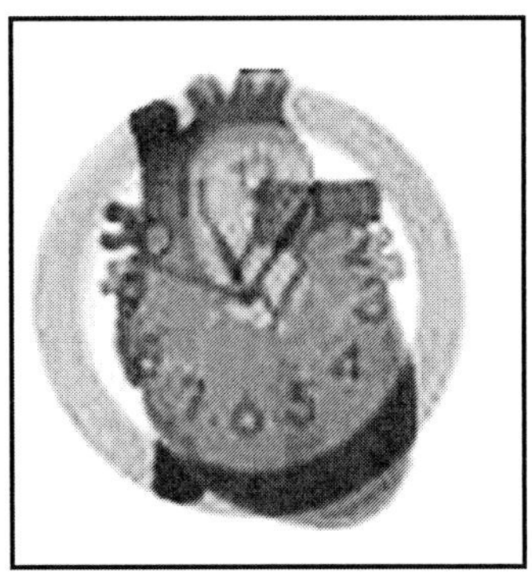

The conduction system includes several components. The first part of the conduction system is the sinoatrial node. Without any neural stimulation, the sinoatrial node rhythmically initiates impulses 70 to 80 times per minute. Because it establishes the basic rhythm of the heartbeat, it is called the pacemaker of the heart. Other parts of the conduction system include the atrioventricular node, atrioventricular bundle, bundle branches, and conduction myofibres. All these components coordinate the contraction and relaxation of the heart chambers.

Cardiac Cycle

The cardiac cycle refers to the alternating contraction and relaxation of the myocardium in the walls of the heart chambers, coordinated by the conduction system, during one heartbeat. Systole is the contraction phase of the cardiac cycle, and diastole is the relaxation phase. At a normal heart rate, one cardiac cycle lasts for 0.8 second.

The cardiac cycle diagram shown to the right depicts changes in aortic pressure, left ventricular pressure, left atrial pressure, and left ventricular volume during a single cycle of cardiac contraction and relaxation. These changes are related in time to the electrocardiogram. Aortic pressure is measure by inserting a pressure catheter into the aorta from a peripheral artery, and the left ventricular pressure is obtained by placing a pressure catheter inside the left ventricle and measuring changes in intraventricular pressure as the heart beats. Left atrial pressure is not usually measured directly, except in investigational procedures. Ventricular volume changes can be assessed in real time using echocardiography or radionuclide imaging, or by using a special volume conductance catheter placed within the ventricle.

A single cycle of cardiac activity can be divided into two basic stages. The first stage is diastole, which represents ventricular filling and a brief period just prior to filling at which time the ventricles are relaxing.

The second stage is systole, which represents the time of contraction and ejection of blood from the ventricles. The cardiac cycle is usually divided into seven phases. The first phase begins with the P wave of the electrocardiogram, which represents atrial depolarization. The last phase of the cardiac cycle ends with the appearance of the next P wave. In order to understand the events of the cardiac cycle, the reader should first review basic cardiac anatomy. The entire cardiac cycle diagram, which contains information on aortic, left ventricular and left atrial pressures, along with ventricular volume, heart sounds and the electrocardiogram, is shown.

AN ELECTROCARDIOGRAM (ECG)

An electrocardiogram (ECG) measures changes in electrical potential across the heart, and can detect the contraction pulses that pass over the surface of the heart. There are three slow, negative changes, known as P, R, and T. Positive deflections are the Q and S waves. The P wave represents the contraction impulse of the atria, the T wave the ventricular contraction. ECGs are useful in diagnosing heart abnormalities.

Heart Sounds

The sounds associated with the heartbeat are due to vibrations in the tissues and blood caused by closure of the valves. Abnormal heart sounds are called murmurs.

Heart Rate

The sinoatrial node, acting alone, produces a constant rhythmic heart rate. Regulating factors are reliant on the atrioventricular node to increase or decrease the heart rate to adjust cardiac output to meet the changing needs of the body. Most changes in the heart rate are mediated through the cardiac centre in the medulla oblongata of the brain. The centre has both sympathetic and parasympathetic components that adjust the heart rate to meet the changing needs of the body. Peripheral factors such as emotions, ion concentrations, and body temperature may affect heart rate. These are usually mediated through the cardiac centre.

Blood

Blood is the fluid of life, transporting oxygen from the lungs to body tissue and carbon dioxide from body tissue to the lungs. Blood is the fluid of growth, transporting nourishment from digestion and hormones from glands throughout the body. Blood is the fluid of health, transporting disease fighting substances to the tissue and waste to the kidneys. Because it contains living cells, blood is alive. Red blood cells and white blood cells are responsible for nourishing and cleansing the body.

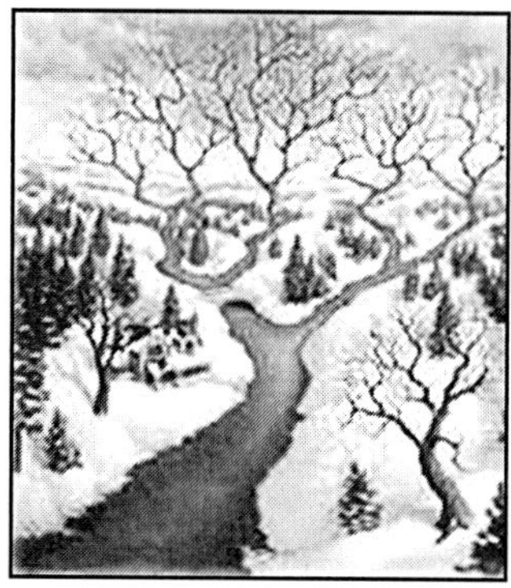

Fig. Without blood, the human body would stop working.

To learn more about blood, select a topic listed below to branch into a sub-section.

- Classification and Structure of Blood Vessels
- Physiology of Circulation
- Circulatory Pathways.

CLASSIFICATION AND STRUCTURE OF BLOOD VESSELS

Blood vessels are the channels or conduits through which blood is distributed to body tissues. The vessels make up two closed systems of tubes that begin and end at the heart. One system, the pulmonary vessels, transports blood from the right ventricle to the lungs and back to the left atrium. The other system, the systemic vessels, carries blood from the left ventricle to the tissues in all parts of the body and then returns the blood to the right atrium. Based on their structure and function, blood vessels are classified as either arteries, capillaries, or veins.

Arteries

Arteries carry blood away from the heart. Pulmonary arteries transport blood that has a low oxygen content from the right ventricle to the lungs. Systemic arteries transport oxygenated blood from the left ventricle to the body tissues. Blood is pumped from the ventricles into large elastic arteries that branch repeatedly into smaller and smaller arteries until the branching results in microscopic arteries called arterioles.

The arterioles play a key role in regulating blood flow into the tissue capillaries. About 10 per cent of the total blood volume is in the systemic arterial system at any given time.

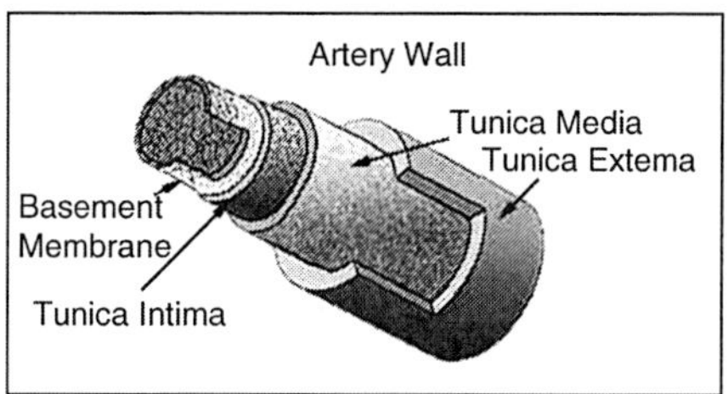

Fig. Artery Wall

The wall of an artery consists of three layers. The innermost layer, the tunica intima (also called tunica interna), is simple squamous epithelium surrounded by a connective tissue basement membrane with elastic fibres. The middle layer, the tunica media, is primarily smooth muscle and is usually the thickest layer.

It not only provides support for the vessel but also changes vessel diameter to regulate blood flow and blood pressure. The outermost layer, which attaches the vessel to the surrounding tissue, is the tunica externa or tunica adventitia. This layer is connective tissue with varying amounts of elastic and collagenous fibres. The connective tissue in this layer is quite dense where it is adjacent to the tunic media, but it changes to loose connective tissue near the periphery of the vessel.

Capillaries

Capillaries, the smallest and most numerous of the blood vessels, form the connection between the vessels that carry blood away from the heart (arteries) and the vessels that return blood to the heart (veins). The primary function of capillaries is the exchange of materials between the blood and tissue cells.

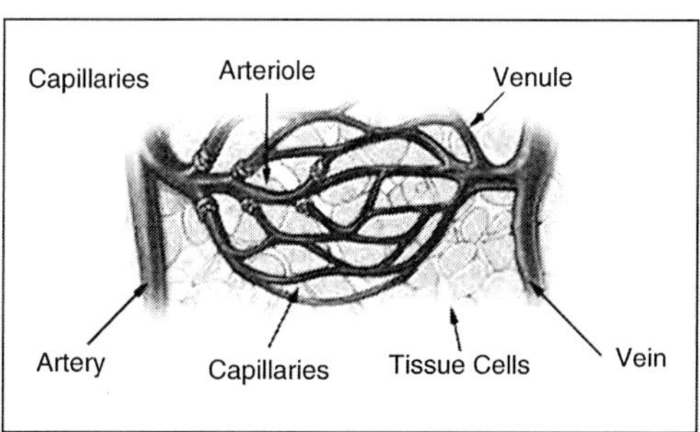

Fig. Capillaries

Capillary distribution varies with the metabolic activity of body tissues. Tissues such as skeletal muscle, liver, and kidney have extensive capillary networks because they are metabolically active and require an abundant supply of oxygen and nutrients. Other tissues, such as connective tissue, have a less abundant supply of capillaries. The epidermis of the skin and the lens and cornea of the eye completely lack a capillary network. About 5 per cent of the total blood volume is in the systemic capillaries at any given time. Another 10 per cent is in the lungs. Smooth muscle cells in the arterioles where they branch to form capillaries regulate blood flow from the arterioles into the capillaries.

Veins

Veins carry blood towards the heart. After blood passes through the capillaries, it enters the smallest veins, called venules. From the venules, it flows into progressively larger and larger veins until it reaches the heart. In the pulmonary circuit, the pulmonary veins transport blood from the lungs to the left atrium of the heart. This blood has a high oxygen content because it has just been oxygenated in the lungs. Systemic veins transport blood from the body tissue to the right atrium of the heart. This blood has a reduced oxygen content because the oxygen has been used for metabolic activities in the tissue cells.

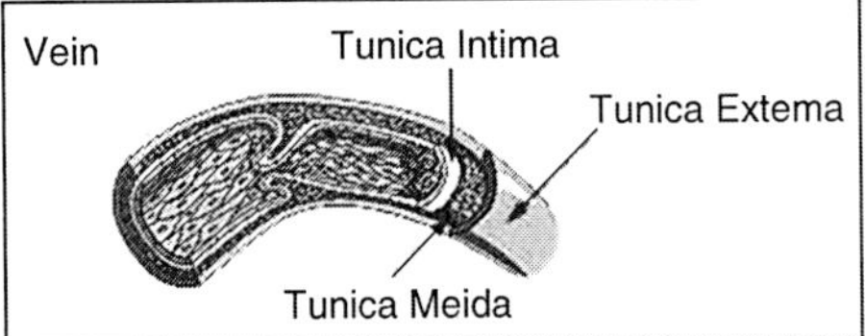

Fig. Vein

The walls of veins have the same three layers as the arteries. Although all the layers are present, there is less smooth muscle and connective tissue. This makes the walls of veins thinner than those of arteries, which is related to the fact that blood in the veins has less pressure than in the arteries. Because the walls of the veins are thinner and less rigid than arteries, veins can hold more blood. Almost 70 per cent of the total blood volume is in the veins at any given time. Medium and large veins have venous valves, similar to the semilunar valves associated with the heart, that help keep the blood flowing towards the heart. Venous valves are especially important in the arms and legs, where they prevent the backflow of blood in response to the pull of gravity.

PHYSIOLOGY OF CIRCULATION

In addition to forming the connection between the arteries and veins, capillaries have a vital role in the exchange of gases, nutrients, and metabolic waste products between the blood and the tissue cells. Substances pass through the capillaries wall by diffusion, filtration, and osmosis. Oxygen and carbon dioxide move across the capillary wall by diffusion. Fluid movement across a capillary wall is determined by a combination of hydrostatic and osmotic pressure. The net result of the capillary microcirculation created by hydrostatic and osmotic pressure is that substances leave the blood at one end of the capillary and return at the other end.

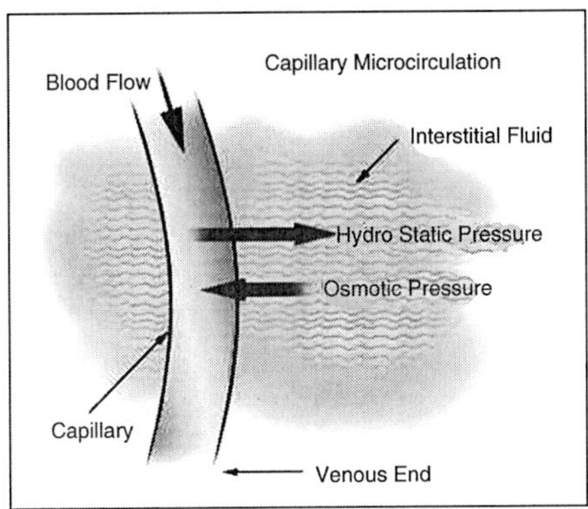

Fig. Capillary Microcirculation

Blood Flow

Blood flow refers to the movement of blood through the vessels from arteries to the capillaries and then into the veins. Pressure is a measure of the force that the blood exerts against the vessel walls as it moves the blood through the vessels. Like all fluids, blood flows from a high pressure area to a region with lower pressure. Blood flows in the same direction as the decreasing pressure gradient: arteries to capillaries to veins. The rate, or velocity, of blood flow varies inversely with the total cross-sectional area of the blood vessels. As the total cross-sectional area of the vessels increases, the velocity of flow decreases. Blood flow is slowest in the capillaries, which allows time for exchange of gases and nutrients.

Resistance is a force that opposes the flow of a fluid. In blood vessels, most of the resistance is due to vessel diameter. As vessel diameter decreases, the resistance increases and blood flow decreases. Very little pressure remains by the time blood leaves the capillaries and enters the venules. Blood flow through the veins is not the direct result of ventricular contraction. Instead, venous return depends on skeletal muscle action, respiratory movements, and constriction of smooth muscle in venous walls.

Pulse and Blood Pressure

Pulse refers to the rhythmic expansion of an artery that is caused by ejection of blood from the ventricle. It can be felt where an artery is close to the surface and rests on something firm. In common usage, the term blood pressure refers to arterial blood pressure, the pressure in the aorta and its branches.

Systolic pressure is due to ventricular contraction. Diastolic pressure occurs during cardiac relaxation. Pulse pressure is the difference between systolic pressure and diastolic pressure. Blood pressure is measured with a sphygmomanometer and is recorded as the systolic pressure over the diastolic pressure. Four major factors interact to affect blood pressure: cardiac output, blood volume, peripheral resistance, and viscosity. When these factors increase, blood pressure also increases.

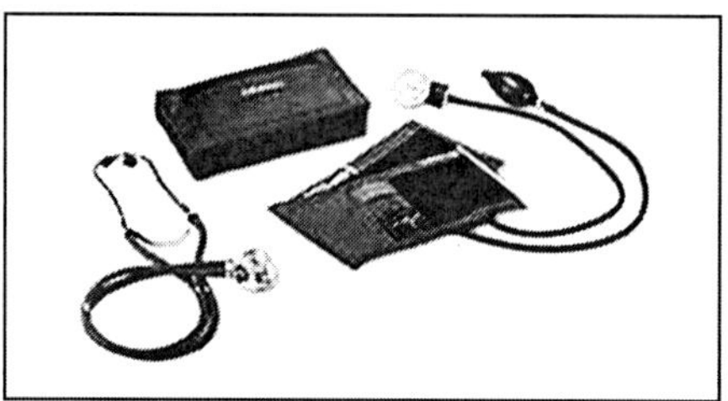

Arterial blood pressure is maintained within normal ranges by changes in cardiac output and peripheral resistance. Pressure receptors (barareceptors), located in the walls of the large arteries in the thorax and neck, are important for short-term blood pressure regulation.

CIRCULATORY PATHWAYS

The blood vessels of the body are functionally divided into two distinctive circuits: pulmonary circuit and systemic circuit. The pump for the pulmonary circuit, which circulates blood through the lungs, is the right ventricle. The left ventricle is the pump for the systemic circuit, which provides the blood supply for the tissue cells of the body.

Pulmonary Circuit

Pulmonary circulation transports oxygen-poor blood from the right ventricle to the lungs where blood picks up a new blood supply. Then it returns the oxygen-rich blood to the left atrium.

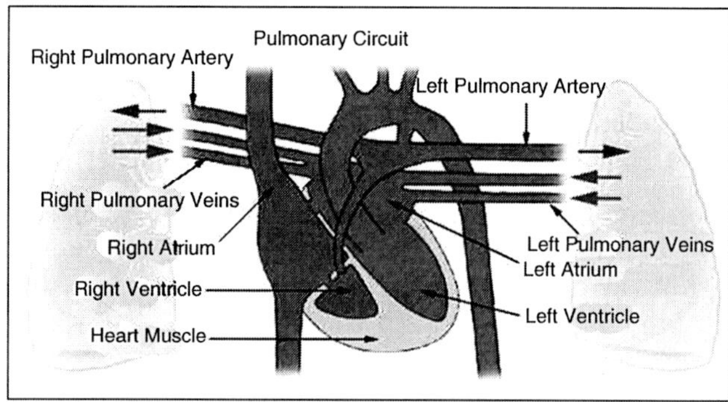

Fig. Pulmonary Circuit

Systemic Circuit

The systemic circulation provides the functional blood supply to all body tissue. It carries oxygen and nutrients to the cells and picks up carbon dioxide and waste products. Systemic circulation carries oxygenated blood from the left ventricle, through the arteries, to the capillaries in the tissues of the body. From the tissue capillaries, the deoxygenated blood returns through a system of veins to the right atrium of the heart.

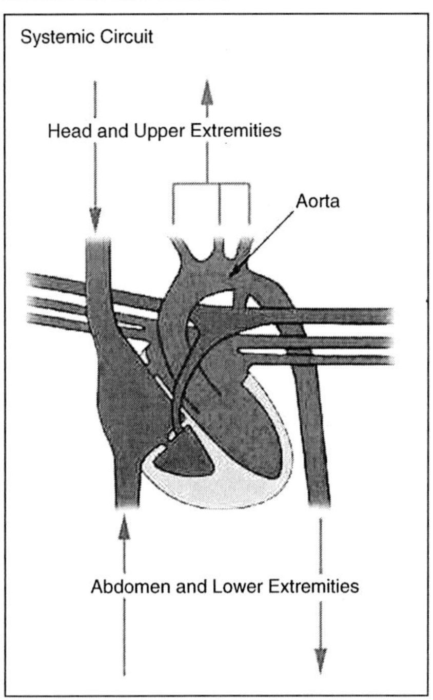

Fig. Systemic Circuit

The coronary arteries are the only vessels that branch from the ascending aorta. The brachiocephalic, left common carotid, and left subclavian arteries branch from the aortic arch. Blood supply for the brain is provided by the internal carotid and vertebral arteries. The subclavian arteries provide the blood supply for the upper extremity.

The celiac, superior mesenteric, suprarenal, renal, gonadal, and inferior mesenteric arteries branch from the abdominal aorta to supply the abdominal viscera. Lumbar arteries provide blood for the muscles and spinal cord. Branches of the external iliac artery provide the blood supply for the lower extremity. The internal iliac artery supplies the pelvic viscera.

Major Systemic Arteries

All systemic arteries are branches, either directly or indirectly, from the aorta. The aorta ascends from the left ventricle, curves posteriorly and to the left, then descends through the thorax and abdomen. This geography divides the aorta into three portions: ascending aorta, arotic arch, and descending aorta. The descending aorta is further subdivided into the thoracic arota and abdominal aorta.

Major Systemic Veins

After blood delivers oxygen to the tissues and picks up carbon dioxide, it returns to the heart through a system of veins. The capillaries, where the gaseous exchange occurs, merge into venules and these converge to form larger and larger veins until the blood reaches either the superior vena cava or inferior vena cava, which drain into the right atrium.

Fetal Circulation

Most circulatory pathways in a fetus are like those in the adult but there are some notable differences because the lungs, the gastrointestinal tract, and the kidneys are not functioning before birth. The fetus obtains its oxygen and nutrients from the mother and also depends on maternal circulation to carry away the carbon dioxide and waste products.

The umbilical cord contains two umbilical arteries to carry fetal blood to the placenta and one umbilical vein to carry oxygen-and-nutrient-rich blood from the placenta to the fetus.

The ductus venosus allows blood to bypass the immature liver in fetal circulation. The foramen ovale and ductus arteriosus are modifications that permit blood to bypass the lungs in fetal circulation.

ANATOMY OF THE HEART

PERICARDIUM

The heart sits within a fluid-filled cavity called the pericardial cavity. The walls and lining of the pericardial cavity are a special membrane known as the pericardium. Pericardium is a type of serous membrane that produces serous fluid to lubricate the heart and prevent friction between the ever beating heart and its surrounding organs. Besides lubrication, the pericardium serves to hold the heart in position and maintain a hollow space for the heart to expand into when it is full. The pericardium has 2 layers—a visceral layer that covers the outside of the heart and a parietal layer that forms a sac around the outside of the pericardial cavity.

STRUCTURE OF THE HEART WALL

The heart wall is made of 3 layers: epicardium, myocardium and endocardium.

- *Epicardium.* The epicardium is the outermost layer of the heart wall and is just another name for the visceral layer of the pericardium. Thus, the epicardium is a thin layer of serous membrane that helps to lubricate and protect the outside of the heart. Below the epicardium is the second, thicker layer of the heart wall: the myocardium.

- *Myocardium.* The myocardium is the muscular middle layer of the heart wall that contains the cardiac muscle tissue. Myocardium makes up the majority of the thickness and mass of the heart wall and is the part of the heart responsible for pumping blood.

- *Endocardium.* Endocardium is the simple squamous endothelium layer that lines the inside of the heart. The endocardium is very smooth and is responsible for keeping blood from sticking to the inside of the heart and forming potentially deadly blood clots.

The thickness of the heart wall varies in different parts of the heart. The atria of the heart have a very thin myocardium because they do not need to pump blood very far—only to the nearby ventricles. The ventricles, on the other hand, have a very thick myocardium to pump blood to the lungs or throughout the entire body. The right side of the heart has less myocardium in its walls than the left side because the left side has to pump blood through the entire body while the right side only has to pump to the lungs.

CHAMBERS OF THE HEART

The heart contains 4 chambers: the right atrium, left atrium, right ventricle, and left ventricle. The atria are smaller than the ventricles and have thinner, less muscular walls than the ventricles. The atria act as receiving chambers for blood, so they are connected to the veins that carry blood to the heart. The ventricles are the larger, stronger pumping chambers that send blood out of the heart. The ventricles are connected to the arteries that carry blood away from the heart.

The chambers on the right side of the heart are smaller and have less myocardium in their heart wall when compared to the left side of the heart. This difference in size between the sides of the heart is related to their functions and the size of the 2 circulatory loops. The right side of the heart maintains pulmonary circulation to the nearby lungs while the left side of the heart pumps blood all the way to the extremities of the body in the systemic circulatory loop.

VALVES OF THE HEART

The heart functions by pumping blood both to the lungs and to the systems of the body. To prevent blood from flowing backwards or "regurgitating" back into the heart, a system of one-way valves are present in the heart. The heart valves can be broken down into two types: atrioventricular and semilunar valves.

- *Atrioventricular valves.* The atrioventricular (AV) valves are located in the middle of the heart between the atria and ventricles and only allow blood to flow from the atria into the ventricles. The AV valve on the right side of the heart is called the tricuspid valve because it is made of three cusps (flaps) that separate to allow blood to pass through and connect to block regurgitation of blood. The AV valve on the left side of the heart is called the mitral valve or the bicuspid valve because it has two cusps. The AV valves are attached on the ventricular side to tough strings called chordae tendineae. The chordae tendineae pull on the AV valves to keep them from folding backwards and allowing blood to regurgitate past them. During the contraction of the ventricles, the AV valves look like domed parachutes with the chordae tendineae acting as the ropes holding the parachutes taut.

- *Semilunar valves.* The semilunar valves, so named for the crescent moon shape of their cusps, are located between the ventricles and the arteries that carry blood away from the heart. The semilunar valve on the right side of the heart is the pulmonary valve, so named because it prevents the backflow of blood from the pulmonary trunk into the right ventricle. The semilunar valve on the left side of the heart is theaortic valve, named for the fact that it prevents the aorta from regurgitating blood back into the left ventricle. The semilunar valves are smaller than the AV valves and do not have chordae tendineae to hold them in place. Instead, the cusps of the semilunar valves are cup shaped to catch regurgitating blood and use the blood's pressure to snap shut.

Conduction System of the Heart

The heart is able to both set its own rhythm and to conduct the signals necessary to maintain and coordinate this rhythm throughout its structures. About 1 per cent of the cardiac muscle cells in the heart are responsible for forming the conduction system that sets the pace for the rest of the cardiac muscle cells.

The conduction system starts with the pacemaker of the heart—a small bundle of cells known as the sinoatrial (SA) node. The SA node is located in the wall of the right atrium inferior to the superior vena cava. The SA node is responsible for setting the pace of the heart as a whole and directly signals the atria to contract. The signal from the SA node is picked up by another mass of conductive tissue known as the atrioventricular (AV) node.

The AV node is located in the right atrium in the inferior portion of the interatrial septum. The AV node picks up the signal sent by the SA node and transmits it through the atrioventricular (AV) bundle. The AV bundle is a strand of conductive tissue that runs through the interatrial septum and into the interventricular septum. The AV bundle splits into left and right branches in the interventricular septum and continues running through the septum until they reach the apex of the heart. Branching off from the left and right bundle branches are many Purkinje fibres that carry the signal to the walls of the ventricles, stimulating the cardiac muscle cells to contract in a coordinated manner to efficiently pump blood out of the heart.

PHYSIOLOGY OF THE HEART

Coronary Systole and Diastole

At any given time the chambers of the heart may found in one of two states:

- *Systole*. During systole, cardiac muscle tissue is contracting to push blood out of the chamber.
- *Diastole*. During diastole, the cardiac muscle cells relax to allow the chamber to fill with blood. Blood pressure increases in the major arteries during ventricular systole and decreases during ventricular diastole. This leads to the 2 numbers associated with blood pressure—systolic blood pressure is the higher number and diastolic blood pressure is the lower number. For example, a blood pressure of 120/80 describes the systolic pressure (120) and the diastolic pressure (80).

The Cardiac Cycle

The cardiac cycle includes all of the events that take place during one heartbeat.

There are 3 phases to the cardiac cycle: atrial systole, ventricular systole, and relaxation.

- *Atrial systole*: During the atrial systole phase of the cardiac cycle, the atria contract and push blood into the ventricles. To facilitate this filling, the AV valves stay open and the semilunar valves stay closed to keep arterial blood from re-entering the heart. The atria are much smaller than the ventricles, so they only fill about 25 per cent of the ventricles during this phase. The ventricles remain in diastole during this phase.
- *Ventricular systole*: During ventricular systole, the ventricles contract to push blood into the aorta and pulmonary trunk. The pressure of the ventricles forces the semilunar valves to open and the AV valves to close. This arrangement of valves allows for blood flow from the ventricles into the arteries. The cardiac muscles of the atria repolarize and enter the state of diastole during this phase.
- *Relaxation phase*: During the relaxation phase, all 4 chambers of the heart are in diastole as blood pours into the heart from the veins. The ventricles fill to about 75 per cent capacity during this phase and will be completely filled only after the atria enter systole. The cardiac muscle cells of the ventricles repolarize during this phase to

prepare for the next round of depolarization and contraction. During this phase, the AV valves open to allow blood to flow freely into the ventricles while the semilunar valves close to prevent the regurgitation of blood from the great arteries into the ventricles.

Blood Flow through the Heart

Deoxygenated blood returning from the body first enters the heart from the superior and inferior vena cava. The blood enters the right atrium and is pumped through the tricuspid valve into the right ventricle. From the right ventricle, the blood is pumped through the pulmonary semilunar valve into the pulmonary trunk. The pulmonary trunk carries blood to the lungs where it releases carbon dioxide and absorbs oxygen. The blood in the lungs returns to the heart through the pulmonary veins.

From the pulmonary veins, blood enters the heart again in the left atrium. The left atrium contracts to pump blood through the bicuspid (mitral) valve into the left ventricle. The left ventricle pumps blood through the aortic semilunar valve into the aorta. From the aorta, blood enters into systemic circulation throughout the body tissues until it returns to the heart via the vena cava and the cycle repeats.

The Electrocardiogram

The electrocardiogram (also known as an EKG or ECG) is a non-invasive device that measures and monitors the electrical activity of the heart through the skin. The EKG produces a distinctive waveform in response to the electrical changes taking place within the heart.

The first part of the wave, called the P wave, is a small increase in voltage of about 0.1 mV that corresponds to the depolarization of the atria during atrial systole. The next part of the EKG wave is the QRS complex which features a small drop in voltage (Q) a large voltage peak (R) and another small drop in voltage (S). The QRS complex corresponds to the depolarization of the ventricles during ventricular systole. The atria also repolarize during the QRS complex, but have almost no effect on the EKG because they are so much smaller than the ventricles.

The final part of the EKG wave is the T wave, a small peak that follows the QRS complex. The T wave represents the ventricular repolarization during the relaxation phase of the cardiac cycle. Variations in the waveform and distance between the waves of the EKG can be used clinically to diagnose the effects of heart attacks, congenital heart problems, and electrolyte imbalances.

Heart Sounds

The sounds of a normal heartbeat are known as "lubb" and "dupp" and are caused by blood pushing on the valves of the heart. The "lubb" sound comes first in the heartbeat and is the longer of the two heart sounds. The "lubb" sound is produced by the closing of the AV valves at the beginning of ventricular systole. The shorter, sharper "dupp" sound is similarly caused by the closing of the semilunar valves at the end of ventricular systole. During a normal heartbeat, these sounds repeat in a regular pattern of lubb-dupp-pause. Any additional sounds such as liquid rushing or gurgling indicate a structure problem in the heart. The most likely causes of these extraneous sounds are defects in the atrial or ventricular septum or leakage in the valves.

Cardiac Output

Cardiac output (CO) is the volume of blood being pumped by the heart in one minute. The equation used to find cardiac output is: CO = Stroke Volume x Heart Rate

Stroke volume is the amount of blood pumped into the aorta during each ventricular systole, usually measured in milliliters. Heart rate is the number of heartbeats per minute. The average heart can push around 5 to 5.5 liters per minute at rest.

THE PHYSIOLOGY OF THE HUMAN HEART

The constant beating of the heart is controlled by the conducting system of the heart, which is a series of specialized nerve tissues that fire through the heart and coordinate the actions of the heart beat:

- Sinoatrial (SA) node: This pacemaker initiates the impulse. It's located anterolaterally just under the epicardium where the superior vena cava enters the right atrium. The impulse from the sinoatrial node spreads through the myocardium of the right and left atria, and it's also quickly transmitted to the atrioventricular node.
- Atrioventricular (AV) node: This node is located in the posterior and inferior portion of the interatrial septum, close to the opening of the coronary sinus in the right atrium. From there the signal is transmitted to the ventricles by a bundle of nerves called the atrioventricular bundle.
- Atrioventricular bundle: This bundle of nerves runs from the atrioventricular node to the ventricles along the interventricular septum. It divides into left and right bundle branches that run deep to the endocardium to become the subendocardial branches (also called the Purkinje fibres):
- Subendocardial branches of the right bundle stimulate the interventricular septum, the papillary muscle, and the wall of the right ventricle.
- Subendocardial branches of the left bundle stimulate the interventricular septum, the papillary muscle, and wall of the left ventricle.

The heart is innervated by the autonomic nerves from superficial and deep cardiac plexuses. The deep cardiac plexus is located on the bifurcation of the trachea, and the superficial cardiac plexus is located on the base of the heart below the arch of the aorta.

The autonomic nervous system is made up of a two-neuron chain (using the presynaptic neuron and the postsynaptic neuron) from the central nervous system to the heart. The presynaptic sympathetic fibres branch off the first five or six thoracic segments of the spinal cord. They enter the sympathetic trunks and synapse with postsynaptic neurons located in the cervical and upper thoracic ganglia. Fibres of the postsynaptic neurons join the cardiac plexus and terminate on the SA node, AV node, cardiac muscle fibres, and coronary arteries.

Sympathetic stimulation increases heart rate, force of contraction, and dilation of coronary arteries. Parasympathetic innervation to the heart is provided by the vagus nerve (CN X).

The presynaptic parasympathetic fibres of the vagus nerve join the postsynaptic sympathetic fibres in the cardiac plexus.

The postsynaptic parasympathetic neurons are located in intrinsic ganglia (within the wall of the heart) and terminate on the SA node, AV node, and coronary arteries. Parasympathetic stimulationhas the opposite effect of sympathetic stimulation.

The cardiac cycle is the sequence of events of each heart beat:

- *Diastole:* During this process, the ventricles fill with blood from the atria. The atrioventricular valves are open, and the pulmonary and aortic valves are closed.
- *Systole:* In this process, the ventricles empty into the aorta and pulmonary arteries. The atrioventricular valves are closed, and the pulmonary and aortic valves are open.

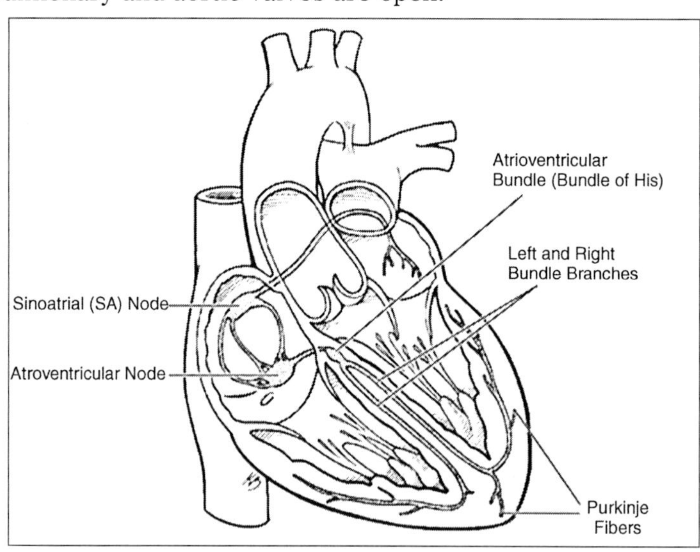

The major blood vessels of the thorax include arteries that branch off the aorta and veins that drain into the vena cava.

Following are the parts of the aorta and its branches:

- *Ascending aorta:* This part of the aorta leaves the left ventricle and ascends up to the sternal angle. It has spaces between the walls of the vessel and the cusps of the aortic valve called aortic sinuses.
- *Arch of the aorta:* Continuing from the ascending aorta, this part arches posteriorly to the left of the trachea and esophagus, above the left primary bronchus
- *Thoracic aorta:* The thoracic aorta continues from the arch and descends in the posteriormediastinum and left of the vertebral column.
- *Posterior intercostal arteries:* These arteries branch off the posterior part of the thoracic aorta and run laterally and anteriorly in the intercostal spaces.
- *Bronchial arteries:* These arteries branch off the anterior part of the aorta or a posterior intercostal artery.
- *Esophageal arteries:* Starting at the anterior part of the thoracic aorta, these arteries run to the esophagus.
- *Superior phrenic arteries:* These arteries start at the anterior part of the thoracic aorta and run to the diaphragm.

Following are the parts of the vena cava and its tributaries:

- *Right and left brachiocephalic veins:* These veins unite to form the superior vena cava near the brachiocephalic trunk (at the level of the 1st costal cartilage).
- *Superior vena cava:* This large vein runs inferiorly to enter the right atrium.
- *Inferior vena cava:* This vein is formed by the union of the iliac. It enters the heart at the lowest part of the right atrium.
- *Azygos vein:* This vein arises from the right ascending lumbar vein and passes through the posterior mediastinum to drain into the superior vena cava.
- *Hemiazygos vein:* This vein starts at the left ascending lumbar vein and crosses the vertebral column around the level of the 8th thoracic vertebra to join the azygos vein.
- *Accessory hemiazygos vein:* This vein is formed by the union of the left fourth to the eighth posterior intercostal veins and joins the azygos vein at the level of the 7th thoracic vertebra.

ELECTRO PHYSIOLOGY OF HUMAN HEART

This chapter defines electro physiology of human heart, blood circulation in both pulmonary and systemic, the components in cardiovascular system and heart sounds. The generation of potential due to mechanical activity of human heart and sounds produced due to closure of valves during blood pumping from atrias to ventricles and to respective parts of the body. This chapter presents a detailed survey on literature focusing on different methods to measure and analyse ECG and PCG.

Electricity plays an important role in medicine. The control and operation of nerves, muscles and organs are functioning by the electricity generated inside the body. The forces of muscles, the action of brain and all nerve signals to and from the brain are caused by the attraction and repulsion of electrical charges. Many electrical signals are generated to carry out the special functions of the body. These signals are the result of electrochemical action of certain type of cells. The best known signals are electrical potentials of nerve transmission and the electrical signals observed in electromyogram (EMG) of the muscle, the electrocardiogram (ECG) of the heart and the electroencephalogram (EEG) of the brain.

One means of obtaining diagnostic information about muscles, heart and brain are to measure their electrical activity. The record of the potential from muscles during movement of is called the electromyogram (EMG). The rhythmical action of the heart is controlled by an electrical signal initiated by spontaneous stimulation of pacemaker cells located at apex of the right atrium *i.e.* sinoatrial node (SA node). The recording of heart's potentials on skin is called electrocardiogram (ECG). The recording of the electric signals due to electrical activity of neurons in the cortex of the brain is called electroencephalogram (EEG). The present study is to study the electrical activity of heart during its mechanical vibrations.

The primary step in investigations of physiological systems requires the appropriate sensors to transducer the phenomenon of interest into a measurable electric signal. The field of biomedical has advanced to the stage of practical application of signal processing and pattern analysis techniques for efficient and improved non- invasive diagnosis.

PHYSIOLOGY OF HEART AND VASCULAR SYSTEM

The analysis of variability in cardiovascular signals is applied widely and many experimental setups were put forward. Spontaneous fluctuations can be observed in cardiovascular function, such as heart rate and blood pressure, even when the environmental parameters are maintained at a constant level as possible and no perturbations influences can be identified.

The observations of heart rate fluctuations is related to various cardiovascular disorders, the analysis of heart rate variability has become widely used tool in the assessment of the regulation of heart rate behaviour (Timo Makikallo 1998). The study of cyclic variations of heart rate plays an important role in the assessment of both physiological and clinical aspects.The heart is actually two separate pumps. A right heart that pumps the blood through the lungs and left heart pumps the blood through the peripheral organs. Each of these composed of 'atrium' and 'ventricle'. Atrium receives the blood and pumps into ventricles. Ventricles supply the main force that circulates the blood either through pulmonary circulation by the right ventricle or through the systemic circulation by the left ventricle.

The blood, blood vessels and heart make up the cardiovascular system (CVS). The blood and its supply of oxygen are so important to the body that the heart is the first major organ to develop in the embryo.

The mechanism in the heart provides cardiac rhythmcity and transmits action potentials through the heart muscle to cause the heart's rhythmical beat. The cardiac event that occurs from the beginning of the next are called the cardiac cycle. Each cycle is initiated by spontaneous generation of an action potential in the' Sino atrious node' or 'Sinus node'.

The cardiac cycle consists of a period of relaxation called 'diastole', during which the heart fills with blood fallowed by a period of contraction called 'systole' together is known as a 'beat'. The heart is composed of three major types of cardiac muscle; atrial muscle, ventricular muscle and specialized excitatory and conductive muscle fibres. Cardiac muscle is a syncytium of many heart muscle cells which are interconnected with "intercalated discs" which are of actually cell membranes separates cardiac muscle cells from one another and offers low resistance to ions to diffuse through cells. If one of these cells is excited, the action potential spreads to all of them.

The heart is composed of two syncytiums the atrial syncytium that consists of walls of two atria and ventricular syncytium consists of the walls of two ventricles. The atria are separated from the ventricles by tissue that surrounds the atrio-ventricular valvular openings. Potentials are conducted from atrial syncytium into ventricular syncytium through the specialized conductive system called A-V bundle a bundle of conductive fibres.

The division of the muscle of the heart into two functional syncytiums allows the atria to contract a short time ahead of ventricular contraction, which is important for effective heart pumping through lungs and peripheral organs. Another importance of the system is that it allows all portions of the ventricles to contract almost simultaneously, which is essential for most effective pressure generation in the ventricular chambers

The cardiac cells present in the heart tissue are individually surrounded with an insulating membrane (supporting a potential mV) containing selective permeable ionic channels. The currents through these channels interact with the membrane potential to regulate the activity of the cell. The flow of various ions (Na,K,Ca...etc) through out the cardiac tissue is responsible for the propagation of the electrical waves through tissue in turn provides the driving force behind the heart's mechanical contraction and its ability to pump blood through the body.

COMPONENTS OF HEART

The heart is a conical, hollow muscular organ placed obliquely behind the body of the sternum and adjoining parts of the body of the costal cartilages, so that 1/3 rd of it lies right and 2/3 rd to the left of the median plane. The heart measures about 12x9cm and weighs 300 gm in males and 250 gm in females. The human heart has four chambers. The upper two chambers, the right and left atria are receiving chambers of blood. Atria collects venous blood from the body and about 75 per cent of the blood flows directly into the ventricle even before atrial contraction. The atrial contraction causes an additional 25 per cent filling the ventricles. The heart's lower chambers right and left ventricles are the powerful pumping chambers. The right and left sides of the heart are separated from each other by a wall of tissue.each side pumps blood through a different circuit of blood vessels.

The Right Atrium

It is the right upper chamber of the heart receives venous blood from the whole body and pumps it to the right ventricle through right atrioventricular (tricuspid) opening. The chamber is elongated vertically, receiving the superior vena cava at the upper end and the inferior vena cava at the lower end. Deoxygenated blood from the whole body feeds into two large veins, the superior vena cava and inferior venecava, which empty into the right atrium of the heart and the same pumps to the right ventricle.

The Right Ventricle

The right ventricle is a triangular chamber which receives blood from the right atrium and pumps it to the lungs through the pulmonary trunk and pulmonary arteries.

Externally, the right ventricle has two surfaces anterior and inferior. The cavity of the right ventricle is crescent in section because of the forward bulge of inter ventricular septum. The wall of the right ventricle is thinner than that of left ventricle in a ratio 1:3.

The left atrium

The left atrium forms the left 2/3 of the base of the heart and is a quadrangular chamber. It receives oxygenated blood from the lungs through four pulmonary veins and pumps it to the left ventricle through Mitral valve.

The Left Ventricle

The left ventricle receives oxygenated blood from the left atrium and pumps it into the aorta, the body's largest artery. Smaller arteries that branch off the aorta distribute blood to the various parts of the body. It forms the apex of the heart.The cavity of the left ventricle is circular in cross section and has the thickest walls nearly half an inch in an adult because it must work the hardest to propel blood to the farthest reaches of the body.

Valves of the Heart

The valves of the heart maintain unidirectional flow of the blood and prevent blood from flowing backward in the heart *i.e.* the valves open easily in the direction of blood flow, but when blood pushes against the valves in the opposite direction the valves close.

There are two pairs of valves in the heart i) atrio ventricular valves ii)Semilunar valves. Atrio-ventricular valves are located between the atria and ventricles. The right atrio-ventricular valve is formed from three cusps of tissue and is called "Tricuspid valve". While the left atrio- ventricular valve has two cusps and is called "Bicuspid or Mitral valve". Both valves are made up of a fibrous ring to which the cusps are connected.The cusps are flat and project into the ventricular cavity. The atrio- ventricular valves kept competent by active contraction of the papillary muscles. Semi lunar valves are located between the ventricles and arteries and each of them consist of three half moon shaped flaps of tissue. They are not attached to fibrous ring but are to the blood vessel.The right semi lunar valve between right ventricle and pulmonary artery is "pulmonary valve " and the valve between left ventricle and aorta is "aortic valve ".These valves are closed during ventricular diastole.

Superior Vena Cava

It is about 7 cm long venous channel which receives blood from the upper half of the body and empties it to the right atrium like other large veins. It has no valves.

The Aorta

The aorta is the great arterial trunk which receives oxygenated blood from the left ventricle and distribute it all parts of the body.

Myocardium

It is the muscle tissue wraps around a scaffolding of tough connective tissue to form the walls of the heart chamber. The atria the receiving chambers of the heart have relatively thin walls than the ventricles, the pumping chambers.

Pericardium

It is a tough, double layered sac which surrounds the heart. The inner layer of the pericardium is known as epicardium rests on top of the heart muscle. The outer layer is attached to the breast bone and other structures in the chest cavity and helps hold the heart in place. The space between the two layers of the pericardium filled with watery fluid which prevents these layers from rubbing against each other during heart beat.

Endocardium

It is the inner surface of the heart's chambers lined with a thin white sheet of shiny tissue. The same type of tissue also lines the blood vessels forming continuous lining throughout the circulatory system. The lining helps blood to flow smoothly and prevents clotting of blood in the circulatory system.

The heart is nourished not by blood passing through, but by the blood vessels also known as "coronary arteries" which encircle the heart like a crown.

About 5 per cent of the blood pumped to the body enters the coronary arteries, which branch from the left ventricle.Three main coronary arteries the right, the left circumflex and the left anterior descending nourish different regions of the heart muscle. From these three arteries small branches arise to provide a constant supply of oxygen.

A DETAILED DESCRIPTION OF VASCULAR SYSTEM

The cardio vascular system is concerned with the transport of blood and lymph through the body. It may be divided into four major components, the heart, the macro circular *i.e.* blood vessels arteries and veins, micro circular *i.e.* capillary and lymph vascular system *i.e.* water and other components of blood plasma. The cardio vascular system (CVS) controls the blood pressure by altering the heart rate and compliance *i.e.* elasticity of blood vessels.

Arteries

Arteries transport blood from high pressure to body tissues as their structure permits them to expand and contract under different pressures due to the presence of elastic fibres. The main artery of the heart is "aorta", which starts from the left ventricle transporting oxygen and nutrients to all body tissues. The presence of elastic fibre enables the arteries to expand when each pulse of blood pumped by the heart and regains its original shape when tension is released. Like all blood vessels the inner layer of arteries is known as "tunica intima", composed of a single layer of flattened endothelial cells fitted together to form a smooth, continuous tube. In large arteries the same layer is supported by thick band of elastic fibres. The middle layer is known as "tunica media" consisting of smooth muscle and elastic fibres. In very large arteries the outer layer is known as "tunica adventitia" also contains elastic fibres and connective tissue.

Veins

Veins transport deoxygenated blood at low pressure towards the heart and act as reservoirs of different capacities to maintain a steady return of blood to heart. The veins of systemic circulation terminate at body's largest veins superior and inferior vena cava which empty into the right atrium of the heart.

The walls of the veins are thinner and contain little elastic fibre with greater internal diameter. These structural properties help them to stretch and store the blood. Since the pressure in veins is low some structural changes is needed to prevent blood from downward pull of gravity. The veins in the lower body contain special one-way valves prevent the accumulation of blood in the legs and feet. During exercise the muscles are in extremities, relaxing and contracting alternately squeezing the veins to force the blood upward towards the heart. The tunica media of veins is thinner and contain less elastic fibre and smooth muscle to function at low pressure and serving as reservoirs to maintain a steady return of blood to the heart.

Arterioles

The functions of arterioles are to distribute the blood and pressure reducing valves. They play an important role in determining the blood pressure. The arterioles have smooth muscle in their walls and do not stretch rather act as pressure reducing valves between the arteries and capillaries. They prevent delicate capillaries from high pressure of blood in the arterial system.

The degree of muscular tension in the walls of arterioles decides their internal diameter in turn changes the resistance of blood flow in arterioles. As they affect the blood pressure because they account for a large component of the peripheral resistance to blood flow. Blood pressure is the product of total peripheral resistance and cardiac output.

Venules

The function of venules is to drain blood from the capillary bed into the venous system.

Capillaries

Capillaries are very small blood vessels their diameter ranges from 4-15 ìm.The sum of the diameters of all capillaries is significantly larger than that of the aorta which results in decrease of blood pressure and flow rate. Capillaries are composed of a single layer of flattened endothelial cells fitted together to form a continuous tube. This results in a very large surface to volume ratio. The low rate of blood and large surface area facilitate the functions are,

- Providing nutrients and oxygen to the surrounding tissue.
- The absorption of nutrients, waste products and carbon dioxide and
- The execution of waste products from the body.

Lymphatic Vessels

Parts of the blood plasma will execute from the blood vessels into the surrounding tissues because of transport across the endothelium. The fluid entering tissues from capillaries adds to the interstitial fluid normally found in the tissue. The surplus of liquid will return to the circulation.Lymph vessels are dedicated to this unidirectional flow of liquid, the lymph. The lymph vessels can be divided into three types depending on their shape and size.

Lymph Capillaries

These are larger than blood capillaries and very irregular on shape. They begin as blind ending tubes in connective tissues.

Lymph Collecting Vessels

They appear almost similar to lymph capillaries but a bit large and form valves. The lymph is moved by the compression of the lymph vessels by surrounding tissues. The direction of lymph flow is determined by the valves

Lymph Ducts

They contain one or two layers of smooth muscle cells in their wall and form valves. The walls of lymph ducts are less elastic and during contractions contribute to the movement of lymph towards the heart in addition to the compression of the ducts by surrounding tissues.

Relations to Other Systems and Organs

The heart and vascular system perform almost the same function to provide oxygen, nutrients and harmonic to the cells of the body tissue. They can be considered as one unit rather than two, because each is equipped to carry out half of that function.

The vascular system is also closely related to the adrenergic receptors and the autonomic nervous system, which together control important aspects of its function.

The alpha adrenergic receptors are the smooth muscle cells in arteries, veins, arterioles and venules. These receptors bind molecules released by cells of the autonomic nervous system and respond by contracting.

BLOOD CIRCULATION -SYSTEMIC AND PULMONARY

The heart basically a double pump provides the force to circulate the blood through two major circulatory systems, the pulmonary circulation in the lungs and the systemic circulation is in organ system that transports substances to and fro from cells.

The blood in normal individual circulates through one system into before being pumped by the other part of the heart to the second system.

The heart is a muscle composed by cells containing small filaments of actin and myosin. These proteins interact in the sense of forming actomyosin during muscle contraction, thus leading to the main purpose of the heart: pumping the blood through the circulatory system.

The synchronous nature of contraction of heart results in the efficient pumping of blood through the pulmonic and systemic circulation. The circulatory system can be thought of as a closed loop circulation system with two pumps. One way valves keep the flow downward through the pumps.

Systemic Circulation

The heart ejects oxygen rich blood under a pressure about 125 mm Hg from main pumping chamber left ventricle, through the largest artery the aorta. Subdivided into smaller arteries in turn divided into even smaller arteries called arterioles and finally into a very fine meshwork of vessels called the capillary bed. Capillaries permit to dissolve oxygen and nutrients from the blood to diffuse across the fluid, known as "interstitial fluid" that fills the gaps between the cells of tissues of organs. The dissolved oxygen and nutrients enter cells through interstitial fluid by diffusion across the cell membranes.

Mean while carbon dioxide and other wastes leave the cell diffuse through the interstitial fluid, cross the capillary bed and enter the blood. The blood collects in small veins called venules gradually join together to form progressively larger veins. Finally the veins converge into two large veins, the superior vena cava and the inferior vena cava bringing blood from upper half and lower half of the body respectively. Both of these main veins join at the right atrium of the heart.

Pulmonary Circulation

The deoxygenated blood returning from the organs and tissues of the body stored momentarily in the reservoir *i.e.* right atrium, during weak contraction (5 to 6 mm Hg) the blood pushed into the right ventricle. On the next ventricular contraction this blood is pumped at a pressure of about 25 mm Hg through pulmonary arteries to the capillary system in the lungs.

At this site microscopic vessels pass adjacent to the "alveoli" or air sacs of the lung where it exchanges oxygen from the membrane to the blood and leaves carbon dioxide from blood to the same membrane. The freshly oxygenated blood then travels through the main veins from the lungs into the left reservoir *i.e.* left atrium of the heart. During weak arterial contraction (7 to 8 mm Hg) blood enters the left ventricle.

On the next contraction of the left ventricle sends blood to the aorta and then to general circulation. On average a typical adult has about 4.5 lts of blood and each section of the heart pumps about 80 ml in each contraction. About 30 sec to 1 min is needed for the average red blood cell to complete a full circuit through both the pulmonary and systemic circulation.

The blood volume is not uniformly divided between the pulmonary and systemic circulation. At any one time 80 per cent of the blood is in the systemic circulation and 20 per cent is in the pulmonary circulation. Of the blood in the systemic circulation about 15 per cent is in the arteries, 10 per cent is in the capillaries and 75 per cent is in the veins.

In the pulmonary circulation about 7 per cent of the blood is in the pulmonary capillaries and the remaining is almost equally distributed between the pulmonary arteries and pulmonary veins.

Additional Functions

In addition to oxygen, the circulatory system also transports nutrients derived from digested food to the body.

These nutrients enter the blood from the walls of the intestine carries the nutrients to the liver for farther metabolic processing.The liver stores variety of substances such as sugar, fats and vitamins and releases glucose to the blood as needed.

The liver also cleans the blood by removing waste products and toxins. After the blood is cleaned, enter the veins converge to form the large vein that joins the vena cava at right atrium.

The circulatory system plays an important role

- In regulating body temperature
- To collect chemical messengers called hormones from hormone producing glands and transports to specific organs and tissues to regulate body's rate of metabolism, growth, sexual development and other functions.
- With immune system and coagulation system, the immune system is a complex system of many disease fighting white blood cells and anti bodies circulate in the blood and are transported to sites of infection. The coagulation system is composed of special proteins called clotting factors which circulate in the blood. When ever blood vessels are cut to torn, the coagulation system works rapidly to stop the bleeding by forming clots.

Other organs support the circulatory system are the brain and the parts of nervous system constantly monitor blood circulation, sending signals to the heart or blood vessels to maintain constant blood pressure.

New blood cells are produced in the bone marrow and old blood cells are broken down in the spleen, where iron and other minerals are recycled. Metabolic waste products are removed from the blood by kidneys which also screen the blood for excess salt and maintain blood pressure and to maintain blood pressure and to balance minerals and fluids of the body.

HEART DISEASES

Heart disease has become very common nowadays due to changes in life style. Many of these diseases are due to either increase the work load of heart or reduce the ability to work at normal rate.

Tachycardia

There are many factors that are responsible for development of heart disease. One such factor is "High blood pressure" (Hypertension) which causes the muscle tension to increase in proportion to the pressure. A fast heart rate (Tachycardia) increases the work load.

Heart Attack

The heart disease that causes most deaths is "heart attack". A Heart attack is caused by blockage of one or more arteries to the heart muscle. During and after heart attack the ability of the heart is seriously impaired.

Bed rest and giving oxygen reduces the work load on heart which increases the oxygen content in the blood so that blood pumped by the heart will be less. Alternate method to reduce risk of heart attack is the regular exercise programme which opens alternate routes in cardiovascular system.

Congestive Heart Failure

Another common disease is congestive heart failure which is due to enlarge in size of the heart reduce the ability for adequate blood circulation.

Applying law of Laplace, if the radius of the heart is doubled, the tension of the heart muscle should be doubled which in turn reduces the efficiency of the heart muscle to maintain the same blood pressure.

Since the heart is stretched it may not be able to produce sufficient force to maintain normal circulation. Stretched heart muscle is less efficient than the normal. It consumes much more O2 for the same amount of work.

Bradycardia

Patients with inadequate electrical signal in the heart muscle will affect the work load of heart. The artrioventricular node *i.e.* between Atria and Ventricles is fatty and does not conduct electric signal and ventricle receive no signal from Atria, but being natural pacing centers which provide a pulse. The resulting heart rate is 30 beat/min *i.e.* Bradycardia results semi invalidism.

Pace Makers

If heart's electrical signals are inadequate to stimulate heart muscles, artificial pace makers are available. To improve the quality of life of faulty atrioventricular nodes, artificial pacemakers are developed.

The pacemaker contains a pulse generator that put out 72 beats/ min. The pace maker is put just below the right collarbone. It lasts for 2 years and impervious to body fluids and do not cause tissue reaction.

Valve Defects

Another heart disease is defective heart valves. These are of two types.

1) The valve either does or opens wide enough (stenosis). In stenosis large amount of work is to be done by heart to obstruct the narrow opening.
2) It does not close well enough (insufficiency).In insufficiency some of the pumped blood flows back and the amount of blood in circulation is reduced.Both types can be replaced by artificial valves.

Cardiovascular Diseases

Aneurysm

Some cardiovascular diseases involve the blood vessels. An aneurysm is a weakening of the wall of an artery which results increase in its diameter in turn increases the tension in the wall proportionately. If it is ruptured in brain, a type called Cerebrovascular accident (CVA).

A more common blood vessel problem is the formation of sclerotic plaques on the walls the artery which causes turbulence in blood flow increases the blood velocity at that point with a decrease in wall pressure due to Bernoulli's theorem.

A Disease in Varicose Vein

Veins with defective valves which allow the blood to flow backward become enlarged or dilated to form the varicose veins. During walking or other exercise, the contraction of the muscle forces the venous blood towards the heart called venous pump. At various points along the veins there are one way flaps or valves that prevent the blood from going back. If these valves become defective blood run backward and pool up in the vein becomes "varicose". The standard treatment for varicose veins is surgical removal of the offending vessels. There are sufficient parallel veins to carry the blood back to the heart.

Stiffness of RBC Membrane

In some cases, mainly in smoking, the membrane of RBC s becomes stiff. There may not be normal flow of blood in the vascular system. Blood may becomc viscous leading to Thrombosis.

ELECTROPHYSIOLOGY OF HEART

The rhythmical action of the heart is considered by an electrical signal initiated by spontaneous stimulation of special muscle cells located in the upper right hand corner of the right atrium near the superior vena cava. This area is known as "sino atrial node".

Cardiac electro physiology is dedicated to the study of the electro chemical activity of the heart. Studies include electrical activation of individual cells as well as the system- level activation, which results in normal or abnormal heart rhythm.

The complex system found by the Autonomous Nervous System (ANS) and the heart is modeled as if it was a modulation system, where the first generates a signal that modulates a sequence of pulses which excite the heart.

The sinus rhythm fluctuates around the mean heart rate, which is due to continuous alteration in the autonomous neural regulation *i.e.* sympathetic and parasympathetic balance. Periodic fluctuations found in heart rate originate from regulation related to respiration, blood pressure (baroreflex) and thermoregulation (Pauli Tikkanen 1999).

Cells in the SA node generate their electrical signal more frequently than cells else where in the heart. These impulses spread rapidly through inter nodal pathways to Atrioventricular node (AV node). At this node the signal is delayed so that all muscle cells of the atria contract virtually in unison. Now the impulse conducts through fibrous connective tissue between atria and ventricles known as "Atrio ventricular bundle "(AV bundle). AV bundle conducts the signal through left and right bundles of "Purkinje fibres" which conduct the cardiac signal to all parts of the ventricles.

Sinoatrial Node

The sinoatrial node is a small, flattened ellipsoid strip of specialized muscle about 3 mm wide, 15 mm long and 1mm long located at the upper right hand corner of the right atrium immediately below and slightly lateral to the opening of the superior vena cava.

The Sinoatrial (SA node), the atrioventricular (AV node) and the Purkinje system can be regarded as potential pacemaker tissues in heart. As the fastest depolarization impulse spreads through the conduction system to other pacemakers before they spontaneously depolarize, the sinoatrial node usually defines heart rate.

The sinus nodal fibres connect directly with the atrial muscle fibres, so that any action potential generates at the sinus node spreads immediately to the atrial muscle wall. For this reason Sinoatrial node is also known as "pace maker" of the heart. It generates the impulse at the rate of about 70/min and initiates the heart beat. However this rate may increase or decrease by the demand of blood supply to the body.

Three types of membrane ion channels play an important role in causing the voltage charges the action potential. They are 1) fast sodium channels 2) slow calcium-sodium channels 3) potassium channels. As the ions move in muscle cells in fractions of second creates action potential at the Sinoatrial node.

This can be observed in spikes and plateau region in the graph plotted between time and membrane potential which is about -55 to -65 mV. This muscle much less negativity compared to ventricular action potential which is -85 to -90 mV is due to slow calcium- sodium channels.

The discharge rate of Sinoatrial node is faster than A-V node or Purkinje fibres. SA node generates impulse before either the A-V node or Purkinje fibres can reach their threshold for self excitation and this process continues on and on. Thus SA node controls the heart beat because its rhythmical discharge rate is greater than any other part of the heart. Therefore, the SA node is the normal "pace maker" of the heart.

Atrioventricular Node

The AV node is located in the posterior wall of the right atrium just behind the tricuspid valve. The cardiac impulse travels from the atria to ventricles relatively slow and this delay allows atria to empty the blood into ventricles before they start contracting.

The reason for delay of impulse is due to presence of connective tissue partition by a small bridge of muscle called atrio ventricular conduction system.

Atrioventricular Bundle (AV Bundle of His)

After making its way through the AV node an impulse passes along a group of muscle fibres called the A.V bundle or bundle of His. The special characteristic of the AV bundle is they prevent re-entry of cardiac impulses from ventricle to atria but from atria to ventricle only.

The Purkinje Fibres

The Purkinje fibres lead from the A-V node through the A-V bundle into the ventricles. The initial part of Purkinje fibres is penetrated through bundle. They are very large fibres, even larger than the normal ventricular muscle fibres and transmit action potential at a velocity of 1.5 to 4.0 m/sec, which is about 6 times the usual ventricular muscle and 150 times that of in some of the AV nodal fibres. Purkinje fibres immediately transmit the cardiac impulse through the entire ventricular muscle.

The rapid transmission of action potential is due to high permeability of the gap junctions at the intercalated between the successive cardiac cells that make up the Purkinje fibres. As a result ions are transmitted easily from one cell to another increase velocity of impulse.

The Purkinje fibres divide into left and right bundle branches that lie under the endocardium on the two respective sides of the ventricular septum. Each branch spreads downward and divides into smaller branches covering ventricular chamber and back towards the base of the heart.

The ends of the Purkinje fibres penetrate into the muscle mass and finally become continuous with the cardiac muscle fibres as the ventricular walls are so thick and massive. The electrical impulse spreads from the SA node through the heart in less than one second.

ELECTROCARDIOGRAM

When the cardiac impulse passes through the heart: electrical current also spreads from the heart into the adjacent tissues surrounding the heart. A small portion of the current spreads all the way to the surface of the body. If electrodes are placed on the body skin on opposite sides of the heart: electrical potentials generated by the current can be recorded. The recording is known as "Electrocardiogram".

Historical Milestones of ECG

1887: Augustus Desire Waller, recorded electric current preceding cardiac contraction.

1903: Einthoven developed string galvanometer

1911: Sir Thomas Lewis published his pioneering paper on ECG

1929: Dock, use of cathode ray oscilloscope for ECG

1932: Wolferth CC and Wood CC introduced chest leads

1942: GoldbergerE, introduced unipolar limb leads.

Nowadays, the HR-ECG is performed through the use of signal mean value estimation technique, based on multiple applications of average operations of the electrocardiographic signs.

Heart rate is obtained by analyzing electrocardiograms (ECG s), which are traces of the electrical activity of the heart measured by leads. Depending on the electrodes involved in taking over the signal, more derivations are obtained and EKG signal is represented as a sequence of sample of variable length. Locating ECG waveform fiducial points (QRS complex,J point, on set and offset of T wave) is crucial step in automated ECG analysis for amplitude and interval measurements. Each beat of the heart can be observed as a series of deflections away from the baseline on the ECG. These deflections reflect the time evolution of electrical activity in the heart which initiates muscle contraction.

When the electric signal generated at Sino atrial node and passes through the heart and the same is spreads to adjacent tissues surrounding the heart. This electrical field passes through numerous other structures including the lungs, blood and skeletal muscle before reaching the body surface. These structures known as transmission factors differ in their electrical properties and perturb the cardiac electrical field as it passes through them. The potentials reaching the skin are then detected by the electrodes placed on specific locations and the electric potentials generated by the current can be identified, amplified, filtered and recorded in different electronic devices known as "Electrocardiogram"

The electrocardiogram as used today is the product of a series of technological and physiological advances. Early demonstrations of the heart's electrical activity reported during the last half of the 19th century. The establishment of the clinical electrocardiogram (ECG) by the Dutch physician Willem Einthoven in 1903 marked the beginning of a new era in medical diagnostic techniques, including the entry of electronics into health care.

Characteristics of the Normal ECG

ECG signals include frequencies from 0.05 Hz to 200 Hz, but up to 100 Hz are adequate for clinical diagnostic purpose. The normal electrocardiogram is composed of a P wave, a QRS complex, a T wave and a U wave.

P wave: - It is caused by electric potential generated when the atria depolarize before atrial contraction begins.

QRS complex: - It is due to potentials generated when the ventricles depolarize before their contraction.

T wave: - It is due to potentials generated when the ventricles recover from the state of depolarization.

U wave: - *I*t fallows T-wave and is due to repolarization of the Purkinje fibres which is occasionally seen.

The heart is activated with each cardiac cycle in a very characteristic manner determined by the anatomy and physiology of working cardiac muscle and the specialized cardiac conduction systems.

P- Wave is generated by activation of the atria, the PR segment represents the duration of atrioventricular conduction (AV conduction), the QRS complex is produced by activation of both ventricles and ST-T wave reflects ventricular recovery.

The voltages measured in ECG depend upon the locations of the electrodes applied to the surface of the body and how closely the electrodes are placed to the heart.

When ECG is recorded from standard combination *i.e.* two arms and one leg or one arm and two legs, the potential of the QRS complex is about 1 mv from the top of the R-wave to the bottom of the S-wave. The voltage of the P-wave is between 0.1 and 0.3 mv and that of T - wave between 0.2 and 0.3 mV.

Electric Events in the Heart

Location in the heart	Event	Time [ms]	ECG-terminology [m/s]	Conduction velocity	Intrinsic frequency [1/min]
SA node					
atrium, Right					
Left					
AV node	impulse generated				
bundle of His	depolarization *)	0			
bundle branches	depolarization	5			
Purkinje fibres	arrival of impulse	85		0.05	
endocardium	departure of impulse	50		0.8-1.0	
Septum	activated	125		0.8-1.0	
Left ventricle	activated	130		0.02-0.05	
epicardium	activated	145		1.0-1.5	
Left ventricle	depolarization	150		1.0-1.5	
Right ventricle	depolarization	175	P	3.0-3.5	
epicardium	depolarization	190	P	0.3 (axial)	
Left ventricle	depolarization	225	P-Q	-	
Right ventricle	repolarization	250	interval	0.8	
endocardium	repolarization	400	QRS	(transverse)	70-80
Left ventricle	repolarization	600	T	0.5	20-40

The relationship between the pumping action of the heart and the electrical potential on the skin reveals the propagation of an action potential in wall of the heart. Before stimulation of syncytial mass of cardiac muscle, all the exteriors of these cells had been positive and the interiors negative. After depolarization of syncytium negative charges leak to the outside of the depolarized muscle fibre making this surface area electronegative and the remaining part of the heart is still positive. The potential distribution for the entire heart when the ventricles are one-half depolarized is shown by the equipotential lines.

The form of potential lines can be represented as electric dipole. The equipotential lines at other times in the heart's cycle can also be represented by electric dipoles of different moments in the cycle would differ in size and orientation. The algebraic averages of all the lines of current flow occur with negativity towards the base of the heart and with positivity towards the apex.

The electrical potential that we measure on the body's surface is merely the instantaneous projection of electric dipole vector in a particular direction. As the vector changes with time so does the projected potential. Electric dipole vector along with the three electrocrdiographic body planes.

The surface electrodes placed on body shows the electrical connections recording electrocardiogram. These electrodes are called standard bipolar leads. The term "bipolar" means that the ECG is recorded from two electrodes located on different sides of the heart. Lead means the combination of two wires and their electrodes to make a complete circuit.

Lead I - The measurement of the potential between right arm and left arm.

Lead II - The potential between right arm and left leg

Lead III- The potential between left arm and left leg.

According to Willem Einthoven, Dutch Physiologist these three leads are called standard limb leads. The potential between any two gives the relative amplitude and direction of the electric dipole vector.

Einthoven's Triangle

This is a diagnostic means of illustrating that the two arms and the left leg form apices of a triangle surrounding the heart. The two pieces at the upper part of the triangle shows the points at which the two arms connect electrically with the fluids around the heart and lower apex is the point at which the leg connects the fluids.

Einthoven's Law

The electrical potential at third is the mathematical sum of the potentials measured between any two bipolar limb leads.

The major electrical events that can be measured using their combination are:

1) the atrial depolarization *i.e.* P-wave
2) the atrial repolarization normally not observed in wave form
3) the ventricular depolarization *i.e.* QRS complex
4) the ventricular repolarization *i.e.* T wave.

These descriptions of the waveforms of the normal ECG represent the patterns most often observed in normal adults. Values for many of the intervals may vary as a function of age, race, gender and body habits and within individuals as a function of autonomic tone and activity level.

ECHOCARDIOGRAM

Echocardiography is an early medical application of ultrasonography. An echocardiogram is a test in which ultra sound is used to examine the heart. A single dimension images known as M - mode echo that allows accurate measurement of heart chambers.

Using a transducer in the form of electrodes placed on the chest (Tran thoracic echocardiogram) gives a two dimensional echo displaying cross-sectional slice of the beating heart including the chambers, valves and the major blood vessels that exit from the right and left ventricles.

By applying Doppler examinations the ultra sound beams will evaluate the flow of blood *i.e.* direction and velocity. Echocardiography evaluates the size of the chambers including the dimension and the thickness of the wall. In patients with long standing hypertension, the test can determine the thickness and stiffness of left ventricle walls.

Pumping function of the heart can also be assessed by echocardiogram. This measure is known as an Ejection fraction or EF. A normal EF is around 55 to 65 per cent. Numbers below 45 per cent show some disease in pumping strength of the heart, while numbers below 30 to 35 per cent represent some major disease. It can also assess the pumping activity of each chamber of heart and also the movement of each wall can be visualized.

Echocardiography reveals the structural thickness and function *i.e.* movement of each heart valve. Along with Doppler it helps to identify abnormal leakage across heart valves and determine their severity. It can also detect the volume status of blood in systemic circulation and also useful in diagnosing of fluid in the pericardium.

Heart Sounds and Phonocardiogram

The sounds from a normal heart rate in the frequency range of 20 to 200 Hz.They are "lub dub lub dub". But only two are ordinarily audible through a stethoscope at optimum positions. "Lub" is associated with closure of AV valve at the beginning of systole and "dub" is associated with closer of semi lunar valves at the end of systole. The human ear is not most sensitive in the heart frequency range, so with electronic amplification the less intense sounds can be detected and recorded graphically as a "Phonocardiogram". This means of registering heart sounds that may be inaudible to the human ear, helps to delineate the precise timing of the heart sounds relative to other events in the cardiac cell. Heart sounds, as heard through a normal stethoscope are produced by a biological membrane in the heart when an event such as the opening or closing of a valve, vibration of the cardiac structure or acceleration or deceleration of blood occurs.

The first heart sound is heard at the onset of ventricular systole and consists of a series of vibrations with low frequencies. It is due to the contraction of the ventricles first causes sudden backflow of blood against the AV valves (tricuspid and mitral valves), causing them to close. The low frequencies are due to vibrations of the adjacent blood, walls of the heart and major vessels around the heart. The vibrations travel through the adjacent tissues to the chest wall, where they can be heard as sound by stethoscope.

The intensity of first sound is a function of the force of ventricular contraction and of the distance between the valve leaflets are farthest apart, as occur when the interval between atrial and ventricular systoles.

The second heart sound occurs from the sudden closure of the semi lunar valves. It is composed of higher pitch with shorter duration of lower intensity and has a more snapping quality than the first heart sound. When semi-lunar valves close, they bulge backward towards the ventricles, which initiates oscillations of the columns of blood and the tensed vessel walls by the stretch and recoil of the closed valve.

Conditions that bring about a more rapid closure of the semi lunar valves such that pulmonary or systemic hypertension increases the intensity of second heart sound.

Phonocardiogram takes simultaneously with ECG as shown in fig, the first sound starts just beyond the peak of R-wave which is composed of irregular waves and is of greater intensity and duration. The second sound which appears at the end of the T-wave.

A third and fourth sound do not appear on this record.

The third heart sound is a week and occurs occasionally, which consists of low intensity, low frequency vibrations heard best in the region of the apex. It occurs at the beginning of the middle third of diastole and is believed to the result of vibrations of the ventricular walls when the ventricles are not filled sufficiently to create even the small amount of elastic tension required for reverberation. The frequency is so low that can not be heard normally but can be recorded using Phonocardiogram.

A fourth is an atrial sound consisting of a few low frequency oscillations is not heard in general but can be recorded using Phonocardiogram. It is caused by oscillation of blood and cardiac chambers created by atrial contraction.

Phonocardiogram

A microphone specially designed to detect low frequency sound is placed on the chest. The heart sounds can be amplified and recorded by a high speed recording apparatus known as Phonocardiogram. Abnormal heart sound due to valvular lesions is known as "heart murmurs". The Phonocardiogram show how the intensity of murmur varies during different portions of systole and diastole.

Photoplethysmography(PPG)

Photoplethysmography (PPG) is a simple and low cost optical techniques that can be used to detect blood volume changes in the microvascular bed of tissue. It is often used non- invasively to make measurements at the skin surface. The PPG waveform comprises a pulsatile(AC) physiological waveform attributed to cardiac synchronous changes in the blood volume with each heartbeat, and is superimposed on a slowly varying (DC) baseline with various lower frequency components attributed to respiration sympathetic nervous system activity and thermoregulation.

Photoplethysmography is based on the determination of the optical properties of a selected skin area. For this purpose IR light is emitted into the skin. Light is absorbed, depending on the blood volume of the skin. Consequently, the backscattered light corresponds with the variation of the blood volume. Blood volume changes can then be determined by measuring the reflected light and using the optical properties of tissue and blood.

There are two different types PPG probes that can be used:

- Reflection probes: This type probe can also be used for the venous test. The light emitting and sensitive parts are located side by side in one probe. The photo sensors detect the light, which is backscattered from the tissue of the skin. Due to the body's anatomy, the PPG sensors can only detect the pulse waves in areas that contain many arteriovenous anastomoses such as fingers, toes, earlobes or some regions of face.
- Transmission probes: In these probes the photo sensors are located on the opposite side as the light emitting parts. The tissue is located between them. This limits the field of application to locations where the light can penetrate all the way through the tissue (fingers, toes, earlobes). In contrast to the reflection probe, the main sources of pulsation also contain the large vessels making these sensors especially useful for peripheral blood pressure measurements.

The arterial photoplethysmography measures and evaluates the shape and size of the pulse waves. The easy application in fingers and toes make this method especially useful in

- Diagnosing arterial disease in fingers and toes by just watching the curve.
- Diagnosing the functional disturbances of blood flow (Raynoulds sunchrome, death finger, fibration syndrome).

- Diagnosing chronic venous diseases such as varicose veins and other disorders that cause by swelling and leg ulcers.
- Measuring peripheral blood pressure even on digits (using transmission probes).

SURVEY OF LITERATURE ON ELECTRO PHYSIOLOGY OF HEART

Manuel Duarte Ortigueira et al (1959) described that a new algorithm can be adopted to study the heart frequency and interpretation of ECG by applying archetypal analysis (prototype analysis). This study helped to clean the ECG waves from noise and isolating them. The isolated waves are normalized and aligned depending upon the average of original beats.

Joseph D. Touch (1986) presented a statistical method for relative peak detection in ECG signal by simple threshold and slope change detection algorithms.

Isla Gilmour (1995) described that a neural sensor called the baroreceptor wasused to obtain the coupled fluctuations of blood pressure and heart rate time series by involving Fourier techniques.

Gianfranco Parati et al (1995) criticized that a concise and critical description of the spectral methods most commonly used (fast Fourier transform versus autoregressive modeling, time varying versus broad band spectral analysis) and an evaluation of their advantage and disadvantages. It also provides insight into the problems that still affect the physiological and clinical interpretation of data provided by spectral analysis of blood pressure and heart rate variability (HRV).

In particular the assessment of blood pressure and heart rate spectra aimed at providing indices of autonomic cardiovascular modulation. Evidence was given that multi variate models which allow evaluation of the interaction between changes in blood pressure, heart rate and other biological signals in the time or frequency domains offer a more comprehensive approach to the assessment of cardiovascular regulation than that represented by the separate analysis of fluctuations in blood pressure or heart rate only.

The European society of cardiology and the North American Society of pacing and Electrophysiology (1996) issued guidelines to measure heart rate variability.

Cosmin Cernazanu et al (1996) described that 15 heart diseases can be diagnosed by using the EKG signal with the help of neural networks. They described how the EKG was initially filtered, how each of the three constituents of the signal. (The P - wave, the QRS complex and the T- wave) had been recognized and interpreted by a neural network, the three interpretation of the constituents and other data had been analyzed by using a neural which established a diagnosis.

Sahambi, et al (1996) proposed an algorithm for ST segment analysis was developed using the multi resolution wavelet approach. The algorithm had been implemented on TMS320C5 based add-on DSP card to PC to provide the on-line analysis and display of ST-segment data. The performance of the system was evaluated using the standard ECG waveforms with different morphologies and heart rates in order to take into account the variability of the data encountered in the clinical environment.

Garrett Stanley et al (1997) presented that age effects on interrelation ships between lung volume and heart rate during standing. Age and position affects and age position interactions were determined by analysis of variance for repeated measures.The spectral estimates were generated using fast Fourier analysis techniques that employ a hamming smoothing window.

Time Makikallio (1998) presented that to assess the clinical applicability of new dynamical analysis methods derived from neo-linear dynamics of heart rate behaviour.

This study covered four different patient populations. Electrocar-diographic recordings of subjects were taken. The data were sampled digitally and transferred to microcomputer for the analysis of heart rate variability. The Fourier transform method was used to estimate the power spectrum densities of heart rate variability.

Clayton and Murray (1998) compared the time frequency analysis of the ECG during human ventricular fibrillation. This chapter focused in using linear and non-linear signal processing techniques to characterize recordings of VF. Time Frequency Distribution (TFD) of the first tens these recordings were estimated with the short time Fourier transform, Wigner-ville, smoothed Wigner -ville and Choi -williams algorithms. Used in tandem with the predictable short time Fourier transform, the smoothed Wigner TFD was a valuable tool for characteriging the TFD of human VF.

Havlin et al (1999) studied in his paper that statistical physics can be applied to heart beat diagnosis. Several studies had revealed that statistical physics concepts that can be used as diagnostic tools for heart failure. They described the sealing exponent characterizing the long range correlations in heart beat time series as well as the multifractal features discovered in heart beat rhythm. It is found that features, the long range correlations and the multifractility are weaker in cases of heart failure.

Piotr Rozentryt et al (1999) presented that amplitude of ECG potentials varies on a beat- to- beat basis. This variability could be seen in different parts of ECG cycles and was usually periodic in nature. In their study they presented a new method allowing analysis which investigates the distribution of variability power in time and frequency domains (spectro temporal maps). A new feature of the method was its ability to attenuate errors in amplitude variability measurements coming from RT interval alterations. They also presented examples of spectro-temporal maps obtained in healthy subjects, surgically denervated patients after heart transplantation and patients with coronary artery disease.

Pauli Tikkanen (1999) reported in his thesis the quantitation of the variability in cardiovascular signals provides information about the autonomic neural regulation of the heart and the circulatory system. An ambulatory measurement setting is in important and demanding condition for the recording and analysis of these signals. In addition to heart rate variability (HRV) measurement using RR intervals, the dynamics of ventricular repolarization duration (VRD) is considered using the invasively obtained action potential duration (APD) and different estimate for QT intervals taken from a surface electrocardiogram (ECG). Further the estimation of the power spectrum is presented on the approach using an autoregressive (AR). The power spectrum analysis is examined by means of wavelet transforms, which are then applied to estimate the non-stationary RR interval variability.

John M.Karemaker (1999) presented that when Fourier analysis was applied to analysis of BP Variability(BPV) and HR Variability(HRV), two frequency peaks stood out; one around the respiratory frequency and one around 0.1 Hz. The respiration -coupled blood pressure oscillations were partly explained by mechanical effects of respiration and possibly by the vagally induced heart period oscillations coupled to respiration known as Respiratory Sinus Arrhythmia(RSA)The Journal of Physiology

Clayton et al (1999) proposed to compare Pseudo-ECGs produced by different configuration of re-entry in a computational model. They initiated single, double and multiple re-entrant waves in a cuboid with Fitz- Hugh Nagumo excitability and estimated one component of the pseudo-ECG and applied linear time frequency and non-linear dimensional analysis. The pseudo -ECG produced by a single re-entrant wave was periodic, where as that produced by a double re-entrant wave was quasiperiodic with slow changes in both frequency content and amplitude. The dimensions of these time series were around 1 and 3 respectively. For pseudo ECG it was more complex and its dimension was around 4. Thus different configurations of re-entrant wave were associated with qualitatively and quantitatively different pseudo-ECG time series.

Szili-Torok, et al (1999) presented that the spectral assessment of HRV and blood pressure variability can be studied with continuous ECG and non-invasive BP recordings on subjects during head-up tilt testing were subjected to analysis. The total spectral power and the power over the low and the high frequency spectral bands were recalculated in an overlapping series with constant time shifting of the initial data - point. Window fast Fourier transformation was applied for assessment of dynamic HR and BP spectral changes during upright tilt testing.

Narayana Dutt and Krishnan (2000) discussed that high performance computing has made a great impact in recent times in achieving practical solutions to problems in health care. Computational efficacy of various techniques had been discussed and examples from critically ill patients of ICCU were taken using real world HRV data were presented. In addition to giving applications to patient care in ICCU, other methods were to also discuss in view of their potential application to critical care medicine.

Malvin C. Teich et al (2000) studied that the statistical behaviour of the sequence of heart beats can be studied by replacing the complex waveform of an individual heart beat recorded in the ECG. They developed a mathematical point process that emulates the human heart beat time series for both normal subjects and heart -failure patients.

Cornelius keyl, et al (2000) discussed that Respiratory Sinus Arrhythmia (RSA) originates mainly from a central coupling between respiration and heart rate or from baroreflex mechanisms. They applied a sinusoidal stimulus to the carotid baroreceptors and generated heart rate fluctuations of the same magnitude as RSA with a frequency similar to, but different from, the breathing frequency. The data were analyzed using discrete Fourier transform and transfer function analysis. Respiratory fluctuations in systolic blood pressure preceded RSA with a time lag equal to that between baroreceptor stimulation and oscillations in RR interval.

Olansen et al (2000) described that the development of a variety of classical biomedical experiments. These are not only reinforcing basic knowledge but also train students in the application of these theories to laboratory research.

Hall et al (2000) discussed that heart sounds can be utilized more efficiently by medical doctors when they are displayed. A system where by a digital stethoscope interface directly to a PC will be described along with signal processing algorithms adopted. The sensor is based on a noise cancellation microphone. They developed a solution using "wavelet denoising". Thus coding of the waveform into the wavelet domain is achieved with relatively few wavelet coefficients in contrast to the many Fourier components that would result from conventional decomposition.

Ranveig Nygaard et al (2001) presented that a time domain algorithm based on the coding of line segments which are used to approximate the signal. These segments are fit in a way that was optimal in the rate of distortion sense. The approach was applicable to any signal but they focused on compression of ECG signals. Evaluation was based on both on percentage root-mean square difference (PRD), performance measure and visual inspection of the reconstructed signals. IEEE Transactions on Biomedical Engineering Vol 48 No 1

Richard P. Sloan et al (2001) discussed that considerable evidence implicates hostility in the development of coronary artery disease; the pathogenic mechanisms remain poorly understood. They developed a psycho physiological model that holds that altered autonomic nervous system function links psychological trails with CAD outcomes. With ambulatory electrocardiographic recording they demonstrated in a predominantly male sample that hostility was inversely associated with HF power, but only during working hours. These findings were consistent with the hypothesis that hostile individual experience multiple stressful interpersonal transactions each day, resulting in overall lower HF power during the day but not at night.

Dash (2002) discussed that good knowledge on the basics with attention to technical details goes to long way. Application of advanced technology in ECG monitoring gives maximum information and should be utilized to its fullest extent.

Seria Mecanica (2002) presented that possibilities of higher order spectral methods in biological signal processing in a concise form were introduced the second order spectrum, the third order spectrum (bisprectrum) and the coherence function of a signal. These transforms were applied to ECG and Phonocardiographic signals.

Patrice E.Mesharry et al (2003) developed a dynamical model based on three coupled ordinary differential equations was introduced which was capable of generating realistic synthetic electrocardiogram (ECG) signals. The operator could specify the mean and standard deviation of the heart rate, the morphology of the PQRST cycle and the power spectrum of the RR-tachogram.

Kalda Sakki, et al (2003) described elaborate efficient and adequate tools for the analysis of human heart rate fluctuations, as it is a complex and non-stationary wave. They classified the measures of heart rate variability as

1. Linear methods- applied Fourier analysis based on standard statistical measures.
2. Non - linear methods
   - Scale -invariant methods
   - Scale -dependent methods.

Naidu and Reddy (2003) developed autoregressive moving average (ARMA) method to study frequency domain representation of a short term heart rate time series (HRTS) signal was used for evaluating the cardiovascular control system. The spectral parameters used were,percentage power in low frequency band(per centPLF), percentage power in high frequency band (per centPHF), power ratio of low frequency to high frequency(PRLH), peak power ratio of low frequency to high frequency (PPRLH) and total power (TP)Results obtained from ARMA - based analysis of heart - rate time series signals were capable of complementing the clinical examination results.

Itrarce A Dachi et al (2003) presented that the ventricular phase angle, a parametric method applied to Fourier phase analysis (FPA) in radionuclide ventriculography, allows the quantitative analysis of ventricular contractile synchrony,FPA reproducibility using gated blood pool SPECT (GBPS) could be improved over that in planar radionuclide angiography(PRNA).

Maarvili, et al (2003) presented an algorithm to detect the first heart sound(S1) and second sound (S2). The algorithm utilizes instantaneous energy of Electrocardiogram (ECG) to estimate the presence of S1 and S2.

Patrick E. Mcshany and Gari D. Clifford (2004) developed software for generating electrocardiogram signals, ECGSYN. A dynamical model that faithfully reproduces the main features of the human electrocardiogram (ECG), including heart rate variability, RR intervals and QT intervals was presented. Details of the underlying algorithm and open -source software implementation in Mat Lab C and Java were described.

Nathan A Wedge, et al (2004) studied the characteristics of excitable cell mathematical models, with the goal of developing new insights and techniques in simulating the electrical behaviour of the human heart.They presented an examination of the Fitz Hugh- Nagumo model and its response to stimulus and in order to move towards the goal of full cardiac simulations. They adopted a method of optimizing single- cell calculations through local interpolation techniques. In addition to it they introduced a separate method of optimizing multi - cell simulations by tracking cellular activations

Lambros V. Skalars et al (2004) presented a new approach in modeling the electrical activity of the human heart. A recurrent artificial neural network was used in order to exhibit a subset of the dynamics of the electrical behaviour of the human heart. The proposed model could also used, when integrated as a diagnostic tool of the human heart system. This diagnostic system aimed to accomplish two major roles.Firstly, become a useful tool for health care practitioners in the area of diagnosis. Secondly it used as a simulator for biological systems used in education and research related to human physiology.

Petra Barthel, et al (2004) studied that heart rate turbulence (HRT) was a measure of the autonomic response to perturbations of arterial blood pressure after single ventricular premature complex. HRT was a simple and non-invasive method to assess baroreflex function. In post infarction patients HRT was a potent risk stratification tool and provides informa of left ventricular function. Esther Pueyo, et al (2004) studied that the QT interval response to RR interval changes was assessed in 24 - hour Holter recordings by considering weighted averages of a history of past RR intervals to characterize the influence of heart rate on each QT measurement. Two main results were found in this study, first the process of QT adaptation to rate changes was highly individual and second RR interval variations some previous minutes to completely characterize the QT response.

Luigi De Ambroggi and Alexander D. Corlan (2004) studied the complexity of T - Wave using multiple thoracic leads or 12-lead ECG. According to them Body surface potential maps (BSPM) ware advantageous over the conventional

12 leads. This could analyze repolarization potentials. They were instantaneous potential distribution QRS-T integral maps, eigenvector analysis, principal component analysis and auto - correlation analysis.

Walid El-Atabamy et al (2004) discussed that cardiac arrhythmias disrupt the normal synchronized contraction sequence of the heart and reduce the pumping efficiency. The detection and classification of such arrhythmias was essential. In this chapter four types of ventricular arrhythmias (PVC, VB, VT and VF) were considered. A no. of features was extracted from ECG signal using a neo-linear dynamical signal analysis technique, recurrence dynamical analysis (RQA). Then three statistical classifiers were used in the classification. Results confirmed the robustness of the new techniques and demonstrate its value as a new diagnostic tool.

Tom Froese (2004) presented classification results of ECG signals with pathological conditions after they had been translated into the wavelet domain. Both the traditional Linear Discriminant Analysis method and the connectionist Multi- Layer Perception classifier were used on the problem and their results compared and contrasted. It was shown that the much simpler signal representation of a few wavelet coefficients obtained through the discrete wavelet transform eases the classification of time-variant signals considerably.

Morteja Moazami, et al (2004) introduced ECG compression algorithm based on two dimensional multi wavelet transform. Multi wavelets offer the possibility of superior performance for image processing applications. They studied SPIHT algorithm to achieve the clinical diagnosis.

Mohammed Pooyam, et al (2004) presented wavelet compression of ECG signals based on Set partitioning in hierarchical trees (SPIHT) coding algorithm. SPIHT is applied to the one dimensional analysis.

Lambros V. skarlas, et al [2004] presented a neural network to exhibit a subset of the dynamics of the electrical behaviour of the human heart. Zoltan German sallo (2005) described that each heart beat is a complex of distinct cardio logical events represented by distinct features in the ECG waveform. The proposed tasks concerning the three topics (preprocessing, parameter extraction and application of soft computing methods) were accomplished with relatively good results with the multi scale feature of wave transforms, various morphologies were excited better at different scales. A comprehensive comparative study to choose the best wavelet function for ECG signal processing purposes, using self synthesized test signals and decomposition - reconstruction error as a criterion.

Geng Hong et al (2005) studied that the measurement of Heart Rate Variability (HRV), provides a non- invasive measurement of the autonomic nervous system (ANS) activity. HRV can be measured with the variation of RR intervals exhibited in a sequence of ECG sample. The measurement results based on three minute and five minute HRVs. Four major measurements were,first the standard deviation of normal -beat to normal-beat intervals (SDNN) second square root of the mean squared difference of successive difference normal-beat to normal-beat intervals(RMSSD),third the proportion of interval difference of successive normal-beat to normal-beat intervals greater than 50ms (Pnn50), fourth the ratio of low frequency energy to high frequency energy (LF/HF) based on Fourier analysis method. Results had shown that the HRV presented by both SDNN and LF/HF using the 3-minute measuring data diffrs significantly from that using 5-minute measuring data.

Alireza Akhbardeh, et al (2005) discussed that among different methods used for analyzing heart conditions and monitoring their body's signals. They proposed a new method Ballistocardiography (BCG) to analyze the same without attaching electrodes on the body during recording. They used shift Invariant Daubochies wavelet transform to extract essential BCG features and Artificial Neural Networks to classify them. They were proved reliable and high performance.

Gari D.clifford (2006) presented that changes in the ECG were quasi periodic, the frequency can be quantified in both statistical terms. In essence, all these statistics quantify the power or degree to which no oscillation was present in a particular frequency band often expressed as a ratio to power in another band. Even for scale frequency approaches the process of features extraction tends to have a bias for a particular scale. ECG statistics were evaluated directly on the ECG signal.

Michal Huptych, et al (2006) presented an overview of a software tool for preprocessing, analysis and visualization of ECG signal. Their work was to automate the task of preprocessing, analysis and visualization, signal frequency, decomposition and map creation by multi - channel measurement from patient body surface (Body surface potential mapping). Signal frequency decomposition was performed by continuous wavelet transform. The software tool had been programmed in Java and tested on the data acquired from the CARDIAC 1122 system which measures signals from 80 unipolar electrodes evenly placed on the body surface.

Ming Jiang (2006) described that the areas of remote ECG feature extraction utilizing wavelet transformation concepts and sensor network system at low cost and Low-power wearable platforms provide continuous ECG monitoring which by measuring potentials between various points on the body using a galvanometer. The system was enabled with integrated RF communication capability that relay the signals wirelessly to a work station monitor.The work station was equipped with ECG signal processing software that performs ECG characteristic extraction via wavelet transformation.

Mirko Degli Esposh et al (2006) discussed a similarity distance function between symbolic strings recently introduced. Application to phylogenetic tree construction and HRV analysis were considered.

Chouhan and Mehta (2006) presented algorithm employs a modified slope of ECG signal as the feature for detection of QRS. A sequence of transformation of the filtered and base line drift corrected ECG signal is used for extraction of a new modified slope feature.

Anirudha Joshi (2006) proposed that a novel hybrid Holder-SVM detection algorithm for arrhythmia classification. The Holder exponents were computed efficiently using the Wavelet Transform Modulus Maxima (WTMM) method.

Debbal and Bereksi-Reguing (2006) studied that the continuous wavelet transform provides enough features of the PCG signals that will help clinics to diagnosis. It was shown that the frequency content of such a signal can be determined by the FFT without difficulties. In their study it was discussed that second heart sound 32 consists of two major components (A2 and P2) with a time delay between them is very important for medical diagnosis.

Yanyan Hao, et al (2007) proposed compression of ECG as a signal with finite rate of innovation (FRI). By modeling the ECG signal as the sum of hand limited and non-uniform linear spline which contains finite rate innovation (FRI). The simulation results had shown the performance of the compression of ECG as a signal with FRI was quite satisfactory in presenting the diagnostic information as compared to the classical sampling scheme which uses the sine interpolation Elena Visotska, et al (2007) presented successful application biorthogonal wavelet transform had allowed statistically characterize not only ECG signal and wavelet components but also to receive with authentic accuracy distinctive characteristics of two compared ECG signals. Decisions of problems during forecasting and early diagnostics of heart attack, also in time revealing of fatal infringements of heart rhythm, the prevention sudden coronary death were considered in this work.

Sinisa S.Ilic (2007) proposed that Continuous Wavelet Transform (CWT) diagram of healthy patients and patients with Left Bundle Branch Block (LBBB) were easy to distinguish. The concentration of CWT coefficients with higher amplitude was at lower frequencies for patients with LBBB to healthy patients. The sequence of segments in the ECG signal can be identified in CWT diagram too. Correlation between specific ECG waveforms and carefully chosen wavelets could be at higher and it might result in better recognition of characteristic segments in ECG signal.

Elif Derya Ubeyl (2007) studied the automated diagnostic systems employing diverse and composite features was analyzed and their accuracies were determined. Combining multiple classifiers with diverse features is viewed as a general problem in various applications areas of pattern recognition. Xanthis et al (2007) developed an improved solution of the non- linear and ill-posed inverse problem of ECG was presented. For this purpose a three dimensional volume conductor model of the human body is constructed based on a classical anatomic atlas.

Swaroop S singh et al (2007) studied on retrospective ECG recordings of patients during cardiac arrest have shown significant changes in heart rate variability indices increases prior to the onset of cardiac arythmia. The Early detection of these changes in HRV indices is for a successful medical intervention to decrease the rate of cardiac arrest.

Debbal and Bereksi - Reguing (2007) had presented the synthesis study of the Fast Fourier transform (FFT) in analyzing the phonocardiogram signal (PCG). It was studied that the spectral analysis van provide enough features of the PCG signals that will help clinicians to obtain qualitative and quantitative measurements of PCG signal characteristics and consequently aid to diagnosis.

Stridh et al (2007) developed a new method for ECG based characterization of atrial fibrillation (AF) which explores the morphology of the f- waves. Fallowing QRST cancellation, the method divides the atrial signal into short blocks and performs a model based analysis of each block. The blocks are then clustered into different waveform patterns.

THE CARDIOVASCULAR SYSTEM

The cardiovascular system is one of the major body systems. It transports oxygen, carbon dioxide, waste products, nutrients and hormones to and from various parts of the body.

The cardiovascular system is made up of the heart, the blood vessels (arteries and veins and capillaries) and blood. The heart has major vessels that supply it with deoxygenated blood (travels back to the heart from the body), and major vessels that carry oxygenated blood away from the heart to all the parts of the body.

The major vessels that carry blood to and from the heart are:

- Nferior vena cava conveys deoxygenated blood (blood low in oxygen) from the lower extremities of the body to the heart
- Superior vena cava coveys deoxygenated blood from the upper extremities of the body to the heart
- Aorta conveys oxygenated blood (blood high in oxygen) away from the heart

This information is important so that you can gain an understanding of how the heart works and some of the conditions that may affect the functioning of the heart.

HEART

The heart is a hollow organ about the size of a fist and is composed of special muscle tissue (cardiac muscle). It lies under the breast bone in the centre of the cardiothoracic cavity. In the average lifetime the heart beats 250 million times and pumps 340 million litres of blood. The heart is a sophisticated pump that is controlled by an electrical current that is initiated in the brain.

The heart is divided into a left and right side by a muscular wall called the septum and has four chambers.

Heart Chambers and Valves

The chambers of the heart include the:

- Right atrium which receives deoxygenated blood (low in oxygen) from all over the body
- Right ventricle receives blood from the right atrium and sends it to the lungs via the pulmonary artery to become oxygenated and get rid of carbon dioxide
- Left atrium receives oxygenated blood from the lungs and sends it to the left ventricle
- Left ventricle receives blood from the left atrium and sends it out to the body via the aorta.

The heart wall consists of three layers - the endocardium is the inner lining, the myocardium is the muscle layer and the pericardium is the outer covering.

The chambers of the heart are separated by valves:

- Tricuspid valve is located between the right atrium and right ventricle
- Bicuspid (mitral) valve is located between the left atrium and left ventricle
- Pulmonary valve is between the right ventricle and the pulmonary artery
- Aortic valve is between the left ventricle and the aorta

The major vessels that carry blood to and from the heart are:

- Inferior vena cava conveys deoxygenated blood (blood low in oxygen) from the lower extremities of the body to the heart
- Superior vena cava coveys deoxygenated blood from the upper extremities of the body to the heart
- Aorta conveys oxygenated blood (blood high in oxygen) away from the heart

BLOOD VESSELS

The cardiovascular system consists of arteries and veins and capillaries. Arteries carry oxygenated blood to the cells of the body, veins carry deoxygenated blood away from the cells.

Arteries

Arteries are tubes that carry oxygenated blood (high in oxygen) away from the heart. Arteries have thick, muscular, elastic walls. They branch off forming arterioles with thinner walls that then become capillaries. Arteries carry blood rich in oxygen and nutrients. Blood that comes from a wound to an artery is bright red and spurts. The aorta is the largest artery and as it leaves the heart it branches into smaller arteries, eventually they become capillaries.

Veins

Veins are tubes that carry deoxygenated blood (low in oxygen) from the cells back to the heart where it is pumped to the lungs so that the blood can pick up more oxygen. The veins have one-way valves that help move the blood towards the heart.

Veins have thinner muscular walls. They carry blood back to the heart that is low in oxygen and high in carbon dioxide, a waste product.

Capillaries

Capillaries are very small vessels that surround the cells of the body and facilitate the movement of oxygen and nutrients into the cells and carbon dioxide and waste products away from the cells.

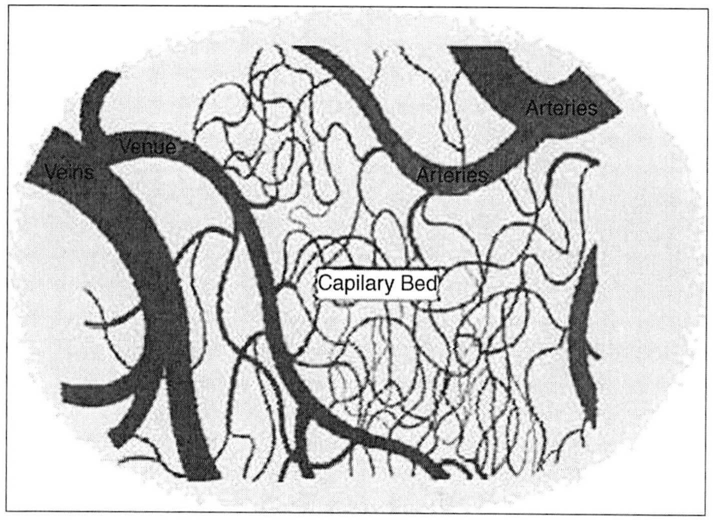

Fig. Capillaries

Plasma

Plasma is a straw coloured watery fluid in which the blood cells are suspended. It contains antibodies (gamma globulin) and antitoxins, plasma proteins, mineral salts, nutrients, waste products such as urea and creatinine, gases such as oxygen and carbon dioxide, hormones and enzymes.

The blood cells float in the plasma. They are produced in the bone marrow and lymphatic tissues of the body. The bone marrow, liver and spleen destroy worn-out blood cells.

Blood

Blood is made up of a liquid (plasma) and cells. Blood is connective tissue, a red body fluid made up of liquid (plasma) and cells. The body contains 5 to 6 litres of blood. Fifty-five percent of the blood is plasma.

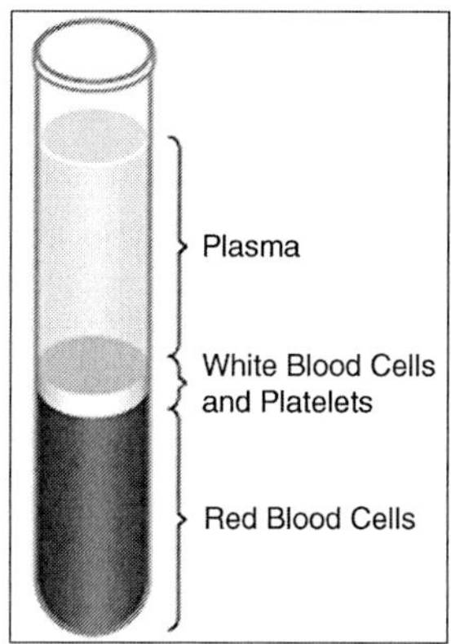

Fig. Components of blood

Blood cells

There are 3 types of blood cells.

1. Erythrocytes or red blood cells (RBC) - carry most of the oxygen and small amounts of carbon dioxide. Haemoglobin carries the oxygen molecule and gives blood its colour. There are approximately 5 million RBC per cubic millimetre of blood and the average life span is 100 - 120 days.

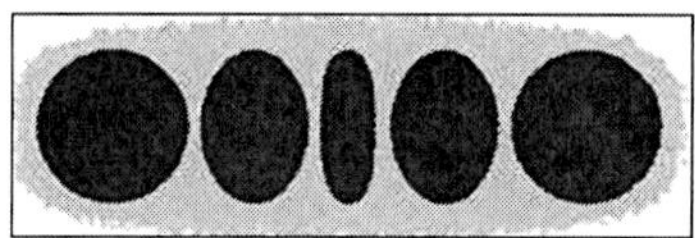

1. 2. Leucocytes or white blood cells (WBC) - help fight infection as they can attack microorganisms. There are 7,000 - 8,000 WBC per cubic millimetre.

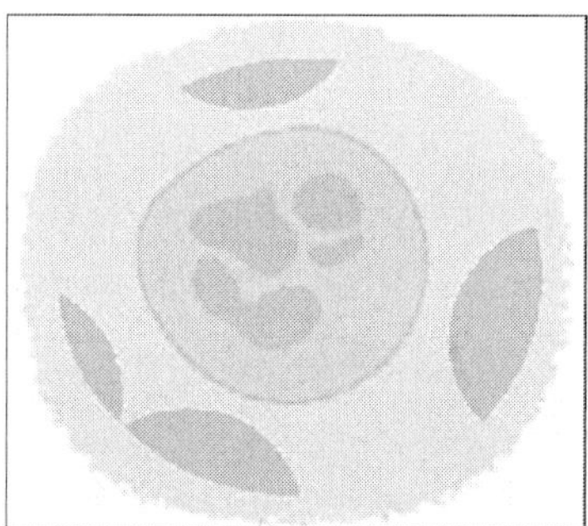

Fig. White blood cells

1. 3. Thrombocytes (platelets) - are parts of cells which plug small leaks in the walls of blood vessels and initiate blood clotting. There are 200,000 to 400,000 per cubic millimetre.

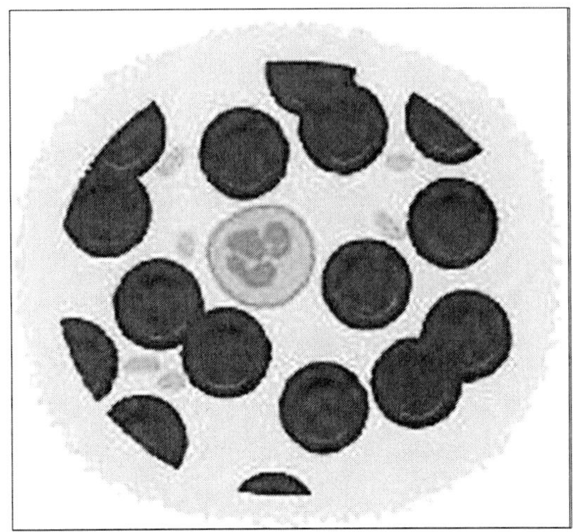

Fig. Platelets

THE FLOW OF BLOOD THROUGH THE HEART

The correct term for contraction of the heart is systole. This is followed by relaxation of the heart called diastole. One systole and diastole form the cardiac cycle. A cardiac cycle takes only 0.8 seconds and during this time the following events occur.

First, the upper chambers, or atria, of the heart relax and fill with blood as the lower ventricles contract, forcing out blood through the aorta and pulmonary arteries. Next the ventricles relax, allowing blood to flow into them from the contracting upper chambers. Then the cycle is repeated; this happens approximately 70 to 80 times per minute.

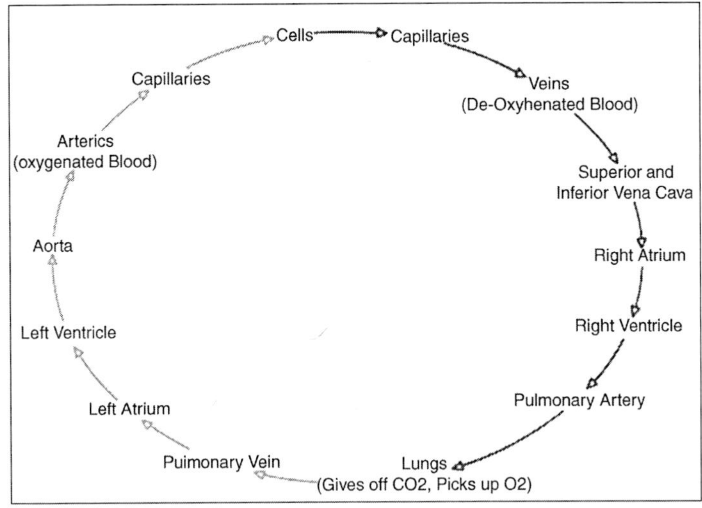

Fig. Diagram of the flow of blood through arteries and veins

The rate and rhythm of the heart is regulated by the conduction system that is made up of specialised neuromuscular tissue that sends out impulses. The impulses begin at the Sino-Atrial (SA) node in the right atrium and spread across the two atria.

The atria then contract and the impulses from the S-A node reach the Atrio-Ventricular (AV) node in the right atrium. Messages from the A-V node then travel down the Bundle of His in the septum and continue through the Purkinje fibres to the walls of the ventricles.

An electrocardiogram, or ECG, is a diagnostic test that records the electrical impulses of the heart.

The blood flows around the body continuously due to the regular beat of the heart. Beginning at cells, the passage of blood is as follows:

Pulse

The pulse is the beat of the heart and the movement of blood through the arteries at various points in the body.

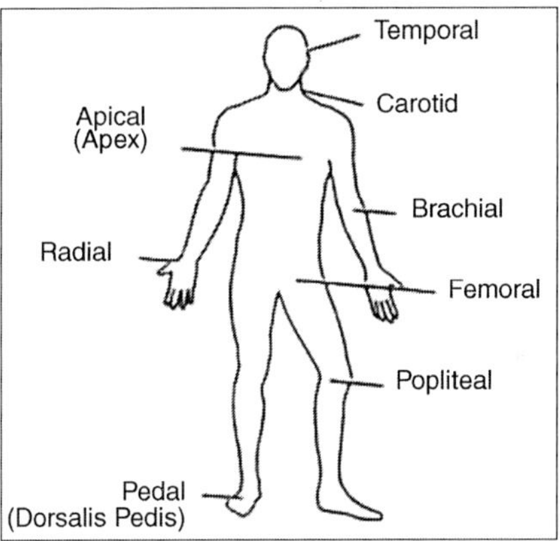

Fig. Where the pulse can be found

Counting a pulse

A pulse is defined as a wave of distension of an artery allowing the contraction of the left ventricle of the heart. When counting a pulse it is important to be aware of the rate, the rhythm and the volume.

The normal pulse rate for an adult is 60-100 beats per minute (BPM)

Terminology

Rate: The number of beats per minute.
Rhythm: The regularity of the beats.
Volume: The strength of the beat.
Bradycardia: Decrease in pulse below 60 b.p.m.
Tachycardia: Increase in beats above 100 b.p.m.

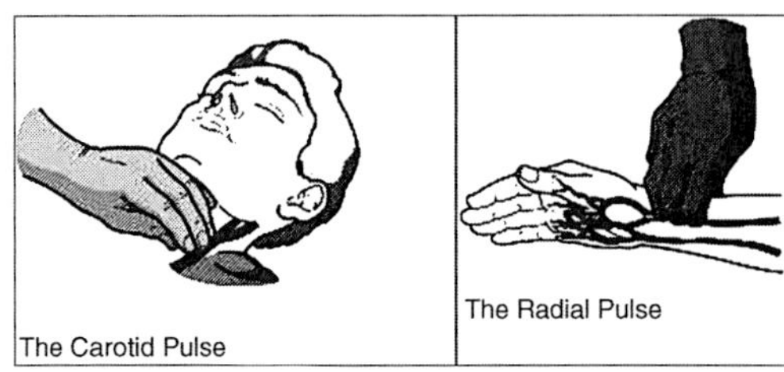

Taking a person's blood pressure

Blood pressure is the amount of force exerted against the walls of an artery by the blood. The heart muscle contracts and relaxes. The period of contraction is called systole and the period of relaxation is called diastole.

Both systolic and diastolic pressure are measured. Blood pressure is measured in millimetres (mm) of mercury (Hg). The systolic pressure is recorded over the diastolic pressure. The average adult has a systolic of 120mm Hg and a diastolic of 80 mm Hg. This is written as 120/80 mm Hg.

The normal blood pressure range for an adult is 100/60 to 135/80

A person is described as having hypertension when they have a reading above 140/90. A reading of below 90/60 is described as hypotension.

THE HEART'S ELECTRICAL CONDUCTION SYSTEM

The heart is primarily made up of muscle tissue. A network of nerve fibres coordinates the contraction and relaxation of the cardiac muscle tissue to obtain an efficient, wave-like pumping action of the heart

CONTROL OF HEARTBEAT

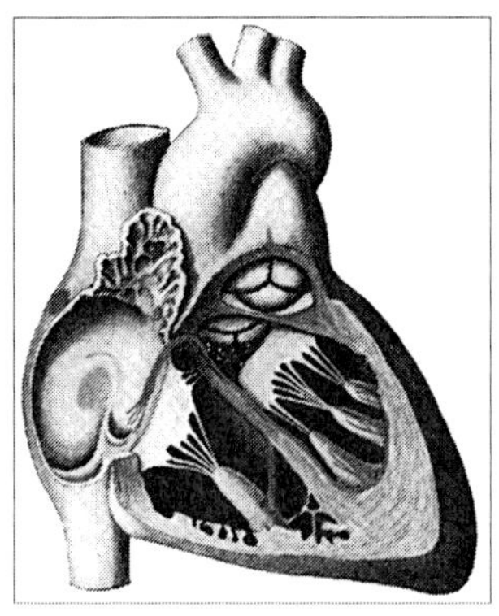

Fig. Schematic representation of the sinoatrial node and the atrioventricular bundle of His. The location of the SA node is shown in blue. The bundle, represented in red, originates near the orifice of the coronary sinus, undergoes slight enlargement to form the AV node. The AV node tapers down into the bundle of HIS, which passes into the ventricular septum and divides into two bundle branches, the left and right bundles. The ultimate distribution cannot be completely shown in this diagram.

The heart contains two cardiac pacemakers that spontaneously cause the heart to beat. These can be controlled by the autonomic nervous system and circulating adrenaline. If the cardiac muscles just contracted and relaxed randomly at a natural rhythm the cycle would become disordered and the heart would become unable to carry on its function of being a pump. Sometimes when the heart undergoes great damage to one part of the cardiac muscle or the person incurs an electric shock, the cardiac cycle can become uncoordinated and chaotic. Some parts of the heart will contract whilst others will relax so that instead of contracting and relaxing as a whole, the heart will flutter abnormally. This is called fibrillation and can be fatal if not treated within 60 seconds.

SA Node

The sinoatrial node (abbreviated SA node or SAN, also called the sinus node) is the impulse generating (pacemaker) tissue located in the right atrium of the heart. Although all of the heart's cells possess the ability to generate the electrical impulses (or action potentials) that trigger cardiac contraction, the sinoatrial node is what normally initiates it, simply because it generates impulses slightly faster than the other areas with pacemaker potential. Because cardiac myocytes, like all nerve cells, have refractory periods following contraction during which additional contractions cannot be triggered, their pacemaker potential is overridden by the sinoatrial node.

The SA node emits a new impulse before either the AV or purkinje fibres reach threshold. The sinoatrial node (SA node) is a group of cells positioned on the wall of the right atrium, near the entrance of the superior vena cava. These cells are modified cardiac myocytes. They possess some contractile filaments, though they do not contract. Cells in the SA node will naturally discharge (create action potentials) at about 70-80 times/minute.

Because the sinoatrial node is responsible for the rest of the heart's electrical activity, it is sometimes called the primary pacemaker. If the SA node doesn't function, or the impulse generated in the SA node is blocked before it travels down the electrical conduction system, a group of cells further down the heart will become the heart's pacemaker. These cells form the atrioventricular node (AV node), which is an area between the right atrium and ventricle, within the atrial septum. The impulses from the AV node will maintain a slower heart rate (about 40-60 beats per a minute). When there is a pathology in the AV node or purkinje fibres, an ectopic pacemaker can occur in different parts of the heart. The ectopic pacemaker typically discharges faster than the SA node and causes an abnormal sequence of contraction. The SA node is richly innervated by vagal and sympathetic fibres. This makes the SA node susceptible to autonomic influences. Stimulation of the vagus nerve causes decrease in the SA node rate (thereby causing decrease in the heart rate). Stimulation via sympathetic fibres causes increase in the SA node rate (thereby increasing the heart rate). The sympathetic nerves are distributed to all parts of the heart, especially in ventricular muscles. The parasympathetic nerves mainly control SA and AV nodes, some atrial muscle and ventricular muscle. Parasympathetic stimulation from the vagal nerves decreases the rate of the AV node by causing the release of acetylcholine at vagal endings which in turn increases the K+ permeability of the cardiac muscle fibre. Vagal stimulation can block transmission through AV junction or stop SA node contraction which is called "ventricular escape." When this happens, the purkinje fibres in the AV bundle develops a rhythm of their own. In the majority of patients, the SA node receives blood from the right coronary artery, meaning that a myocardial infarction occluding it will cause ischemia in the SA node unless there is a sufficiently good anastomosis from the left coronary artery. If not, death of the affected cells will stop the SA node from triggering the heartbeat

AV Node

The atrioventricular node (abbreviated AV node) is the tissue between the atria and the ventricles of the heart, which conducts the normal electrical impulse from the atria to the ventricles. The AV node receives two inputs from the atria: posteriorly via the crista terminalis, and anteriorly via the interatrial septum. An important property that is unique to the AV node is decremental conduction. This is the property of the AV node that prevents rapid conduction to the ventricle in cases of rapid atrial rhythms, such as atrial fibrillation or atrial flutter. The atrioventricular node delays impulses for 0.1 second before spreading to the ventricle walls. The reason it is so important to delay the cardiac impulse is to ensure that the atria are empty completely before the ventricles contract (Campbell *et al.*, 2002). The blood supply of the AV node is from a branch of the right coronary artery in 85 per cent to 90 per cent of individuals, and from a branch of the left circumflex artery in 10 per cent to 15 per cent of individuals. In certain types of supraventricular tachycardia, a person could have two AV Nodes; this will cause a loop in electrical current and uncontrollably-rapid heart beat. When this electricity catches up with itself, it will dissipate and return to normal heart-beat speed.

AV Bundle

The bundle of HIS is a collection of heart muscle cells specialized for electrical conduction that transmits the electrical impulses from the AV node (located between the atria and the ventricles) to the point of the apex of the fascicular branches. The fascicular branches then lead to the Purkinje fibres which innervate the ventricles, causing the cardiac muscle of the ventricles to contract at a paced interval. These specialized muscle fibres in the heart were named after the Swiss cardiologist Wilhelm His, Jr., who discovered them in 1893. Cardiac muscle is very specialized, as it is the only type of muscle that has an internal rhythm; *i.e.*, it is myogenic which means that it can naturally contract and relax without receiving electrical impulses from nerves. When a cell of cardiac muscle is placed next to another, they will beat in unison. The fibres of the Bundle of HIS allow electrical conduction to occur more easily and quickly than typical cardiac muscle.

They are an important part of the electrical conduction system of the heart as they transmit the impulse from the AV node (the ventricular pacemaker) to the rest of the heart. The bundle of HIS branches into the three bundle branches: the right left anterior and left posterior bundle branches that run along the intraventricular septum. The bundles give rise to thin filaments known as Purkinje fibres. These fibres distribute the impulse to the ventricular muscle. Together, the bundle branches and purkinje network comprise the ventricular conduction system. It takes about 0.03-0.04s for the impulse to travel from the bundle of HIS to the ventricular muscle. It is extremely important for these nodes to exist as they ensure the correct control and co-ordination of the heart and cardiac cycle and make sure all the contractions remain within the correct sequence and in sync.

Purkinje Fibres

Purkinje fibres (or Purkyne tissue) are located in the inner ventricular walls of the heart, just beneath the endocardium. These fibres are specialized myocardial fibres that conduct an electrical stimulus or impulse that enables the heart to contract in a coordinated fashion. Purkinje fibres work with the sinoatrial node (SA node) and the atrioventricular node (AV node) to control the heart rate. During the ventricular contraction portion of the cardiac cycle, the Purkinje fibres carry the contraction impulse from the left and right bundle branches to the myocardium of the ventricles. This causes the muscle tissue of the ventricles to contract and force blood out of the heart — either to the pulmonary circulation (from the right ventricle) or to the systemic circulation (from the left ventricle). They were discovered in 1839 by Jan Evangelista Purkinje, who gave them his name.

Pacemaker

The contractions of the heart are controlled by electrical impulses, these fire at a rate which controls the beat of the heart. The cells that create these rhythmical impulses are called pacemaker cells, and they directly control the heart rate. Artificial devices also called pacemakers can be used after damage to the body's intrinsic conduction system to produce these impulses synthetically.

4Fibrillation

Fibrillation is when the heart flutters abnormally. This can be detected by an electrocardiogram which measures the waves of excitation passing through the heart and plotting a graph of potential difference (voltage) against time. If the heart and cardiac cycle is functioning properly the electrocardiogram shows a regular, repeating pattern. However if there is fibrillation there will be no apparent pattern, either in the much more common 'Atrial Fibrillation', or the less likely but much more dangerous 'Ventricular Fibrillation'. In a hospital during VF the monitor would make a sound and alert the doctors to treat the fibrillation by passing a huge current through the chest wall and shocking the heart out of its fibrillation. This causes the cardiac muscle to stop completely for 5 seconds and when it begins to beat again the cardiac cycle would have resumed to normal and the heart will be beating in a controlled manner again. Fibrillation is an example of "circus movement" of impulses through the heart muscle. Circus movement occurs when an impulse begins in one part of the heart muscle and spreads in a circuitous pathway through the heart then returns to the originally excited muscle and "re-enters" it to stimulate it once more. The signal never stops. A cause of circus movement is long length pathway in which the muscle is no longer in a refractory state when the stimulus returns to it. A "flutter" is a circus movement in coordinated, low frequency waves that cause rapid heart rate. If the Bundle of HIS is blocked, it will result in dissociation between the activity of the atria and that of the ventricles, otherwise called a third degree heart block. The other cause of a third degree block would be a block of the right, left anterior, and left posterior bundle branches. A third degree block is very serious medical condition that will most likely require an artificial pacemaker.

ANATOMY AND PHYSIOLOGY OF THE HEART

LOCATION OF THE HEART

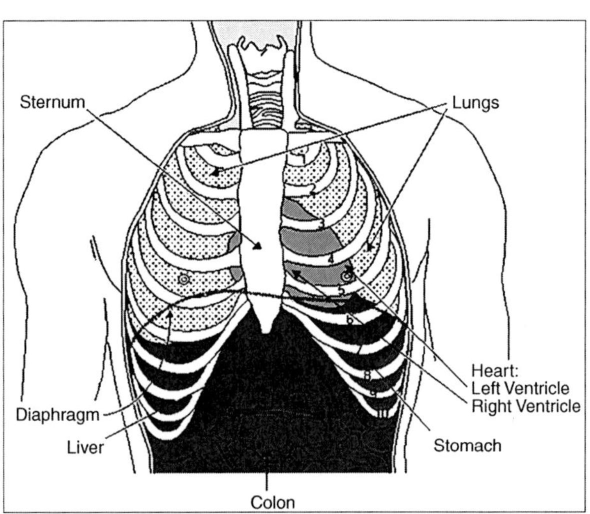

Fig. Location of the heart in the thorax. It is bounded by the diaphragm, lungs, esophagus, descending aorta, and sternum.

The heart is located in the chest between the lungs behind the sternum and above the diaphragm. It is surrounded by the pericardium. Its size is about that of a fist, and its weight is about 250-300 g. Its center is located about 1.5 cm to the left of the midsagittal plane. Located above the heart are the great vessels: the superior and inferior vena cava, the pulmonary artery and vein, as well as the aorta. The aortic arch lies behind the heart. The esophagus and the spine lie further behind the heart.

ANATOMY OF THE HEART

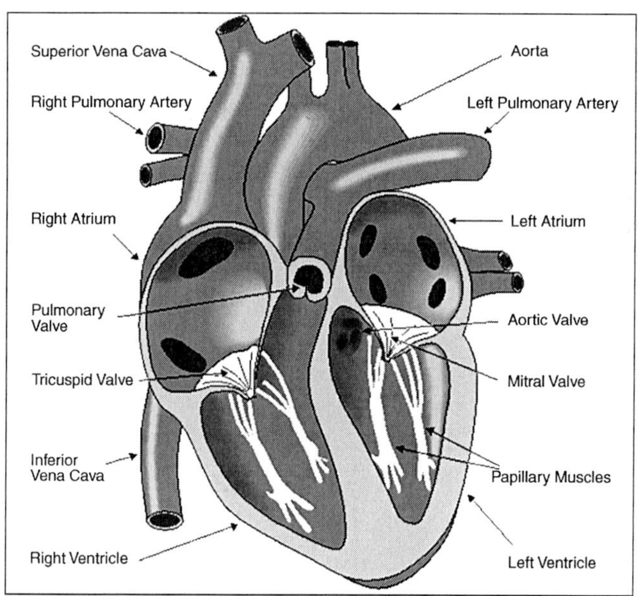

Fig. The anatomy of the heart and associated vessels.

The walls of the heart are composed of cardiac muscle, called *myocardium*. It also has *striations* similar to skeletal muscle. It consists of four compartments: the *right* and *left* atria and *ventricles*. The heart is oriented so that the anterior aspect is the right ventricle while the posterior aspect shows the left atrium. The atria form one unit and the ventricles another. This has special importance to the electric function of the heart. The left ventricular free wall and the *septum* are much thicker than the right ventricular wall. This is logical since the left ventricle pumps blood to the systemic circulation, where the pressure is considerably higher than for the pulmonary circulation, which arises from right ventricular outflow.

The cardiac muscle fibres are oriented spirally and are divided into four groups: Two groups of fibres wind around the outside of both ventricles. Beneath these fibres a third group winds around both ventricles. Beneath these fibres a fourth group winds only around the left ventricle. The fact that cardiac muscle cells are oriented more tangentially than radially, and that the resistivity of the muscle is lower in the direction of the fibre has importance in electrocardiography and magnetocardiography.

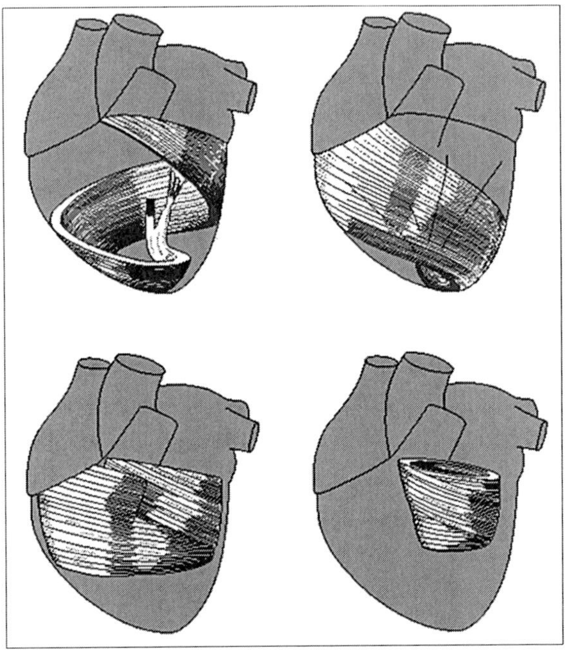

Fig. Orientation of cardiac muscle fibres.

The heart has four valves. Between the right atrium and ventricle lies the *tricuspid* valve, and between the left atrium and ventricle is the *mitral valve*. The *pulmonary* valve lies between the right ventricle and the pulmonary artery, while the *aortic valve* lies in the outflow tract of the left ventricle (controlling flow to the aorta). The blood returns from the systemic circulation to the right atrium and from there goes through the tricuspid valve to the right ventricle. It is ejected from the right ventricle through the pulmonary valve to the lungs. Oxygenated blood returns from the lungs to the left atrium, and from there through the mitral valve to the left ventricle. Finally blood is pumped through the aortic valve to the aorta and the systemic circulation..

ELECTRIC ACTIVATION OF THE HEART

CARDIAC MUSCLE CELL

In the heart muscle cell, or *myocyte*, electric activation takes place by means of the same mechanism as in the nerve cell - that is, from the inflow of sodium ions across the cell membrane. The amplitude of the action potential is also similar, being about 100 mV for both nerve and muscle. The duration of the cardiac muscle impulse is, however, two orders of magnitude longer than that in either nerve cell or skeletal muscle.

A *plateau phase* follows cardiac depolarization, and thereafter repolarization takes place. As in the nerve cell, repolarization is a consequence of the outflow of potassium ions.

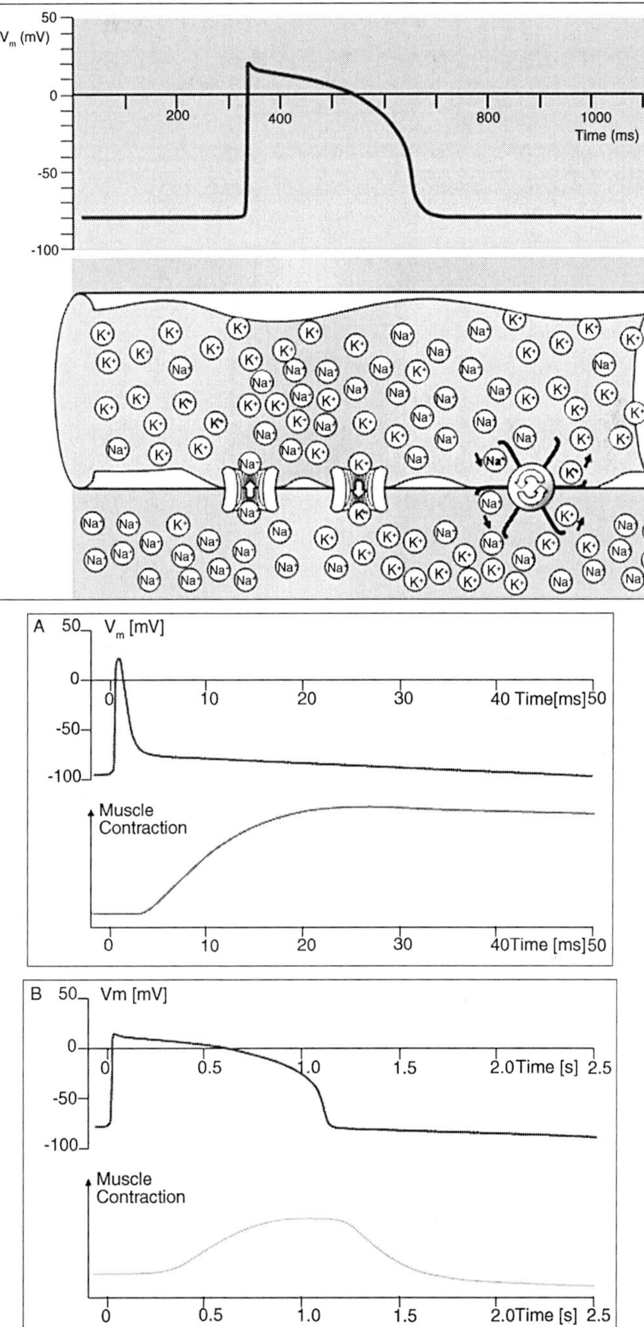

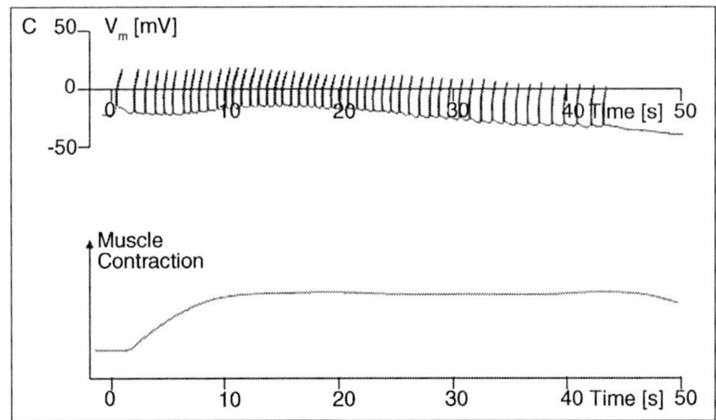

Fig. Electric and mechanical activity in

The duration of the action impulse is about 300 ms. Associated with the electric activation of cardiac muscle cell is its mechanical contraction, which occurs a little later. For the sake of comparison, the electric activity and mechanical contraction of frog sartorius muscle, frog cardiac muscle, and smooth muscle from the rat uterus. An important distinction between cardiac muscle tissue and skeletal muscle is that in cardiac muscle, activation can propagate from one cell to another in any direction.

As a result, the activation wavefronts are of rather complex shape. The only exception is the boundary between the atria and ventricles, which the activation wave normally cannot cross except along a special conduction system, since a neo-conducting barrier of fibrous tissue is present..

(A) frog sartorius muscle cell,

(B) frog cardiac muscle cell, and

(C) rat uterus wall smooth muscle cell.

In each section the upper curve shows the transmembrane voltage behaviour, whereas the lower one describes the mechanical contraction associated with it.

THE CONDUCTION SYSTEM OF THE HEART

Located in the right atrium at the superior vena cava is the *sinus node* (*sinoatrial* or *SA node*) which consists of specialized muscle cells. The sinoatrial node in humans is in the shape of a crescent and is about 15 mm long and 5 mm wide. The SA nodal cells are self-excitatory, *pacemaker cells*. They generate an action potential at the rate of about 70 per minute. From the sinus node, activation propagates throughout the atria, but cannot propagate directly across the boundary between atria and ventricles.

The *atrioventricular node* (AV node) is located at the boundary between the atria and ventricles; it has an intrinsic frequency of about 50 pulses/min. However, if the AV node is triggered with a higher pulse frequency, it follows this higher frequency. In a normal heart, the AV node provides the only conducting path from the atria to the ventricles. Thus, under normal conditions, the latter can be excited only by pulses that propagate through it. Propagation from the AV node to the ventricles is provided by a specialized conduction system. Proximally, this system is composed of a common bundle, called the *bundle of His* (named after German physician Wilhelm His, Jr., 1863-1934). More distally, it separates into two *bundle branches* propagating along each side of the septum, constituting the *right* and *left bundle branches*.

(The left bundle subsequently divides into an anterior and posterior branch.) Even more distally the bundles ramify into *Purkinje fibres* (named after Jan Evangelista Purkinje (Czech; 1787-1869)) that diverge to the inner sides of the ventricular walls. Propagation along the conduction system takes place at a relatively high speed once it is within the ventricular region, but prior to this (through the AV node) the velocity is extremely slow.

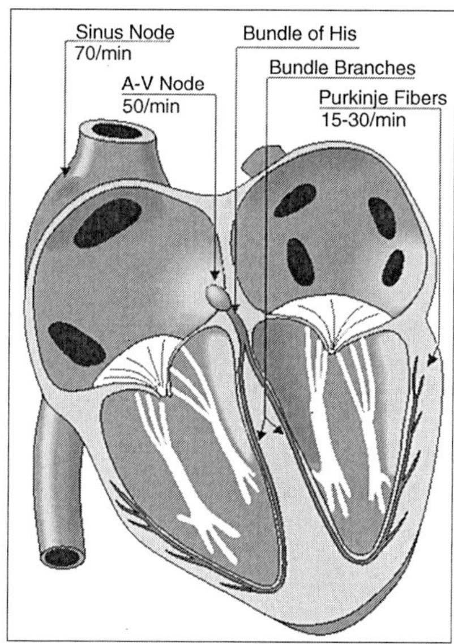

Fig. The conduction system of the heart.

From the inner side of the ventricular wall, the many activation sites cause the formation of a wavefront which propagates through the ventricular mass towards the outer wall. This process results from cell-to-cell activation. After each ventricular muscle region has depolarized, repolarization occurs.

Repolarization is not a propagating phenomenon, and because the duration of the action impulse is much shorter at the *epicardium*(the outer side of the cardiac muscle) than at the *endocardium* (the inner side of the cardiac muscle), the termination of activity appears as if it were propagating from epicardium towards the endocardium.

Because the intrinsic rate of the sinus node is the greatest, it sets the activation frequency of the whole heart. If the connection from the atria to the AV node fails, the AV node adopts its intrinsic frequency. If the conduction system fails at the bundle of His, the ventricles will beat at the rate determined by their own region that has the highest intrinsic frequency. The electric events in the heart. The waveforms of action impulse observed in different specialized cardiac tissue. Atrial repolarization occurs during the ventricular depolarization; therefore, it is not normally seen in the electrocardiogram.

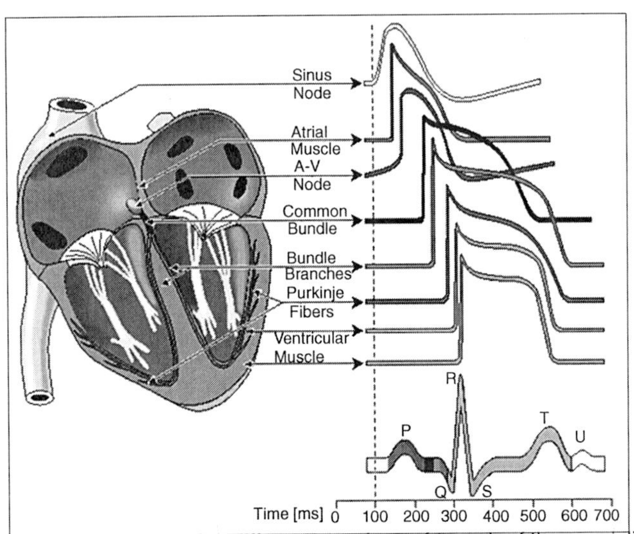

Fig. Electrophysiology of the heart.The different waveforms for each of the specialized cells found in the heart are shown. The latency shown approximates that normally found in the healthy heart.

A classical study of the propagation of excitation in human heart was made by Durrer and his co-workers. They isolated the heart from a subject who had died of various cerebral conditions and who had no previous history of cardiac diseases.

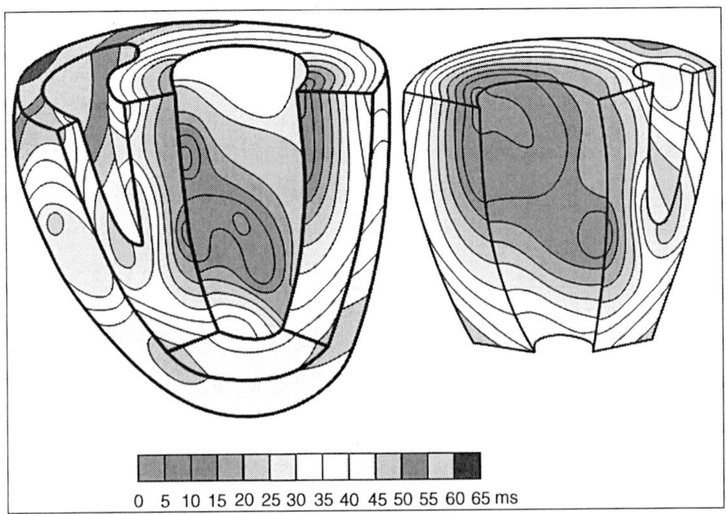

Fig. Isochronic surfaces of the ventricular activation.

The heart was removed within 30 min post mortem and was perfused. As many as 870 electrodes were placed into the cardiac muscle; the electric activity was then recorded by a tape recorder and played back at a lower speed by the ECG writer; thus the effective paper speed was 960 mm/s, giving a time resolution better than 1 ms. The ventricles are shown with the anterior wall of the left and partly that of the right ventricle opened.

The isochronic surfaces show clearly that ventricular activation starts from the inner wall of the left ventricle and proceeds radially towards the epicardium. In the terminal part of ventricular activation, the excitation wavefront proceeds more tangentially. This phenomenon and its effects on electrocardiogram and magnetocardiogram signals.

THE GENESIS OF THE ELECTROCARDIOGRAM

Activation Currents in Cardiac Tissue

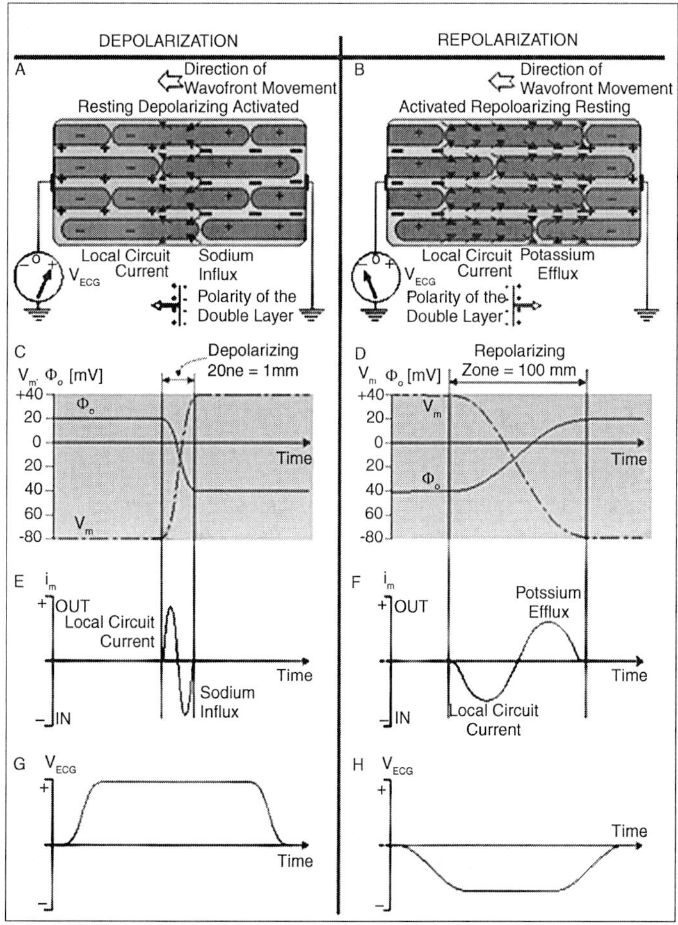

Fig. The genesis of the electrocardiogram.

The cardiac electric events on an intracellular level. Such electric signals may be recorded with a microelectrode, which is inserted inside a cardiac muscle cell. However, the electrocardiogram (ECG) is a recording of the electric potential, generated by the electric activity of the heart, on the surface of the thorax. The ECG thus represents the extracellular electric behaviour of the cardiac muscle tissue. In this section we explain the genesis of the ECG signal via a highly idealized model.

A segment of cardiac tissue through which propagating depolarization (A) and repolarization (B) wavefront planes are passing. In this illustration the wavefronts move from right to left, which means that the time axis points to the right. There are two important properties of cardiac tissue that we shall make use of to analyze the potential and current distribution associated with these propagating waves. First, cells are interconnected by low-resistance pathways (gap junctions), as a result of which currents flowing in the intracellular space of one cell pass freely into the following cell. Second, the space between cells is very restrictive (accounting for less than 25 per cent of the total volume). As a result, both intracellular and extracellular currents are confined to the direction parallel to the propagation of the plane wavefront.

The aforementioned conditions are exactly those for which the linear core conductor model, fully applies; that is, both intracellular and extracellular currents flow in a linear path. In particular when using the condition $I_i + I_o = 0$ and

$$\frac{\partial \Phi i}{\partial x} = -I_i r_i \quad \frac{\partial \Phi o}{\partial x} = -I_o r_o$$

one obtains

$$\frac{\partial \Phi i}{\partial x} = I_o r_i \quad \frac{\partial \Phi_o}{\partial x} = -I_o r_o$$

Integrating from $x = -\infty$, to $x = x$ gives

$$\Phi_i = r_i \int I_o dx \quad \Phi_o = -r_o \int I_o dx$$

ing the second of Equations above from the first and applying $V_m = \Phi_i - \Phi_o$, the definition of the transmembrane potential, we obtain:

$$V_m = \left(r_i + r_o\right) \int I_o dx$$

From Equation above we obtain the following important relationships valid for linear core conductor conditions, namely that

$$\Phi_i = \frac{r_i}{r_i + r_o} V_m$$

and

$$\Phi_o = -\frac{r_o}{r_i + r_o} V_m$$

These equations describe "voltage divider" conditions and were first pointed out by Hodgkin and Rushton (1946). Note that they depend on the validity of Equation 3.36 which, in turn, requires that there be no external (polarizing) currents in the region under consideration.

DEPOLARIZATION WAVE

We may now apply Equation 6.5 to the propagating wave under investigation. The variation in the value of $V_m(x)$ is easy to infer since in the *activated* region it is at the plateau voltage, generally around +40 mV, whereas in the *resting* region it is around -80 mV. The *transition* region is usually very narrow (about 1 mm, corresponding to a depolarization of about 1 ms and a velocity < 1 m/s), as the figure suggests. Application of Equation 6.4 results in the extracellular potential (Φ_o) behaviour (solid line). The ratio $r_o/(r_o + r_i) =$ 0.5 has been chosen on the basis of experimental evidence for propagation along the cardiac fibre axis. The transmembrane current I_m can be evaluated from $V_m(x)$ applying the general cable equation:

$$\Phi_o = -\frac{r_o}{r_i + r_o} V_m$$

The equation for the transmembrane current im is thus

$$i_m = \frac{1}{r_i + r_o} \frac{\partial^2 V_m}{\partial x^2}$$

This current is confined to the depolarization zone. The right of the centerline it is inward (thick arrows), and just to the left it is outward (thin arrows). The inward portion reflects the sodium influx, triggered by the very large and rapid rise in sodium permeability. An examination of the extracellular potential Φ_O shows it to be uniform except for a rapid change across the wavefront. Such a change from plus to minus is what one would expect at a double layer source where the dipole direction is from right to left.

So we conclude that for the depolarization (activation) of cardiac tissue a double layer appears at the wavefront with the dipole orientation in the direction of propagation. One can also approximate the source as proportional to the transmembrane current - estimated here by a lumped negative point source (on the right) and a lumped positive point source (on the left) which taken together constitute a dipole in the direction of propagation (to the left). Finally, a double layer, whose positive side is pointing to the recording electrode (to the left), produces a positive (ECG) signal.

REPOLARIZATION WAVE

The nature of the repolarization wave is in principle very different from that of the depolarization wave. Unlike depolarization, the repolarization is not a propagating phenomenon. If we examine the location of repolarizing cells at consecutive time instances, we can, however, approximate the repolarization with a proceeding wave phenomenon. As stated previously, when a cell depolarizes, another cell close to it then depolarizes and produces an electric field which triggers the depolarization phenomenon. In this way, the depolarization proceeds as a propagating wave within cardiac tissue.

The recovery of cardiac cells is relatively slow, requiring approximately 100 ms (compare this with the time required to complete activation - roughly 1 ms). For this reason, we have depicted the recovery interval as much wider than the activation interval. The polarity of $V_m(x)$ decreases from its plateau value of +40 mV on the left to the resting value of -80 mV on the right. Again, Equation 6.5 may be applied, in this case showing that the extracellular potential Φ_o (solid line) increases from minus to plus. In this case the double layer source is directed from left to right. And, it is spread out over a wide region of the heart muscle. (In fact, if activation occupies 1 mm, then recovery occupies 100 mm, a relationship that could only be suggested, since in fact, it encompasses the entire heart!) The transmembrane current I_m can be again evaluated from $V_m(x)$ by applying Equation previous. To the right of the centerline it is outward (thick arrows) and just to the left it is inward (thin arrows). The outward portion reflects the potassium efflux due to the rapid rise of potassium permeability. The current inflow is again the "local circuit" current. The course of the transmembrane current during repolarization.

Thus, during repolarization, a double layer is formed that is similar to that observed during depolarization. The double layer in repolarization, however, has a polarity opposite to that in depolarization, and thus its negative side points towards the recording electrode; as a result, a negative (ECG) signal is recorded.

In real heart muscle, since the action potential duration at the epicardium is actually shorter than at the endocardium, the recovery phase appears to move from epicardium to endocardium, that is, just the opposite to activation (and opposite the direction in the example above). As a consequence the recovery dipole is in the same direction as the activation dipole. Since the recovery and activation dipoles are thus in the same direction one can explain the common observation that the normal activation and recovery ECG signal has the same polarity..

Bibliography

A Complete Book on Yoga : The Step-by-Step Guide to Yoga for Health *and Beauty for Everybody*, Mahaveer Publication, 2006.

A. Sahoo and R.K. Singh: *Animal Health and Production* , Satish Serial Publishing House, 2013.

Ashok Birbal Jain and Aruna A Birbal Jain: *A To Z Of Health* Challenges After Thirty : A Practical Guide To Your Health *Needs*, Macmillan India, 2006.

Ashok Birbal Jain and Aruna A Birbal Jain: *A to Z of Health Problems* After Thirty : A Practical Guide to Become a Well-Informed *Patient*, MacMillan India, 2006.

C S Jain: *A Complete Book on Health and Nutrition*, Cyber Tech, 2009.

C. Shanthi Johnson and S. Irudaya Rajan: *Ageing and Health in India,* Rawat Pub, 2010.

C.P. Prakasam and S. Siva Raju: *Adolescents Reproductive Health Perspectives* , B R Publication, 2006.

Debashis Basu; B Francis Kulirani and B Datta Ray: *Agriculture Food Security Nutrition and Health in North East India* : , Mittal Publication, 2006.

Dharam Vir Mangla: *Art of Yoga : Herbs for Health* , Global Books Organisation, 2010.

Esmw Floyd: *1001 Little Health Miracles*, Carlton Publishing, 2009.

G.S. Lavekar and M.M. Padhi: *A Hand Book of Common Siddha Kayakalpa (Rasayana) Herbs for Healthy Life*, Central Council for Res, 2008.

George K. Mathews: *Assessment of Health And Physical Education* , Crescent Publishing, 2009.

Hans H. Rhyner: *Ayurveda : The Gentle Health System*, Motilal Banarsidass, 1998.

Indrani Gupta, Mayur Trivedi and Subodh Kandamuthan: *Adoption* 292 Health and Diseases Food Science and Factors of Health Technologies in India : Implications for the AIDS *Vaccine* , Sage, 2007, pbk.

Ishrat Syed and Kalpana Swaminathan: *A Compendium of Family Health* , Rupa, 2005.

Jagdamba Dixit: *Be Healthy : The Dimensions of Positive Health: A Family Health Guide,* , B R Pub, 2006.

John Humphrey, J. Richard: *Aquatic Animal Quarantine and Health Certification in Asia*, Rohana P. Subasinghe and Michael J. Philips, Daya, 2005.

K.V. Rajendran, P.N. Pandey and B.N. Pandey: *Aquatic Resources and Health Management* , Narendra, 2010.

Mandeep Singh Nathial: *Basics of Health and Physical Education* , Khel Sahitya Kendra, 2008.

Manju Gupta: *A-Z Handbook of Women Health* , Khel Sahitya Kendra, 2006.

Mark Bunn: *Ancient Wisdom for Modern Health : Rediscover the Simple Timeless Secrets of Health and Happiness*, Macmillan Publishers India, 2011.

Mukul Singh and Sujata K. Dass: *Anatomy Physiology and Health Education*, Shree Pub, 2009.

Paraddi Kusuma Mallapa and Ganesh Shankar: *Ashtanga Yoga in Relation to Holistic Health*, Satyam Pub, 2006.

Pradeep Kapoor: *101 Health Problems of Children* , Rupa Publications, 2011.

R S Chauhan and Kuldeep Dhama: *Aflatoxicosis in Animals and Its Public Health Significance* , International Book, 2008.

Rajesh Jani: *Basics of Wildlife Health Care and Management*, Narendra Publishing House, 2012.

Ramesh Bijlani: *Back To Health Through Yoga*, Rupa Publications, 2008.

S B Singh and O P Charasia: *Advances In Agriculture Environment and Health* Satish Serial Publication, 2009.

S. Siva Raju: *Ageing Health and Development* , Ulimiri V. Somayajulu and C.P. Prakasam, B.R. Publishing Corporation, 2013.

S. Waseem A. Ashraf: *Agricultural Environment and Health*, Concept, 2006.

Satish Sonkar: *World History of Physical and Health Education: Ancient Period* , ABD, 2005.

Satyawan: *Administration of Health Agencies*, Regal, 2008.

Shanti Gowans: *Ayurveda for Health and Well-Being* , Jaico, 2000.

Sieger, Robin: *42 Days to Wealth, Health and Happiness* , Random House India, Jan-06.

Sinku Kumar Singh: *Anatomy Physiology Kinesiology and Health Education*, Khel Sahitya Kendra, 2011.

Sita Ram Sharma: *A Handbook Of Health Education,* Sarup Book Publishers, 2009.

Subodh K. Singh: *Animal Health*, Bio-Green Books, 2012.

T.L. Devaraj: *Ayurveda for Health and Family Welfare* , Chaukhambha Orientalia, 2011.

T.L. Devaraj: *Ayurveda for Perfect Health* , UBSPD, 2002.

Index

A

Abnormalities 142, 166
Active Transport 201, 205
Adaptive 1, 3, 5, 7, 8, 9, 11, 12, 14, 15, 16, 17, 19, 21, 26, 30, 31, 32, 33, 51, 76, 77, 78, 139
Adrenal Glands 179
Allergen 86, 89, 91, 98, 99, 100, 101, 102, 105, 106, 107, 108, 109
Anatomical Terminology 178
Anatomy of the Heart 220, 267
Antimicrobial 3, 4, 10, 18, 39, 72, 73, 80, 81
Antiviral 4, 66, 109, 110, 113, 114, 115, 116, 117, 123, 126
Attenuated 1, 2, 16, 22, 23, 24, 25, 55, 112, 134
Autoimmunity 1, 5, 16, 17, 20

B

Blood Cells 189, 191, 209, 210, 214, 236, 258, 259
Blood Vessels 179, 202, 208, 209, 214, 215, 217, 218, 227, 229, 230, 232, 233, 236, 238, 244, 256, 259
Body Cavities 179, 186, 208, 210
Body Functions 179
Body Membranes 211
Body Tissues 214, 215, 224, 248

C

Cardiac Cycle 212, 213, 223, 224, 226, 229, 242, 260, 263, 265, 266
Cardiac Output 213, 218, 225, 233
Cell Organelles 190, 192, 193
Central Nervous System 189, 226
Cloning 147, 152, 157, 158, 159, 160, 162, 164, 166, 169, 170, 173, 174
Components of Heart 230
Conduction System 212, 222, 239, 240, 242, 261, 263, 265, 270, 271
Congestive Heart Failure 237
Control of Heartbeat 262
Counting a Pulse 261

D

Depolarization Wave 275
Digestive System 209

E

Epithelial Transport 208
Epitopes 2, 3, 5, 8, 21, 22, 33, 34, 105

F

Facilitated Diffusion 201, 205
Fetal Circulation 220

G

Growth and Development 182

H

Heart Attack 224, 237, 255
Heart Diseases 236
Heart Sounds 213, 224, 227, 244, 245

Histocompatibility 149
Hormonal 164
Human Body Structure 177

I

Immunotherapy 93, 105, 106, 107, 109
Inadequate 24, 26, 127
Inflammatory 4, 10, 15, 20, 43, 45, 47, 48, 49, 53, 54, 57, 61, 63, 68, 73, 74, 78, 80, 83, 86, 87, 92, 93, 94, 95, 96, 97, 98, 101, 102, 103, 104, 119, 122, 125, 127, 133, 134, 136, 137
Inhibition 26, 54, 121
Innate 1, 3, 4, 7, 8, 9, 10, 11, 12, 13, 14, 16, 18, 19, 21, 31, 32, 34, 40, 59, 79, 100, 126, 134, 137, 138, 139
Integumentary System 208
Interferons 13, 33, 44, 66, 113, 114, 120, 127

L

Life Process 179, 180
Location of the Heart 266
Lymphatic Vessels 233

M

Major Systemic Veins 220
Membrane Junctions 191
Mutagenesis 147, 165

N

Nervous System 189, 202, 210, 226, 234, 236, 246, 251, 253, 263
Nervous Tissue 202

O

Organ Systems 208

P

Permeability 13, 43, 64, 73, 74, 95, 96, 98, 99, 101, 103, 104
Phagocytosis 3, 14, 26, 28, 29, 34, 39, 42, 66, 67, 69, 73, 74, 77, 78, 81, 84, 116, 118, 120, 121, 122, 123, 138, 139
Physiology of Circulation 214, 216
Planes of the Body 178
Pulmonary Circuit 218

R

Recombinant 24, 111, 114
Relation Directions 183, 184
Reproductive System 210
Respiratory System 209

S

Scrapie 141, 142, 143, 144, 145, 146
Sinoatrial Node 212, 213, 225, 228, 239, 262, 263, 265, 270
Skeletal Muscle 191, 210, 216, 228, 229, 254, 275
Structural Organization 181
Subsequently 1, 14, 30, 62, 124, 130, 134, 136, 137
Susceptibility 143, 144, 145
System of the Heart 212, 225, 265, 271
Systemic Circulation 211, 218, 224, 229, 232, 234, 235, 244, 265, 267, 268

T

The Electrocardiogram 212, 213, 228, 266, 272, 273, 274
Tissues and Organs 202
Types of Glands 208

V

Valves of the Heart 221, 231
Vulnerability 144

X

Xenotransplantation 163, 168, 169, 175, 176